CLINICAL DECISION MAKING IN COLORECTAL SURGERY

CLINICAL DECISION MAKING IN COLORECTAL SURGERY

Steven D. Wexner, M.D., F.A.C.S., F.A.S.C.R.S.
Chairman, Department of Colorectal Surgery
Cleveland Clinic Florida
Fort Lauderdale, Florida

Anthony M. Vernava III, M.D., F.A.C.S., F.A.S.C.R.S
Chief, Section of Colon and Rectal Surgery
Director, Residency Training Program in
Colon and Rectal Surgery
Associate Professor of Surgery
Saint Louis University Health Sciences Center
Department of Surgery
St. Louis, Missouri

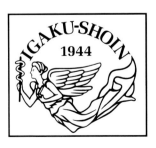

IGAKU-SHOIN   NEW YORK • TOKYO

This book is dedicated to the Caporella family whose philanthropy and generosity will hopefully one day allow us to find better treatments and cures for the diseases discussed within this textbook.

Published and distributed by

IGAKU-SHOIN Medical Publishers, Inc.
One Madison Avenue, New York, New York 10010

IGAKU-SHOIN Ltd.,
5-24-3 Hongo, Bunkyo-ku, Tokyo 113-91

ISBN: 0-89640-262-2   (New York)
ISBN: 4-260-14262-3   (Tokyo)

Printed and bound in the U.S.A.
10 9 8 7 6 5 4 3 2 1

ACKNOWLEDGMENTS

Obviously, such an extensive textbook could not be developed and written solely by the two editors. We are both extremely indebted to numerous individuals who have assisted and corroborated along the way. Firstly, Gene Kearn, Vincent Polk and their associates at Igaku-Shoin were very helpful with the administrative and technical details of the development and execution of this textbook. Secondly, our secretaries Elektra McDermott and Jody Brown are to be commended for the persistence with which they ensured timely completion of the work. It is certainly no mean feat to have insured that over 125 authors followed the guidelines and produced appropriate material in a timely fashion. Similarly, we would like to thank each chapter author for their excellent contributions contained in the pages of this book. Lastly, and most importantly, we owe a debt of gratitude to our loving families, specifically our wives Pamela Rosen Wexner and Rene Vernava as well as our children, as it was precious time spent away from them which allowed completion of this textbook.

FOREWORD

It is always a privilege and honor to be asked to write a foreword for a new text. This is especially so, given the close ties between the editors, fellow members of the colorectal surgical fraternity, and myself. Steve Wexner and Tony Vernava, have much in common. Both received their colorectal training simultaneously under the tutelage of Stanley Goldberg and his colleagues at the University of Minnesota—a program that has nurtured many young surgeons and molded current and future leaders of the specialty. Both Drs. Wexner and Vernava possess the talent, passion and boundless enthusiasm and energy that attracted the interest in authorship of so many national and international opinion setters in colorectal surgery.

Many of these contributors are academic surgeons, yet all share the the distinction of being busy, active clinicians, many of whom hold a major teaching role. Both authors lead busy training programs in colorectal surgery, programs that are among the most productive in clinical research of disorders of the large intestine.

Professor John Goligher once wrote that the author of a foreword serves two main functions—"to say something by way of introduction about the author(s)" and "to offer some words of explanation and commendation about the book itself." Both authors, although young, enjoy a national and international reputation and need no further introduction.

The book itself is unusual—one might say, unique—amongst the array of general and specialized texts on the large intestine. The algorithmic approach to how clinical decisions are made in colorectal surgery is attractive on many scores. The first of these is brevity. By its very nature, this has an attractiveness to the reader. Where else can you find, for example—a three (manuscript) paged comprehensive treatise on how to treat rectovaginal fistula. The second is clarity. Because of its brevity, there has been an enforced discipline of and by the chapter author, to cut to the chase and encompass the "good stuff" in a reasonably comprehensive and readable form. Thirdly, the approach follows closely the way in which those experienced clinicians go about addressing a problem. That is, they provide a method.

In all texts, there are trade offs—in this case, a fully comprehensive text is not attempted and the reader would be referred to several ones extant. The multi-authored chapters here may have drawbacks in terms of commonality of style. However, having edited a multi-authored text myself, I feel such productions have a certain value in that they come to print much sooner; they are, therefore, more contemporary with current thinking; and, the spectra of expertise of the authors are more encompassing than that of just a few producing a general text.

Those especially likely to find this book rewarding, and a valuable addition to their library or office, include the following: residents in general and colorectal surgery (especially just before the Board exams); gastroenterologists at all levels; family practitioners who will have a ready source for telling patients what to expect upon referral. Some colorectal surgeons will also find this text valuable— especially for conditions not frequently encountered—or simply to check that the approach they are using parallels that of the expert author being reviewed. On both these scores, this colorectal surgeon will be including this book in his library.

Victor W. Fazio, M.D.
Professor of Surgery, Ohio State University
   School of Medicine at Cleveland Clinic
Rupert B. Turnbull, Jr. Chairman,
   Department of Colorectal Surgery,
   Cleveland Clinic Foundation,
   Cleveland, Ohio

PREFACE

Many excellent textbooks already exist in the field of colorectal surgery. Therefore, it is not the intention of the authors to be redundant or repetitious with the myriad of excellent published material already readily available. This textbook was instead designed as a problem focused approach to colorectal surgery. Instead of the reader needing to digest countless paragraphs of text to find the few pertinent sentences relative to the particular problem at hand: rather each problem is presented as a separate algorithm. The structure of this textbook is there are 97 algorithm scenarios presented which are common to the colon and rectal surgeon. In each case, the algorithm includes a letter coded guide with each letter referenced by textual explanatory material and supported by a list of suggested readings. The 97 chapters have been divided into eight sections. The first section includes general problems such as evaluation of the anus, rectum and colon, physiologic evaluation, bowel preparation and preoperative assessment. The second section includes evaluation of anorectal complaints. Since multiple approaches exist to the evaluation of melena, two separate algorithms have been included to give the readers the two most commonly accepted methods of evaluation of this complaint. The third section presents the evaluation of systemic symptoms and complaints while sections four through seven present the evaluation and management of specific pathologic conditions. These disorders are classified by topography within the lower gastrointestinal tract. Specifically, section 4A includes the evaluation and management of non-neoplastic anorectal pathology while section 4B presents the diagnosis and management of neoplastic anorectal conditions. Section five, colonic pathology, is subdivided into inflammatory conditions, miscellaneous non-neoplastic conditions, and neoplastic conditions. Similarly, section six presents small bowel disorders and is subdivided into non-neoplastic and neoplastic disorders. Section seven includes five chapters which discuss and evaluate stomal disorders while section eight presents the evaluation and management of common intraoperative and postoperative complications.

The editors have consciously included much overlap and cross-referencing within the book because, in clinical practice, many conditions and evaluations do indeed overlap. Therefore, rather than excluding or "pigeon-holing" very specific evaluations and treatment schemes, continuity exists throughout the book. The editors have made great efforts to include numerous world-recognized authorities to author the chapters within this book. Specifically, authors have been included from North and South America, Europe, the United Kingdom, Australia, Asia, and the Mideast. This type of global approach is unique to a textbook of colorectal surgery.

In summary, this globally authored, in-depth, problem focused book, offers the reader the opportunity to rapidly review the evaluation and management of specific colorectal complaints and conditions. The inclusion of authors from throughout the world helps lend a global perspective to the evaluation and management processes. The deliberate overlap of each algorithm will insure that no details are overlooked during perusal of a given subject area.

CONTRIBUTORS

Herand Abcarian, M.D., F.A.C.S., F.A.S.C.R.S.
Turi Josefson Professor and Head
Department of Surgery
University of Illinois
Chicago, Illinois

Gary J. Anthone, M.D.
Assistant Professor of Surgery
Department of Surgery
University of Southern California
School of Medicine
Los Angeles, California

H. Randolph Bailey, M.D., F.A.C.S., F.A.S.C.R.S.
Clinical Professor of Surgery and Chief,
Division of Colon and Rectal Surgery
Colon and Rectal Surgery Residency
Training Program
University of Texas at Houston
Houston, Texas

Sanjiv Bais, M.D.
Division of Colon and Rectal Surgery
Sansum Clinic/Santa Barbara
Medical Foundation Clinic
Santa Barbara, California

Garth H. Ballantyne, M.D., F.A.C.S., F.A.S.C.R.S.
Director, Center for Advanced
Laparoscopic Surgery
Chief, Division of Laparoscopic Surgery
St. Luke's Roosevelt Hospital Center
New York, New York

John U. Bascom, M.D., PhD.
Attending and Consulting Staff
Sacred Heart General Hospital
Eugene, Oregon

Robert W. Beart, Jr., M.D., F.A.C.S., F.A.S.C.R.S.
Professor of Surgery
University of Southern California
Los Angeles, California

David E. Beck, M.D., F.A.C.S., F.A.S.C.R.S.
Chairman, Department of Colon
and Rectal Surgery
Ochsner Clinic
New Orleans, Louisiana

Paul Belliveau, M.D., F.R.C.S.C., F.A.C.S., F.A.S.C.R.S
Associate Professor of Surgery
McGill University and
Assistant Surgeon, Royal Victoria Hospital
and St. Mary's Hospital
Montreal, Quebec
Canada

Anne Berger, M.D.
Department of Surgery
Hôpital Saint Antoine
Paris, France

Douglas D. Berglund, M.D.
Division of Colon and Rectal Surgery
University of Minnesota
Minneapolis, Minnesota

Mitchell Bernstein, M.D.
Department of Colorectal Surgery
Cleveland Clinic Florida
Fort Lauderdale, Florida

Thomas B. Blake III, M.D.
Division of Colon and Rectal Surgery
Orlando Regional Medical Center
Orlando, Florida

Mans Bohe, M.D.
Associated Professor
Lund University
Department of Surgery
Malmö General Hospital
Malmö, Sweden

E. L. Bokey, M.D., F.R.A.C.S.
Professor of Colon and Rectal Surgery
Sydney Central Department of Colon
and Rectal Surgery at Concord Hospital
Sydney, Australia

Gregory F. Bonner, M.D.
Staff Physician
Department of Gastroenterology
Cleveland Clinic Florida
Fort Lauderdale, Florida

J. Brian Boyd, M.D.
Chairman, Department of Plastic
and Reconstructive Surgery
Cleveland Clinic Florida
Fort Lauderdale, Florida

Mary Lou Boyer, B.S., R.N., C.E.T.N.
Chief of Enterostomal Therapy
Department of Colorectal Surgery
Cleveland Clinic Florida
Fort Lauderdale, Florida

Douglas A. Brewer, M.D.
Department of Colon and Rectal Surgery
Lahey Clinic
Burlington, Massachusetts

Patrick Brillant, M.D.
Section of Colon and Rectal Surgery
Mayo Clinic
Rochester, Minnesota

David Caminer, M.D.
Department of Plastic and
Reconstructive Surgery
Cleveland Clinic Florida
Fort Lauderdale, Florida

**Philip F. Caushaj, M.D., F.A.C.S.,
F.A.C.G., F.A.S.C.R.S.**
Chief, Department of Surgery
The Medical Center of Central
Massachusetts
Worcester, Massachusetts and
Associate Professor of Surgery
University of Massachusetts
Medical School
Worcester, Massachusetts

John D. Cheape, M.D.
Colorectal Surgeon
University Hospital
Augusta, Georgia

David A. Cherry, M.D., F.R.C.S.(C)
Assistant Clinical Professor of Surgery
University of Connecticut
Hartford, Connecticut

**Mark A. Christensen, M.D., F.A.C.S.,
F.A.S.C.R.S.**
Chief, Section of Colon and Rectal Surgery
Department of Surgery
Creighton University School of Medicine
Omaha, Nebraska

James M. Church, M.D.
Staff Surgeon and Head
Inherited Colorectal Cancer Registries
Department of Colorectal Surgery
Cleveland Clinic Foundation
Cleveland, Ohio

José R. Cintron, M.D.
Assistant Professor of Surgery
University of Illinois College of Medicine
Attending Surgeon West Side VA
Medical Center
Chicago, Illinois

Stephen M. Cohen, M.D.
Department of Colorectal Surgery
Cleveland Clinic Florida
Fort Lauderdale, Florida

**Zane Cohen, M.D., F.R.C.S.(C),
F.A.S.C.R.S.**
Chairman, Department of Surgery
Professor of Surgery
University of Toronto
Mount Sinai Hospital
Toronto, Ontario, Canada

Thomas H. Dailey, M.D., F.A.C.S.
Director, Division of Colon
and Rectal Surgery
Professor of Clinical Surgery
Columbia University College of Physicians
and Surgeons
New York, New York

Eli D. Ehrenpreis, M.D.
Staff Physician
Department of Gastroenterology
Cleveland Clinic Florida
Fort Lauderdale, Florida

Göran Ekelund, M.D.
Associate Professor
Lund University
Chairman, Department of Surgery
Malmö General Hospital
Malmö, Sweden

Ian G. Finlay, F.R.C.S., F.R.C.S.(Glas.)
Consultant Colorectal Surgeon
Glasgow Royal Infirmary
Glasgow, Scotland

Charles O. Finne III, M.D., F.A.C.S., F.A.S.C.R.S.
Clinical Assistant Professor of Surgery
Division of Colon and Rectal Surgery
Department of Surgery
University of Minnesota Medical School
Minneapolis, Minnesota

James W. Fleshman, M.D., F.A.C.S., F.A.S.C.R.S.
Assistant Professor of Surgery
Director, Residency Training Program
Washington University School of Medicine
St. Louis, Missouri

Pascal Frileux, M.D.
Staff Surgeon
Department of Surgery
Hôpital Laennec
Paris, France

Francis A. Frizelle, M.B., Ch.B., M.Med.Sci., F.R.A.C.S.
Department of Colon and Rectal Surgery
Mayo Clinic
Rochester, Minnesota

G. Ching Ger, M.D.
Chairman, Section of Colon and
Rectal Surgery
803 Army Hospital
Taiching, Taiwan
Republic of China

David H. Gibbs, M.D.
Department of Colon and Rectal Surgery
Ochsner Clinic
New Orleans, Louisiana

Stanley M. Goldberg, M.D., F.A.S.C., F.A.S.C.R.S., F.R.C.S. (Hon.), F.R.A.C.S. (Hon.)
Clinical Professor of Surgery
Division of Colon and Rectal Surgery

University of Minnesota
Minneapolis, Minnesota

Lester Gottesman, M.D., F.A.C.S., F.A.S.C.R.S
Division of Colorectal Surgery
St. Luke's Hospital
New York, New York and
Assistant Professor of Clinical Surgery
Columbia University College of
Physicians and Surgeons
New York, New York

Mark K. Grove, M.D.
Staff Surgeon
Department of General and Vascular
Surgery
Cleveland Clinic Florida
Fort Lauderdale, Florida

Angelita Habr-Gama, M.D.
Associate Professor of Surgery
Director, Division of Colon and Rectal
Surgery
São Paulo University School of Medicine
São Paulo, Brazil

R. J. Heald, F.R.C.S.
Chief, Colorectal Surgery
Colorectal Research Unit
Baskingstoke District Hospital
Baskingstoke, Hampshire, England

Friedrich Herbst, M.D.
Assistant Professor of Surgery
University of Vienna
Vienna, Austria

Terry C. Hicks, M.D., F.A.C.S., F.A.S.C.R.S.
Vice-Chairman
Department of Colon and Rectal Surgery
Ochsner Clinic Foundation
New Orleans, Louisiana

Kari-Matti Hiltunen, M.D.
Consultant Colorectal Surgeon
Department of Surgery
Tampere University Hospital
Tampere, Finland

Karen D. Horvath, M.D.
Department of Surgery
Columbia University and Presbyterian
Hospital
College of Physicians and Surgeons
New York, New York

Philip Huber Jr., M.D., F.A.C.S.
Associate Professor of Surgery
University of Texas Southwest
Medical Center
Dallas, Texas

Leif Hulten, M.D., Ph.D.
Professor of Surgery
Göteborg University
Department of Surgery
The Colorectal Unit
Göteborg, Sweden

Charles L. Jackson, M.D.
Chairman, Department of Urology
Cleveland Clinic Florida
Fort Lauderdale, Florida

Jonathan E. Jensen, M.D., F.A.C.P.
Staff Physician
Department of Gastroenterology
Cleveland Clinic Florida
Fort Lauderdale, Florida

Douglas R. E. Johnson, M.D., F.R.C.S.C.
Division of Colon and Rectal Surgery
Univeristy of Minnesota
Minneapolis, Minnesota

J. Marcio N. Jorge, M.D.
Director, Anorectal Physiology
Laboratory
Colorectal Division
University of São Paulo
São Paulo, Brazil

Michael R. B. Keighley, M.S., F.R.C.S.
Chairman and Barling Professor
of Surgery
University of Birmingham
Queen Elizabeth Hospital
Birmingham, England

Bruce A. Kerner, M.D., F.A.C.S., F.A.S.C.R.S.
Clinical Associate Professor
Department of Surgery
Ohio State University
Columbus, Ohio

Karamjit S. Khanduja, M.B.B.S., F.A.C.S., F.A.S.C.R.S.
Chief, Division of Colorectal Surgery
Mount Carmel Health
Columbus, Ohio

Indru T. Khubchandani, M.D., F.A.C.S., F.R.C.S.
Professor of Surgery
Hahnemann Hospital
Philadelphia, Pennsylvania and
Staff, Colon and Rectal Surgery
Health East Teaching Hospitals
Allentown, Pennsylvania

Mark Killingback, M.D., F.R.A.C.S.
Colorectal Surgeon
Sydney Adventist Hospital
Sydney, Australia

Kent A. Kirby, M.D.
Department of Urology
Cleveland Clinic Florida
Fort Lauderdale, Florida

Witold A. Kmiot, M.S., F.R.C.S. (Gen.)
Lecturer of Surgery
University of Birmingham
Queen Elizabeth Hospital
Birmingham, England

Michael M. Krausz, M.D.
Professor of Surgery
Director, Department of Surgery B
Lady Davis "Carmel" Hospital
Haifa, Israel

Han Kuijpers, M.D.
Professor of Surgery
Department of Surgery
Academisch Ziekenhuis
Nijmegen, Netherlands

Sergio W. Larach, M.D., F.A.C.S., F.A.S.C.R.S.
Clinical Assistant Professor of Surgery
Chairman and Residency Program Director
Division of Colorectal Surgery
Orlando Regional Medical Center
Orlando, Florida

Walter E. Longo, M.D.
Assistant Professor of Surgery
Head of Research,
Section of Colon & Rectal Surgery
St. Louis University Medical Center
St. Louis, Missouri

Ann C. Lowry, M.D., F.A.C.S., F.A.S.C.R.S.
Clinical Assistant Professor of Surgery
University of Minnesota

Department of Surgery
Minneapolis, Minnesota

**Martin A. Luchtefeld, M.D., F.A.S.C.,
F.A.S.C.R.S.**
Assistant Clinical Professor
Michigan State University
College of Human Medicine
East Lansing, Michigan and
Staff Colorectal Surgeon and
Residency Program Director
Colon and Rectal Surgery
Ferguson Clinic
Grand Rapids, Michigan

**John M. MacKeigan, M.D., F.R.S.C.(C),
F.A.C.S., F.A.S.C.R.S.**
Associate Clinical Professor of Surgery
Michigan State University
College of Human Medicine
East Lansing, Michigan and
Staff Colorectal Surgeon
Ferguson Clinic
Grand Rapids, Michigan

**Findlay A. MaCrae, M.D., F.R.A.C.P.,
M.R.C.P**
Department of Colorectal Surgery
Royal Melbourne Hospital
Melbourne, Australia

**Robert D. Madoff, M.D., F.A.C.S.,
F.A.S.C.R.S.**
Clinical Assistant Professor of Surgery
Director of Research
Division of Colon and Rectal Surgery
University of Minnesota
Minneapolis Minnesota

Martti Matikainen, M.D.
Chief of Gastroenterology
Surgeon, Department of Surgery
Tampere University Hospital
Tampere, Finland

**Robin S. McLeod, M.D., F.R.C.S.(C),
F.A.S.C.R.S.**
Associate Professor of Surgery
Department of Surgery
Residency Program Director in
Colon and Rectal Surgery
University of Toronto and
Staff Surgeon
Mount Sinai Hospital

Toronto, Ontario
Canada

Victor L. Modesto, M.D., F.A.C.S.
Division of Colon and Rectal Surgery
St. Luke's Hospital Center
New York, New York and
Clinical Assistant Professor of Surgery
Uniformed Services University of
the Health Sciences
Bethesda, Maryland

Harry K. Moon, M.D.
Staff Surgeon
Department of Plastic and
Reconstructive Surgery and
Chief of Staff
Cleveland Clinic Florida
Fort Lauderdale, Florida

Pedro J. Morgado, M.D., F.A.C.S.
Professor Titular
Faculty of Medicine
Central University of Caracas and
Colorectal Surgeon
Centro Medico de Caracas
San Bernardino, Caracas
Venezuela

Pedro J. Morgado Jr., M.D.
Colorectal Surgeon
Centro Medico de Caracas
San Bernardino, Caracas
Venezuela

**Heidi Nelson, M.D., F.A.C.S.,
F.A.S.C.R.S.**
Assistant Professor of Surgery
Mayo Clinic
Rochester, Minnesota

Graham L. Newstead, M.D.
Chairman, Colorectal Unit
Associate Director, Division of
Surgery
Prince of Wales Hospital
University of New South Wales
Sydney, Australia

R. J. Nicholls, M. Chir., F.R.C.S.
Consultant Surgeon and Dean of
the Academic Institute
St. Mark's Hospital
London, England

Juan J. Nogueras, M.D.
Staff Surgeon
Department of Colorectal Surgery
Cleveland Clinic Florida
Fort Lauderdale, Florida

P. Ronan O'Connell, M.D., F.R.C.S.I.
Clinical Lecturer in Surgery
University College of Dublin and
Consultant Surgeon,
Mater Misericordiae Hospital
Dublin, Ireland

**Gregory C. Oliver, M.D., F.A.C.S.,
F.A.S.C.R.S.**
Assistant Clinical Professor of Surgery
Residency Program Director
Division of Colon and Rectal Surgery
The Robert Wood Johnson School of
Medicine
Plainfield, New Jersey

**Frank G. Opelka, M.D., F.A.C.S.,
F.A.S.C.R.S.**
Staff Surgeon
Ochsner Clinic
Department of Colon and Rectal Surgery
New Orleans, Louisiana

Alejandro González Padrón, M.D.
Department of Colorectal Surgery
Cleveland Clinic Florida
Fort Lauderdale, Florida

Lars Påhlman, M.D., Ph.D.
Associate Professor
Department of Surgery, Colorectal Unit
Akademiska Sjukhuset
Uppsala University
Uppsala, Sweden

**Russell K. Pearl, M.D., F.A.C.S.,
F.A.S.C.R.S.**
Associate Professor of Surgery
University of Illinois College of Medicine
Attending Surgeon, Division of Colon
and Rectal Surgery
Cook County Hospital
Chicago, Illinois

**John H. Pemberton, M.D., F.A.C.S.,
F.A.S.C.R.S.**
Professor of Surgery
Mayo Medical School
Consultant, Division of Colon and
Rectal Surgery

Mayo Clinic and Mayo Foundation
Rochester, Minnesota

Walter R. Peters, M.D.
Staff Surgeon
Columbia Surgical Associates
Columbia, Missouri

Robin Phillips, M.S., F.R.C.S.
Consultant Surgeon
St. Mark's Hospital
London, England

Marcelo F. Piccirillo, M.D.
Department of Colorectal Surgery
Cleveland Clinic Florida
Fort Lauderdale, Florida

Richard M. Pitsch Jr., M.D., F.A.C.S.
Colorectal Surgeon
Chairman, Section of General Surgery
Lincoln General Hospital
Assistant Clinical Professor
Department of Surgery, Division
of Colon and Rectal Surgery
Creighton University School of Medicine
Omaha, Nebraska

Elliot Prager, M.D.
Sansum Medical Clinic
Santa Barbara, California

W. Terence Reilly, M.D.
Division of Colon and Rectal Surgery
Mayo Clinic and Mayo Foundation
Rochester, Minnesota

Petachia Reissman, M.D.
Department of Colorectal Surgery
Cleveland Clinic Florida
Fort Lauderdale, Florida

**Patricia L. Roberts, M.D., F.A.C.S.
F.A.S.C.R.S.**
Staff Surgeon
Department of Colon and Rectal Surgery
Lahey Clinic
Burlington, Massachusetts and
Clinical Assistant Professor of Surgery
Boston University
Boston, Massachusetts

Guillermo O. Rosato, M.D.
Chairman, Department of Colorectal
Surgery
Hospital Evita
Buenos Aires, Argentina

Lester Rosen, M.D., F.A.C.S., F.A.S.C.R.S.
Professor of Surgery
Allentown Affiliated Hospitals and
Hahnemann University
Residency Program Director
Division of Colorectal Surgery
Allentown, Pennsylvania

David A. Rothenberger, M.D., F.A.C.S., F.A.S.C.R.S.
Clinical Professor of Surgery
Director, Division of Colon and Rectal
Surgery
University of Minnesota
Minneapolis, Minnesota

William B. Ruderman, M.D.
Chairman, Department of Gastroenterology
Cleveland Clinic Florida
Fort Lauderdale, Florida

Theodore J. Saclarides, M.D., F.A.C.S., F.A.S.C.R.S.
Associate Professor of Surgery
Head, Section of Colon and Rectal Surgery
Rush Medical College
Chicago, Illinois

Carlos Sardiñas, M.D.
Instructor in Surgery
Caracas University Hospital
Caracas, Venezuela

Stephanie L. Schmitt, M.D.
Chief, Colon and Rectal Surgery
Director, Surgical Research
The Medical Center of Central
Massachusetts
Worcester, Massachusetts and
Assistant Professor of Surgery
University of Massachusetts
Medical School
Worcester, Massachusetts

Anthony J. Senagore, M.D., M.S.
Department of Surgery
Michigan State University
School of Human Medicine
East Lansing Michigan
Staff Colorectal Surgeon
Ferguson Clinic
Grand Rapids, Michigan

Stephen M. Sentovich, M.D.
Section of Colon and Rectal Surgery

Creighton University
Omaha, Nebraska

Mark E. Sesto, M.D., F.A.C.S.
Chairman, Department of General
and Vascular Surgery
Cleveland Clinic Florida
Fort Lauderdale, Florida

Susan A. Sgambati, M.D.
University of Connecticut
and Yale University Schools of Medicine
Division of G.I. Surgical Research
New Haven, Connecticut

M. J. Solomon, M.D.
Director of Research
Sydney Central Department of Colon
and Rectal Surgery at
Royal Prince Alfred Hospital
Sydney, Australia

Marco Sorgi, M.D.
Staff, Department of Surgery
Domingo Luciani Hospital
Caracas, Venezuela

Barry L. Stein, M.D.
Department of Colon and Rectal Surgery
Lahey Clinic
Burlington, Massachusetts

Scott Strong, M.D.
Staff Surgeon
Department of Colorectal Surgery
Cleveland Clinic Foundation
Cleveland, Ohio

Steven J. Stryker, M.D.
Associate Professor of Clinical Surgery
Northwestern University
Chicago, Illinois

Alan G. Thorson, M.D., F.A.C.S., F.A.S.C.R.S.
Associate Professor of Surgery and
Program Director
Section of Colon and Rectal Surgery
Creighton University School of Medicine
Clinical Associate Professor of Surgery
University of Nebraska College of Medicine
Omaha, Nebraska

Alan E. Timmcke, M.D., F.A.C.S., F.A.S.C.R.S.
Staff Surgeon
Department of Colon and Rectal Surgery

Ochsner Clinic Foundation
New Orleans, Louisiana

Magaly Gemio Teixeira, M.D.
Assistant Professor of Surgery
Division of Colon and Rectal Surgery
São Paulo University School of Medicine
São Paulo, Brazil

**Joe J. Tjandra, M.D., F.R.A.C.S.,
F.R.C.S., F.R.C.P.S.**
Department of Colorectal Surgery
Royal Melbourne Hospital
Melbourne, Australia

Thomas Troeng, M.D.
Lund University
Department of Surgery
Malmö, Sweden

Tina Ure, M.D.
St. Louis University Health Sciences Center
St. Louis, Missouri

Joji Utsunomiya, M.D., Ph.D.
Second Department of Surgery
Hyogo College of Medicine
Nishinomiya, Hyoga
Japan

**Carol-Ann Vasilevsky, M.D., C.M.,
F.R.C.S., F.A.C.S., F.A.S.C.R.S.**
Assistant Professor of Surgery
McGill University
Attending Surgeon, Department of
Colorectal Surgery
Sir Mortimer B. Davis Jewish General
Hospital
Montreal, Quebec
Canada

**Anthony M. Vernava III, M.D., F.A.C.S.,
F.A.S.C.R.S.**
Chief, Section of Colon and Rectal Surgery
Director, Residency Training Program in
Colon and Rectal Surgery
Associate Professor of Surgery
Saint Louis University Health Sciences
Center
St. Louis, Missouri

James Weick, M.D.
Chairman, Department of Hematology and
Oncology
Cleveland Clinic Florida
Fort Lauderdale, Florida

Eric G. Weiss, M.D.
Staff Surgeon
Department of Colorectal Surgery
Cleveland Clinic Florida
Fort Lauderdale, Florida

**Steven D. Wexner, M.D., F.A.C.S.,
F.A.S.C.R.S.**
Chairman and Residency Program Director
Department of Colorectal Surgery and
Chairman, Continuing Medical Education
Cleveland Clinic Florida
Fort Lauderdale, Florida

**Richard L. Whelan, M.D., F.A.C.S.,
F.A.S.C.R.S.**
Assistant Professor of Surgery
Director, Division of Colon and Rectal
Surgery and Director, Anorectal Physiology
Laboratory
Department of Surgery
Columbia University and Presbyterian
Hospital
College of Physicians and Surgeons
New York, New York

Gregory Weiner, M.D.
Instructor, General Surgery
Rush Medical College
Chicago, Illinois

Paul R. Williamson, M.D., F.A.C.S.
Assistant Professor of Surgery and
Co-Program Director
Colon and Rectal Fellowship Program
Orlando, Florida

**W. Douglas Wong, M.D., F.A.C.S.,
F.R.C.S.(C)**
Clinical Assistant Professor of Surgery
Director, Residency Training Program
Division of Colorectal Surgery
University of Minnesota Medical School
Minneapolis, Minnesota

T. Yamamura, M.D., Ph.D.
Second Department of Surgery
Hyogo College of Medicine
Nishinomiya, Hyogo
Japan

Yung Kang Yang, M.D.
Division of Colorectal Surgery
Tri-Service General Hospital
Taipei, Taiwan
Republic of China

CONTENTS

CLINICAL DECISION MAKING IN COLORECTAL SURGERY

SECTION 1

General

CHAPTER 1

Anorectal Evaluation

Anthony M. Vernava, III, M.D. and Walter E. Longo, M.D.

Refer to Algorithm 1–1.

ANORECTAL EVALUATION

A. Although most patients with complaints referrable to the anorectum attribute their symptoms to "hemorrhoids," the astute physician can usually diagnose the pathology on the basis of a good history. The chief complaint, duration of symptoms and whether they are improving, and what measures the patient has already taken should be elucidated. Rectal bleeding should be characterized as either melena, hematochezia, or outlet type. The character, location, and duration of anorectal pain should be discovered. Queries should be made as to whether the patient has any systemic symptoms such as fever and chills or diarrhea. Specific areas of questioning related to specific disorders appear in their respective algorithms throughout the text.

B. Knowledge of several aspects of the patient's past medical history and systems review are essential to the safe and effective management of anorectal disease since these coexisting pathologies can affect therapy. All patients should be asked whether they have a personal history of inflammatory bowel disease including Crohn's disease or mucosal ulcerative colitis. A sexually transmitted disease history should be taken. Both personal and family histories of colorectal neoplasia should be elucidated since patients with such histories are at higher risk for colorectal cancer than is the general population.

C. The initial part of the physical exam assesses the patient's ability to cooperate since this exam is uncomfortable and embarrassing. The prone position is preferred for routine anorectal examination since it provides excellent expo-

Paragraph identifiers A, B, etc. appearing throughout text refer to corresponding elements in numbered algorithm displays labeled with superscript letters (e.g., paragraph A in Chapter 1 text corresponds to History[A] element in Algorithm 1–1).

3

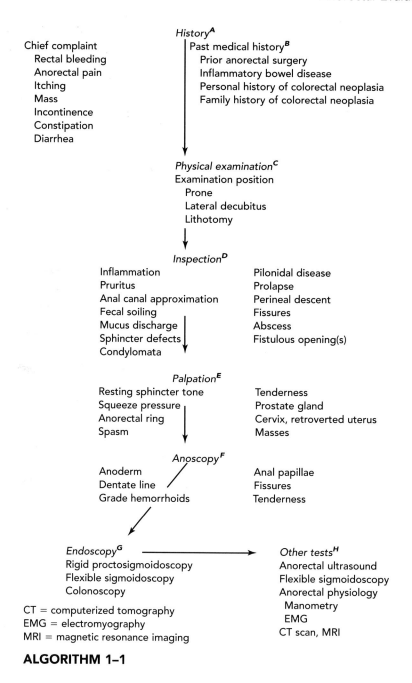

History^A

Chief complaint
  Rectal bleeding
  Anorectal pain
  Itching
  Mass
  Incontinence
  Constipation
  Diarrhea

Past medical history^B
  Prior anorectal surgery
  Inflammatory bowel disease
  Personal history of colorectal neoplasia
  Family history of colorectal neoplasia

Physical examination^C
Examination position
  Prone
  Lateral decubitus
  Lithotomy

Inspection^D
Inflammation   Pilonidal disease
Pruritus   Prolapse
Anal canal approximation   Perineal descent
Fecal soiling   Fissures
Mucus discharge   Abscess
Sphincter defects   Fistulous opening(s)
Condylomata

Palpation^E
Resting sphincter tone   Tenderness
Squeeze pressure   Prostate gland
Anorectal ring   Cervix, retroverted uterus
Spasm   Masses

Anoscopy^F
Anoderm   Anal papillae
Dentate line   Fissures
Grade hemorrhoids   Tenderness

Endoscopy^G ⟶ Other tests^H
Rigid proctosigmoidoscopy   Anorectal ultrasound
Flexible sigmoidoscopy   Flexible sigmoidoscopy
Colonoscopy   Anorectal physiology
                                  Manometry
CT = computerized tomography   EMG
EMG = electromyography   CT scan, MRI
MRI = magnetic resonance imaging

ALGORITHM 1–1

sure. Some elderly or otherwise incapacitated patients are unable to tolerate this position, and an alternative includes the lateral decubitus position. Lithotomy is generally not a good option.

D. Visual *inspection* of the perineum and perianal skin is performed prior to digital rectal exam and anoscopy or endoscopy. The buttocks should be gently separated to facilitate the exam. The condition of the perianal skin should be noted along with any pruritus, inflammation, fecal soiling, or mucus discharge. Any pruritus should be graded as either mild, moderate, or severe. Notation should be made as to whether the anal canal is approximated or patulous; the presence of any sphincter defect should be noted. The presence and precise location of any fissures, abscesses, or external fistulous openings and the extent of perineal descent should be specifically evaluated and recorded. Any prolapsed tissue will be seen. All abnormal findings should be recorded and illustrated in the medical record.

E. The next step in a complete anorectal exam is gentle *palpation:* A well-lubricated, gloved index finger should be used to palpate the perianal skin for any subcutaneous lesions or tenderness. Next, a gentle but thorough digital rectal exam should be done with the tip of the examining finger reaching above the anorectal ring. The entire circumference of the anorectum should be palpated by gentle circumanal rotation of the examining finger. The examiner specifically should note the resting sphincter tone, the squeeze pressure, the mobility of the puborectalis, and the presence of any spasm or tenderness. The presence of any mass should be noted along with its character (fixed or mobile), and precise location. In men, the prostate gland and in women, the cervix, and any retroverted uterus, should be specifically evaluated and noted.

F. After the digital rectal exam is completed, an *anoscopy* is performed with a well-lubricated anoscope. The condition of the anal canal mucosa should be evaluated and any inflammation noted; hemorrhoids should be graded. Any fissures should be further evaluated and the presence or absence of any hypertrophied anal papillae should be recorded. Tenderness elicited on the placement of the anoscope should prompt further evaluation for an occult, postanal abscess or fissure.

G. Finally, endoscopy is performed. The patient should have been prepped with one or more cleansing enemas. Flexible sigmoidoscopy is preferred to rigid proctosigmoidoscopy for the initial evaluation because of patient comfort and length of insertion. The average length of insertion of a rigid proctosigmoido-scope is only 20 cm; thus flexible sigmoidoscopy has a 3–6 times higher yield. However, rigid proctosigmoidoscopy is a more accurate method of measuring distance from the anal verge. Whether colonoscopy is indicated depends on specific patient complaints, family history, and the findings on anorectal examination. The presence of isolated benign anorectal disease is not an indication for colonoscopy.

H. In difficult cases other tests may be indicated. For patients with incontinence or constipation, anorectal physiologic testing is helpful in defining etiology and planning therapy. Intraanal ultrasound is an excellent method of identifying and documenting external and internal sphincter disruption. Chronic anal pain may indicate a postanal abscess or a retrorectal tumor, and a computerized tomography (CT) scan or magnetic resonance image (MRI) can be diagnostic.

BIBLIOGRAPHY

1. Allan A, Keighley MRB: Management of perianal Crohn's disease. *World J Surg* 12:198–202, 1988.

2. Baker WN, Milton-Thompson GJ: The anal lesion as the sole presenting symptom of intestinal Crohn's disease. *Gut* 12:165, 1971.

3. Binderow S, Wexner SD: Anorectal complaints. In: Barkin JS, Rogers AL (eds). Difficult decisions in digestive diseases (2nd ed). St. Louis: Mosby-Yearbook, Inc. 1994; 289–306.

4. Law PJ, Kamm MA, Bartram CI: A comparison between electromyography and anal endosonography in mapping external anal sphincter defects. *Dis Colon Rectum* 33:370–373, 1990.

5. Longo WE, Dean PA, Virgo KS, et al: Colonoscopy in patients with benign anorectal disease. *Dis Colon Rectum* 36:368–371, 1993.

6. Nivatvongs S, Frud DS: How far does the proctosigmoidoscope reach? A prospective study of 1000 patients. *N Engl J Med* 303:380–382, 1980.

7. Vernava AM, Longo WE, Daniel GL: Pudendal neuropathy and the importance of EMG evaluation of fecal incontinence. *Dis Colon Rectum* 36:23–27, 1993.

8. Winnan G, Berci G, Parish J, et al: Superiority of the flexible to the rigid sigmoidoscopy in routine proctosigmoidoscopy. *N Engl J Med* 302:1011–1012, 1980.

See also Chapters 6, 8, 10, 11, 12A, 12B, 13, 15.

CHAPTER 2

Colonic Evaluation

Eric G. Weiss, M.D. and Steven D. Wexner, M.D.

Refer to Algorithm 2-1.

A. A detailed history allows formation of a differential diagnosis based on questions relating to rectal bleeding, pain, bowel habits, systemic symptoms, and significant past medical history.

B. Inspection requires adequate lighting and positioning of the patient in the prone jackknife position. Inspect for abnormal masses or tissue, color and condition of the perianal skin, any scars, and abnormal shape of the external opening of the anus. Anal position at rest (open versus closed) and during coughing should be noted. Any soiling of either the perianal skin or the undergarments should be noted. All skin tags and other irregularities should be described and ultimately all of the information gleaned from inspection should be diagrammed in the medical record. (See Figure 2-1.)

C. Digital exam includes a prostate exam in males and examination of the posterior vaginal wall in females. The exam includes a full 360° sweep of the anal canal and the lower rectum. Resting and squeeze tone should be noted, as should puborectalis tone and motion. The patient should be asked to bear down to bring any midrectal lesions into contact with the fingertip.

D. Anoscopy evaluates the anal canal; anoderm, dentate line, hemorrhoidal area, and the lowermost rectal mucosa. A side-viewing instrument is optimal as any enlarged hemorrhoids prolapse into sight. Conversely, end viewing instruments, such as a retroflexed flexible sigmoidoscope, reduce tissue away from the anal orifice. Each quadrant, including the three major hemorrhoidal sites as well as potential anterior and posterior fissure sites, should be evaluated. As well as a written description of any findings, a diagrammatic representation is helpful both to other physicians and for subsequent reevaluations. In particular, nonoperative hemorrhoid therapy can be quantifiably monitored. (See Fig. 2-1.)

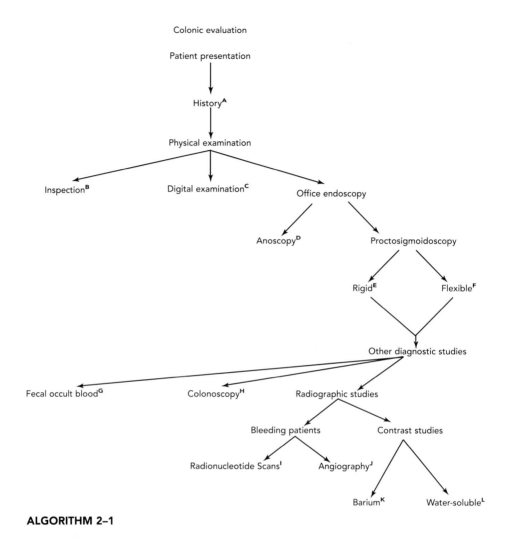

Colonic evaluation

Patient presentation

History^A

Physical examination

Inspection^B   Digital examination^C   Office endoscopy

Anoscopy^D   Proctosigmoidoscopy

Rigid^E   Flexible^F

Other diagnostic studies

Fecal occult blood^G   Colonoscopy^H   Radiographic studies

Bleeding patients   Contrast studies

Radionucleotide Scans^I   Angiography^J

Barium^K   Water-soluble^L

ALGORITHM 2–1

FIGURE 2–1 A simple circle can be used to depict the anus with the letter "p" to denote posterior. Pathology can be drawn in the medical record as appropriate.

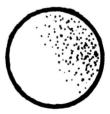

E. Rigid sigmoidoscopy allows visualization of the distal 20–25 cm of colon. Its best use is for measurement of the distance from the anal verge or dentate line of rectal tumors.

F. Flexible proctosigmoidoscopy allows inspection of an additional 40 cm of proximal sigmoid and descending colon. It requires more specialized training and equipment than does rigid examination. However, the ability to use video or a teaching head are added advantages. As well as a written description of any findings, a diagrammatic representation may be helpful to other physicians and for subsequent reevaluation. Specifically, the response to topical therapy for proctitis can be quantifiably monitored. (See Fig. 2–2.)

G. Hemoccult testing may be used to document heme positive stool or in conjunction with proctosigmoidoscopy as a screening tool for colorectal neoplasia. It is important to avoid certain food products and medications during the testing period as described in the specific instructions accompanying the cards, as a false-positive or false-negative test may result. The overall sensitivity is in the range of 50%.

H. Colonoscopy allows complete visualization of the colon. It is useful when lesions are noted by radiographic studies or by proctosigmoidoscopy; also useful in patients with a personal or family history of neoplasia, patients with rectal bleeding or hemoccult positive stools, and patients with a history of inflammatory bowel disease.

I. Technetium-labeled scans are useful only in the actively bleeding patient for localization or lateralization of the bleeding. The study has no therapeutic benefit, but is noninvasive and allows detection of $\geq 0.5–1$ mL/min of blood loss.

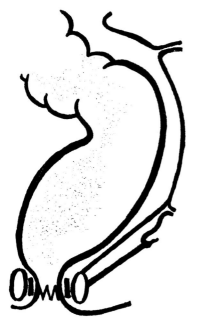

FIGURE 2–2 This cross-sectional diagram of the rectum is useful for diagramatic representation of anorectal pathology.

J. Selective visualization via mesenteric vessels is an invasive procedure that requires arterial catheterization. It allows detection of ≥0.5 mL/min of blood loss. The technique very accurately localizes bleeding and may also be therapeutic with either vasopressin infusion or embolization.

K. Air-contrast study is superior to the single-column study.

L. A water-soluble agent is used when colonic obstruction, an acute inflammatory process, or an anastamotic leak is suspected. However, these agents provide less detail than does barium.

BIBLIOGRAPHY

1. deRoos AD, Hermans J, Shaw PC, et al: Colon polyps and carcinomas: Prospective comparisons of the single and double contrast examination in the same patient. *Radiology* 154:11–13, 1985.

2. Markisz JA, Front D, Royal HD, et al: An evaluation of 99mTC-labeled red blood cell scintigraphy for determination and localization of gastrointestinal bleeding sites. *Gastroenterology* 83:394–398, 1982.

3. Wexner SD, Brabbee GW, Wichern WA Jr.: Sensitivity of hemoccult testing in patients with colorectal carcinoma. *Dis Colon Rectum* 27(12):775–776, 1984.

4. Wexner SD, Dailey TH: The intial management of left lower quadrant peritonitis. *Dis Colon Rectum* 29:635–638, 1986.

See also Chapters 10, 11, 12A, 12B, 13, 15.

CHAPTER 3

Physiologic Evaluation

J. Marcio N. Jorge, M.D. and Steven D. Wexner, M.D.

Refer to Algorithm 3–1.

A. Exclusion of both intestinal and systemic organic etiology is mandatory before referring the patient with functional symptoms to the physiology lab. Specific tests are dictated by history and physical exam. Barium enema and/or colonoscopy is usually indicated and, if found, primary pathology is treated.

B. The initial therapeutic schema usually includes dietary assessment, and when indicated, psychological evaluation. A high-fiber diet and a diary of defecation and symptoms are helpful, as the symptoms can be better evaluated or even improved, when diet-related. Patients referred to the lab, therefore, usually have refractory, severe idiopathic symptoms. This step is, however, optional in patients with severe symptoms and obvious etiology, such as traumatic incontinence.

C. Functional anorectal disorders often present clinically as constipation and/or incontinence, and these symptoms have complex and multifactorial etiology. Therefore, a combination of tests is usually necessary. A more complete list of tests is displayed in Table 3–1.

D. The major importance of colonic transit times resides in excluding factitious constipation. Colonic transit times, in fact, provide a definition for constipation, by converting an otherwise hopelessly subjective symptom to an objective part of the medical record.

E. In a patient with severe and chronic persistent symptoms of constipation and a normal colonic transit time, or if use of laxatives, enemas or other medications affecting gastrointestinal (GI) motility during the test is suspected, colonic transit times should be repeated.

F. The importance of assessment of segmental colonic transit time remains as a controversial issue. This assessment may involve either multiple ingestion of markers or multiple abdominal radiographs. From a practical point of view, however, x-rays taken on days 3 and 5 after ingestion of a single marker may help in the stratification of motility patterns: colonic inertia and outlet obstruction (Figs. 3–1, 3–2).

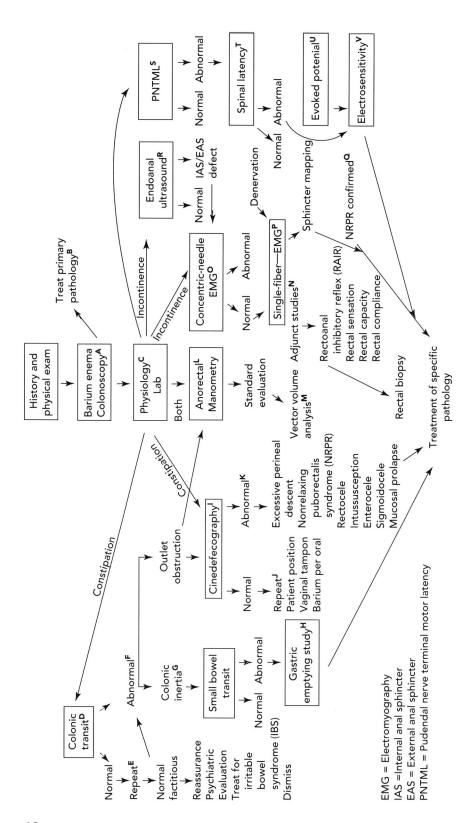

History and physical exam

Barium enema Colonoscopy[A]

Treat primary pathology[B]

Physiology[C] Lab

Constipation

Both

Incontinence

Incontinence

Colonic transit[D]

Constipation

Normal
Repeat[E]
Normal
factitious
Reassurance
Psychiatric
Evaluation
Treat for
irritable
bowel
syndrome (IBS)
Dismiss

Abnormal[F]

Colonic inertia[G]

Outlet obstruction

Small bowel transit

Normal   Abnormal

Gastric emptying study[H]

Cinedefecography[I]

Normal

Repeat[J]
Patient position
Vaginal tampon
Barium per oral

Abnormal[K]

Excessive perineal
descent
Nonrelaxing
puborectalis
syndrome (NRPR)
Rectocele
Intussusception
Enterocele
Sigmoidocele
Mucosal prolapse

Anorectal Manometry[L]

Standard evaluation

Vector volume analysis[M]

Adjunct studies[N]

Rectoanal
inhibitory reflex (RAIR)
Rectal sensation
Rectal capacity
Rectal compliance

Rectal biopsy

Treatment of specific pathology

Concentric-needle EMG[O]

Normal   Abnormal

Single-fiber—EMG[P]

Denervation

Sphincter mapping

NRPR confirmed[Q]

Endoanal ultrasound[R]

Normal   IAS/EAS defect

PNTML[S]

Normal   Abnormal

Spinal latency[T]

Normal   Abnormal

Evoked potenial[U]

Electrosensitivity[V]

Treatment of specific pathology

EMG = Electromyography
IAS =Internal anal sphincter
EAS = External anal sphincter
PNTML = Pudendal nerve terminal motor latency

Algorithm 3-1

12

TABLE 3–1 ANORECTAL PHYSIOLOGIC TESTING

Manometry	Spinal latency
Adjunct manometric studies	Perineal latency
Sensory threshold	Sensory evoked potentials
Rectoanal Inhibitory Reflex (RAIR)	Anal mucosal electrosensitivity
Rectal capacity	Anal mucosal thermal sensitivity
Rectal compliance	Anal endosonography
Colonic transit study	Tests of continence
Cinedefecography	Enema retention
Electromyography (EMG)	Saline infusion test
Concentric needle—EMG	Solid sphere test
Single-fiber—EMG	
Pudendal nerve terminal motor latency	

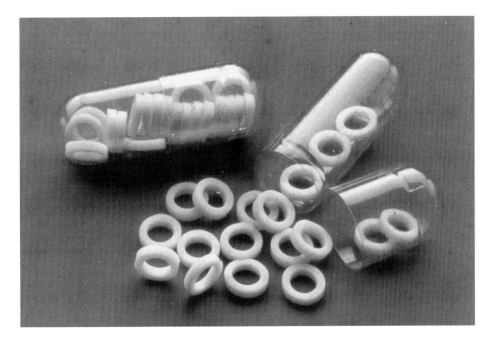

FIGURE 3–1 The sitz mark™ (Konsyl Pharmaceuticals Inc., Fort Worth, TX) capsule contains 24 radiopaque rings for colonic transit studies.

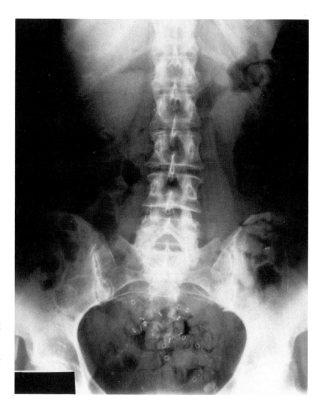

FIGURE 3–2A This transit study reveals a pelvic outlet obstruction pattern as all markers are in the rectosigmoid on day 5.

G. In patients with colonic inertia, evaluation for colectomy includes reassessment of severity of symptoms (history, transit times, and response to trials of therapy with laxatives and prokinetics), exclusion of small bowel dysmotility (lactulose breath H_2 test), and exclusion of pelvic floor dysfunction.

H. If dyspeptic symptoms, such as nausea, vomiting, heartburn, and bloating are present, gastric emptying studies are indicated in order to exclude a generalized gastrointestinal stasis.

I. Cinedefecography permits radiologic visualization of the dynamics of defecation (Fig. 3–3). Specifically, pelvic dynamic measurements, anatomical abnormalities and rectal emptying can all be assessed. Evaluation of both absolute and dynamic (evacuation–rest) values of anorectal angle, perineal descent and puborectalis length allows diagnosis of excessive perineal descent and paradoxical puborectalis syndrome. Comparison of an absolute measurement, such as the anorectal angle, in a patient against a group of controls is frequently a frustrating endeavor; therefore, evaluation of isolated parameters remains of uncertain value. More value is obtained from comparing resting, squeezing, and pushing values in a single patient. Cinedefecography also permits the diagnosis of causative or associated anatomical abnormalities such as nonrelaxing puborectalis (Fig. 3–4), rectocele, occult rectoanal intussusception, sigmoidocele, and enterocele. The conventional method using barium paste of similar consistency of stool is preferred to balloon proctography. Although balloon proctography requires less irradiation, it does not assess either anatomical abnormalities or completeness of evacuation. Furthermore, displacement of the balloon results in inaccurate and dubious measurements.

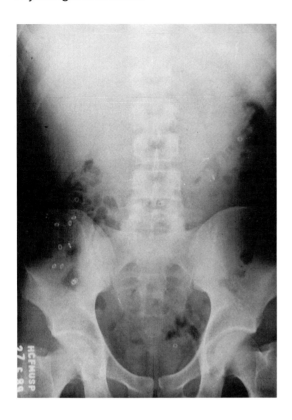

FIGURE 3–2B This transit study reveals colonic inertia as the markers are present diffusely through the abdominal colon on day 5.

J. Although patient position does not affect dynamic pelvic measurements, absolute values are higher in the seated position when compared to the left lateral decubitus, and the former is, therefore, more sensitive for the diagnosis of increased fixed perineal descent. Posteranterior proctography also has been revealed to be helpful as a supplementary examination to validate the diagnosis of rectoanal intussusception. Ingestion of 150 mL of barium contrast orally 1 hour prior to the examination assists with delineation of intrapelvic small bowel loops. Other technical variants that may enhance diagnostic capability of cinedefecography include placement of radiopaque markers on the ischial tuberosities to permit more accurate quantification of perineal descent and introduction of a barium-soaked tampon into the vagina (isolated method), or combined with voiding cystography (colpocystodefecography) in order to better delineate rectoceles and enteroceles.

K. Anatomic defecographic findings, particularly small rectoceles and intussusception, may be found in 25–77% of asymptomatic individuals. Failure to recognize these deviations from the norm can easily lead to overdiagnosis and overtreatment. Therefore, decisions should be based on clinical history and evaluation, during cinedefecography, of rectal emptying.

L. Manometry is useful in the evaluation of common functional disorders, such as fecal incontinence and idiopathic constipation. Additionally, abdominal (low colorectal, coloanal, and ileoanal anastomosis) and anal procedures (fistula and fissure surgery), in patients in whom the continence status is endangered, surgery can be planned in a more objective basis. Specifically, preoperative manometry may be indicated when preoperative history and physical exam-

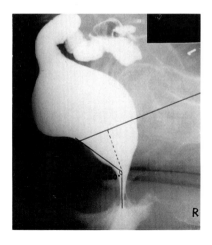

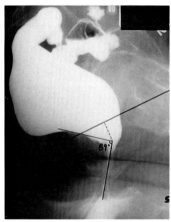

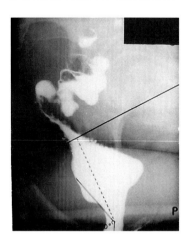

FIGURE 3–3 This normal cinedefogram shows the evacuatory sequence during rest (R), squeeze (S), and push (P).

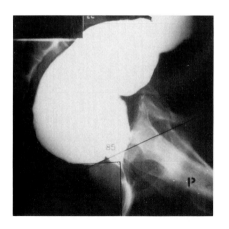

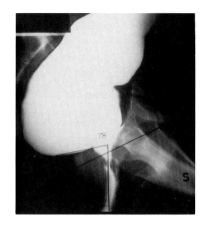

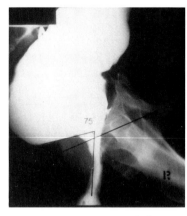

FIGURE 3–4 This cinedefogram shows marked nonrelaxing puborectalis. Note that the anorectal angles during rest, squeeze, and push are not significantly different.

ination suggest clinical or subclinical incontinence (multiparity, excessive perineal descent, a borderline anal tone) or in light of the risk of incontinence related to the procedure itself (complex and recurrent fistula, recurrent fissure after sphincterotomy). Figure 3–5A shows a resting pressure profile, and Fig. 3–5B shows a squeezing pressure profile.

M. Vector volume analysis represents a more detailed assessment of both internal anal and external anal sphincter pressures. However, its role in determining sphincteric symmetry and, therefore, detecting sphincter defects has been questioned. Correlations with anal ultrasound and electromyography mapping is indicated when subclinical defects are suspected in incontinent patients.

N. Adjunct manometric studies include the rectoanal inhibitory reflex (RAIR), rectal sensory threshold, rectal capacity, and rectal compliance. Except for the RAIR, these studies seldom are strictly diagnostic themselves, but they do permit better comprehension of pathophysiology involving constipation or incontinence. The RAIR, characterized by transient external anal sphincter (EAS) contraction followed by pronounced internal anal sphincter (IAS) relaxation, enables rectal contents to "be sampled" by the sensory area of the anal canal (Fig. 3–6). Patients with Hirschsprung's disease, Chagas' disease, der-

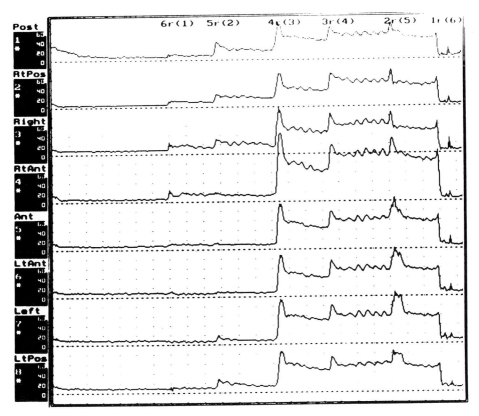

FIGURE 3–5A Resting pressure profile in eight quadrants at 45° intervals from 6 to 1 cm above the dentate line. These pressures are largely reflective of the internal anal sphincter basal tone.

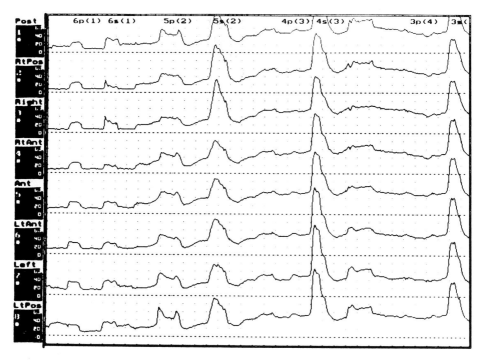

FIGURE 3–5B Squeezing pressure profile in eight quadrants at 45° intervals from 6 to 3 cm above the dentate line reflect the activity of the external anal sphincter and puborectalis during contraction.

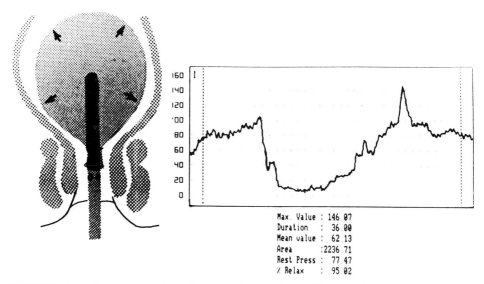

Max. Value : 146.07
Duration : 36.00
Mean value : 62.13
Area :2236.71
Rest Press : 77.47
% Relax : 95.02

FIGURE 3–6 The rectoanal inhibitory reflex is elicited by rapid intrarectal balloon insufflation. The manometric pressure profile shows the normal transient decrease in resting pressure, reflective of internal anal sphincter relaxation.

matomyositis and scleroderma all have abnormal RAIR. Failure of the reflex to occur at any volume is strong evidence of Hirschsprung's disease. However, factors such as the rectal volume may affect results. Therefore, transanal rectal myectomy is indicated in a patient with constipation and an absent RAIR. Diseases may selectively reduce conscious sensation and awareness of rectal fullness even with intact autonomic pathways. This problem results in either fecal impaction, fecal incontinence, or both. Younger and constipated patients tend to have larger capacity rectums than do older and incontinent patients. The nondiseased rectum is highly compliant; it accepts a tremendous increase in volume with a very small change in pressure. Rectal compliance is impaired in diseases such as ulcerative colitis, chronic rectal ischemia, radiation, and Hirschsprung's disease.

O. Electromyography (EMG) is especially valuable in the assessment of fecal incontinence, by providing quantification of motor unit potentials, mapping external anal sphincter defects, and assessing reinnervation patterns (Fig. 3-7).

P. Single-fiber electromyography is a quantitative method for assessing denervation in incontinence. It provides a better assessment of reinnervation, especially extensive muscle atrophy, which results in insufficient motor unit potentials, to be well evaluated by concentric-needle EMG. However, this study is more uncomfortable for the patient, and it does not seem to alter clinical decisions. Its use, therefore, is largely as a research tool.

Q. In patients with idiopathic constipation, electromyography may corroborate the diagnosis of nonrelaxing puborectalis syndrome, when doubt persists after cinedefecography (CD) (Fig. 3-8). Both EMG and CD have comparable sensitivity and specificity, which are individually suboptimal. However, CD is indicated first, as it is pain-free and provides useful data on rectal emptying.

R. Anal endosonography has been shown to be useful for mapping IAS and EAS defects. High correlation with EMG have been demonstrated in patients with traumatic fecal incontinence. Although unable to assess denervation, anal endosonography, by locating the EAS defect, may reduce the number of needle insertions required for EMG mapping. Additionally, anal endosonography may be useful in detecting small perineal abscess in patients with idiopathic anal pain.

S. Pudendal nerve terminal motor latency (PNTML) is particularly important in suspected neurogenic incontinence and in parous women prior to sphincter repair. PNTML is the most significant predictor of functional outcome after sphincter repair, as neuropathy, even when unilateral, is associated with poor postoperative functional results. However, this test does not seem to predict functional results after biofeedback. Although prolonged PNTML indicates pudendal neuropathy, normal latencies do not exclude nerve injury, since only the fastest remaining conducting fibers are recorded in this test.

T. Spinal latency enables exclusion of cauda equina injury as a cause of incontinence. Of patients with fecal incontinence and prolonged PNTML, 23% present conduction delay in the cauda equina between L1 and L4.

U. Since temperature sensation plays a role in discriminating among gas, liquid, and solid, a water-perfused thermode can be used in the assessment of incontinence. The anal canal is highly sensitive to temperature changes, and incontinent patients are significantly less sensitive than are controls.

1. NORMAL

2. MINIMAL
   REDUCTION
   OF MUP's

3. MODERATE
   REDUCTION
   OF MUP's

4. SEVERE
   REDUCTION
   OF MUP's

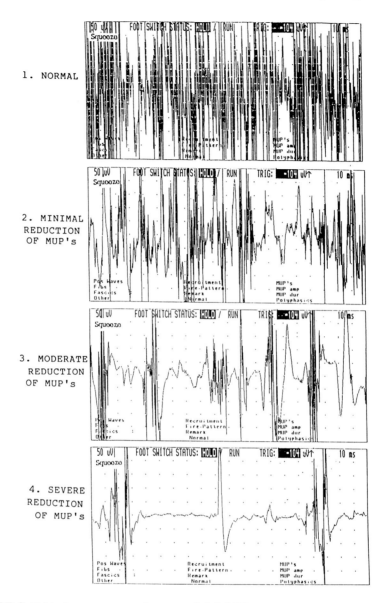

FIGURE 3-7 Various motor unit potential (MUP) recruitment patterns are seen.

V. Cortical somatosensory-evoked potentials are electrical responses of the nervous system to sensory stimulation and, therefore, constitute an alternative method to evaluate the functional integrity of the nerve supply of the anorectum and sphincter.

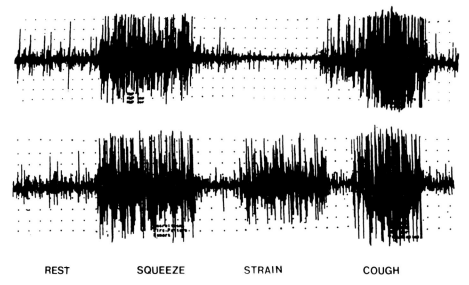

| REST | SQUEEZE | STRAIN | COUGH |

FIGURE 3–8 The top shows a normal external sphincter and puborectalis EMG. Note the electrical quiescence during attempted evacuation (straining). The bottom shows that in a patient with nonrelaxing puborectalis syndrome, electrical activity during attempted evacuation (strain) does not abate.

BIBLIOGRAPHY

1. Farouk R, Duthie GS, Bartolo DCC: Functional anorectal disorders and physiological evaluation. In Beck DE, Wexner SD (eds): *Fundamentals of Anorectal Surgery.* New York: McGraw-Hill, 1992.

2. Hock D, Lombard R, Jehaes C, et al: Colpocystodefecography. *Dis Colon Rectum* 36:1015–1021, 1993.

3. Jorge JMN, Wexner SD: A practical guide to basic anorectal physiology. *Contemp Surg* 43:214–224, 1993.

4. Jorge JMN, Wexner SD: Etiology and management of fecal incontinence. *Dis Colon Rectum* 36:77–97, 1993.

5. Jorge JMN, Wexner SD, Ger GC, et al: Cinedefecography and EMG in the diagnosis of nonrelaxing puborectalis syndrome. *Dis Colon Rectum* 36:668–676, 1993.

6. Jorge JMN, Wexner SD, Marchetti F, et al: How reliable are currently available methods of measuring the anorectal angle? *Dis Colon Rectum* 35:332–338, 1992.

7. Karulf RE, Coller JA, Bartolo DCC, et al: Anorectal physiology testing: a survey of availability and use. *Dis Colon Rectum* 34:464–468, 1991.

8. Law PJ, Kamm MA, Bartram CI: A comparison between electromyography and anal endosonography in mapping external anal sphincter defects. *Dis Colon Rectum* 33:370–373, 1990.

9. McGee SG, Bartram CI: Intra-anal intussusception: diagnosis by posteroanterior stress proctography. *Abdom Imag* 18:136–140, 1993.

10. Wexner SD, Marchetti F, Jagelman DG: The role of sphincteroplasty for fecal incontinence reevaluated: a prospective physiologic and functional review. *Dis Col Rectum* 34:22–30, 1991.

11. Wexner SD, Marchetti F, Salanga VD, et al: Neurophysiologic assessment of the anal sphincters. *Dis Colon Rectum* 34:606–612, 1991.

See also Chapters 17, 18, 19, 21, 33, 34, 61.

CHAPTER 4

Bowel Preparation

Stephen M. Cohen, M.D. and Steven D. Wexner, M.D.

Refer to Algorithm 4-1.

A. The major risk of sepsis from colorectal resections is due to colonic bacterial contamination. Therefore, preoperative preparation to adequately "clean" the colon has become the standard of practice for both colon and rectal surgery.

B. In order to reduce the incidence of septic complications after elective colorectal resections, preoperative preparation of the large intestine includes both mechanical cleansing and the administration of antibiotics.

C. Traditional bowel preparations involving starvation with a variety of purgatives and enemas are time-consuming, costly, and exhausting for the patients. This technique is no longer employed.

D. Elemental diets both maintain nitrogen balance and reduce fecal residue; however, they must be used for at least 5-7 days. A rectal washout is still necessary to improve the quality of the prep (preoperative preparation), and many patients find the elemental solution unpalatable.

E. Irrigation of the large bowel with an electrolyte solution was first used for the treatment of cholera in the early 1970s. This technique was altered as a method to clean the colon. Between 10 and 12 liters of fluid is used, and the procedure takes 4-6 hours. Advantages include the elimination of enemas, dietary restrictions and the entire preparation can be completed the day prior to the operation. Patients, however, do not like this form of bowel regimen as frequent side effects include fatigue, embarrassment, nausea, and vomiting. The use of the nasogastric tube is also quite distressing for most patients although very useful in patients who cannot ingest a large-volume preparation.

F. Electrolyte solutions can cause fluid and sodium retention and are contraindicated in elderly patients with renal, cardiac, or hepatic failure unless used with furosemide.

G. The oligosaccharide mannitol was introduced in 1979. Since it is not absorbed or digested it results in a rapid transit through the small bowel acting as an osmotic cathartic. However, mannitol is associated with dehydration and

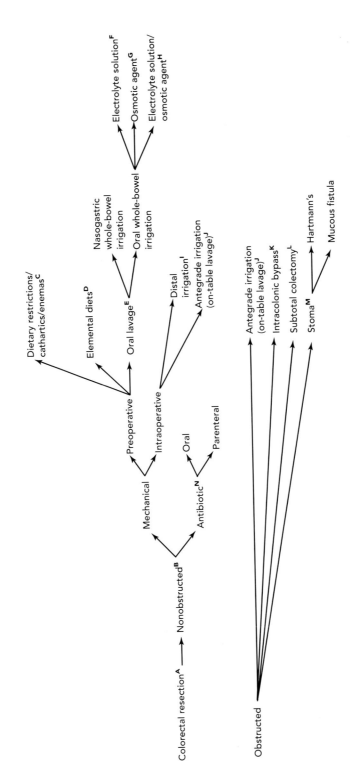

Colorectal resection[A] → Nonobstructed[B]

Mechanical

Preoperative

Dietary restrictions/
cathartics/enemas[C]

Elemental diets[D]

Oral lavage[E]

Nasogastric
whole-bowel
irrigation

Electrolyte solution[F]

Oral whole-bowel
irrigation

Osmotic agent[G]

Electrolyte solution/
osmotic agent[H]

Intraoperative

Distal
irrigation[I]

Antegrade irrigation
(on-table lavage)[J]

Antibiotic[N]

Oral

Parenteral

Obstructed

Antegrade irrigation
(on-table lavage)[J]

Intracolonic bypass[K]

Subtotal colectomy[L]

Stoma[M]

Hartmann's

Mucous fistula

ALGORITHM 4–1

24

sodium loss. Furthermore, there have been reports of fatal explosion with mannitol due to methane production as a result of fermentation by *Escherichia coli*.

H. A combination of an electrolyte solution with an osmotic agent was introduced in 1981 as polyethylene glycol in order to decrease the amount of fluid and electrolyte loss. Sodium sulfate replaced the sodium chloride and mannitol was replaced by polyethylene glycol, an inert, nonabsorbable, nonfermentable compound that acts as an osmotic agent. This agent also included other agents to prevent acidosis and minimize potassium loss. The most acceptable preparation at the present time is phosphate soda. (CB Fleet Co, Lynchburg VA) The two doses of 45 cc each are easier for patients to tolerate than is the 4 liter polyethylene glycol purge. Furthermore despite statistically significantly better patient preference endoscopic visualization is superior. Thus, like mannitol and wholegut nasogastric tube (NGT) lavage, the rather inhumane 4 liter polyethylene glycol prep is being rapidly relegated to the role of an historical footnote.

I. For left-sided colonic and rectal resections, distal irrigation is a useful adjunct for the removal of any retained fecal material in the rectum prior to commencement of the operation. Saline irrigation can be performed until the return is clear and betadine can be instilled if desired.

J. Since staged procedures are associated with a high mortality rate, the concept of intraoperative irrigation for large bowel obstruction has gained popularity. The idea is to resect diseased bowel and perform a primary anastomosis after removing all fecal material from the proximal bowel. A catheter is placed either through the appendiceal stump or the terminal ileum, and after full mobilization of the colon, several liters of saline are infused to remove all fecal material.

K. Others have found the above technique cumbersome and have placed an intraluminal sleeve across the anastomosis in the lumen of the bowel. This allows a path of egress for the stool and prevents direct contact of the stool to the suture line.

L. A subtotal colectomy and ileoproctostomy obviate the need for a bowel prep as the prep is "excised" rather than purged.

M. A stoma is still standard care in severely ill patients with purulent or fecal peritonitis. Either a mucous fistula or a Hartmann pouch can be created with the distal end. No bowel preparation is indicated and the formation of an anastomosis in the face of sepsis is contraindicated.

N. Mechanical cleansing of the bowel reduces the amount of stool and bacteria but does not alter the concentration of bacteria that remains in the colon. Prospective studies have demonstrated a reduction in infectious complications associated with colonic resection from 40–50% to approximately 5–10%. The antibiotics must cover the spectrum of both Gram-negative and anaerobic bacteria, and must be administered before bacterial contamination to provide adequate intraluminal and tissue levels. Furthermore the duration of use must be short to reduce the possibility of resistant bacterial strains. Both luminal and parenteral antibiotics are indicated.

BIBLIOGRAPHY

1. Cohen SM, Binderow SR, Wexner SD, et al: A prospective randomized endoscopist-blinded trial comparing precolonoscopy bowel cleansing methods. *Dis Colon Rectum.* 1994; 37:689–96.

2. Keighley MR, Williams NS: *Surgery of the Anus, Rectum and Colon.* London: Saunders, 1993.

3. Wexner SD, Beck DE: Sepsis prevention in colorectal surgery. In Fielding LP, Goldberg SM (eds): *Operative Surgery: Colon, Rectum, and Anus,* 5th ed. London: Butterworth, pp 41–46, 1993.

See also Chapter 62.

CHAPTER 5

Preoperative Assessment

John D. Cheape, M.D.

Refer to Algorithm 5-1.

A. When elective colorectal surgery has been recommended, a careful patient assessment should be performed. The first steps in this process are the clinical history and physical exam.
B. The assessment of the patient's status can be organized by evaluating the major body systems.
C. The cardiovascular evaluation should encompass the heart as well as the major arteries and veins. The heart should be assessed for myocardial function, coronary blood flow, as well as electrical abnormalities. Correlating findings from the history and physical with basic tests such as electrocardiogram (ECG) and chest x-ray can assist in determining potential cardiac abnormalities such as coronary artery disease, congestive heart failure, and cardiac dysrhythmias. A history of recent myocardial infarction is important. Abnormalities in these basic tests may necessitate further cardiac investigations such as exercise stress test, heart catheterization, or echocardiogram. A careful peripheral vascular exam should be performed with special attention to the carotid arteries. Patients with carotid bruits or symptoms potentially resulting from carotid stenosis may require further assessment usually in the form of noninvasive vascular tests. Cardiology consultation is wise if the history or any cardiac evaluations are suggestive of coronary artery disease or valvular or myocardial dysfunction.
D. Disturbances in pulmonary function may lead to major perioperative morbidity. Abnormalities gleaned from history and physical exam should be correlated with chest x-ray findings. Further evaluations may be necessary in the form of arterial blood gases and pulmonary function tests. Potentially, patients with pulmonary abnormalities may require medical management to optimize their pulmonary function. Where indicated, preoperative bronchodilators can be instituted. Patients receiving such therapy as a baseline need to have serum levels assessed and dosages regulated as necessary.
E. Accurate assessment of the patient's renal status is important in the management of the fluids, electrolytes, and medications that are eliminated by the

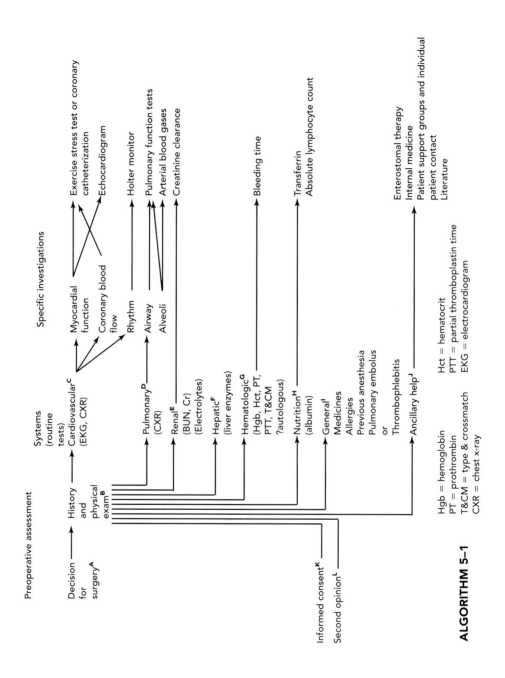

ALGORITHM 5-1

28

kidneys. Particular care should be used when using medications that are potentially nephrotoxic. Elevated blood urea nitrogen (BUN) or creatinine (CR) levels may warrant nephrology consultation or preoperative creatinine clearance assessment. Drug dosage adjustments may be necessary, as might special attention to pre- and postoperative intravenous fluid replacement rates.

F. The liver serves as the major site of metabolism and excretion of anesthetic and narcotic agents. Basic assessment of the hematologic status centers on laboratory assessment of hemoglobin, hematocrit, platelets, and coagulation studies. Most surgeons will have several units of typed and cross-matched blood available prior to major operations. The alternative of using autologous or donor-directed blood has become very popular. The logistics of such preparations should be carefully considered when planning elective surgery. It is certainly reasonable to prescribe iron supplements to patients who are planning autologous donations.

G. Abnormal prothrombin time (PT) and partial thromboplastin time (PTT) need to be thoroughly evaluated and corrected. Oral anticoagulation needs to be discontinued to allow normalization of PT. Contingent on the indication for anticoagulation and the type of surgery planned, perioperative intravenous heparin may be utilized. Abnormal liver function tests should be pursued, especially in patients with a history of neoplasia as the abnormalities may be secondary to metastatic disease. Adjustments in anesthetic requirements may be indicated. Furthermore, if hepatitis is discovered, the blood bank may not wish to process autologous units, and the surgical team may wish to enforce universal precautions.

H. Malnutrition may adversely affect wound healing. Nutritional assessment may be made from specific signs and symptoms noted during the physical exam as well as levels of certain proteins such as albumin or transferrin. Recent weight loss from chronic illness is particularly important. The patient with a history of diarrhea and weight loss—particularly if due to chronic inflammatory bowel disease—may benefit from preoperative total parenteral nutrition (TPN).

I. Current medications and allergies should be considered. The history should include questions about the intake of agents that cause specific perioperative problems. Aspirin can lead to platelet inhibition and difficulties with hemostasis. Aspirin-containing products and all nonsteroidal antiinflammatory drugs (NSAIDS) should be discontinued 10–14 days prior to surgery. Where indicated, a preoperative bleeding time is a useful tool. Recent use of corticosteroids may result in a relative adrenal insufficiency and thus requires perioperative supplementation. It is important to determine difficulties that have occurred with previous operative procedures, particularly problems in airway management or complications with anesthetic agents. A history of previous thrombophlebitis or pulmonary embolus warrants consideration for aggressive prophylaxis. Specific serious abnormalities in a major system will likely require assessment by a specialist in that particular field. It is important to carefully discuss the indications for the surgical procedure as well as the potential risks and complications. It is important to inform the patient of both immediate postoperative and long-term expectations. Expectations about postoperative activity, sexual function, and the ability to return to work should be discussed. Reassurance about future follow-up and accessibility to future questions is important.

J. Ancillary help should be sought whenever indicated. Specifically, preoperative stoma therapy consultation allows proper stoma siting and addresses any physiologic issues. Wherever possible, written literature and informational (not promotional) videos should be provided for patients. The patient should be referred to any available support groups composed of similar patients. If no such groups exist, then the patient should be encouraged to discuss expectations with individual patients of the same sex and similar age who have had the same operation for the same disease. Such ancillary measures greatly reduce normal preoperative anxiety and may well smooth recovery. Where indicated, internal medicine or subspecialty consultation is helpful. If any doubt exists as to the patient's comprehension of the planned procedure, psychiatric consultation may be valuable. Such expert assistance is especially valuable for patients with functional bowel disorders or inflammatory bowel disease. Finally, a detailed informed consent is mandatory. The various risks, benefits, alternatives, and complications should be discussed with the patient and with family members.

K. Informed consent should include a discussion with the patient and the patient's family. All of the various risks, benefits, alternatives and complications should be described.

L. A second opinion, if desired by the patient and family should be encouraged rather than discouraged.

BIBLIOGRAPHY

1. Cerra FB. *Pocket Manual of Surgical Nutrition.* C. V. Mosely Company, St. Louis, Missouri, 1984.

2. Ross AF, Tinker JH. Anesthesia risk. In: *Anesthesia,* Vol. 1. Miller, RD, (ed). Churchill Livingston, New York, NY, 1990.

3. Schouten WR, Gordon PH. Preoperative and Postoperative Management. In: *Principles and Practice of Surgery for the Colon, Rectum, and Anus.* Gordon PH, Nivatvongs S, (eds). Quality Medical Publishers, St. Louis, Missouri, 1992.

See also Chapters 1, 2, and 3.

SECTION 2

Symptoms, Anorectal

CHAPTER 6

Anorectal Pain

Gregory C. Oliver, M.D.

Refer to Algorithm 6–1. See also Table 6–1.

A. The history should delineate the duration of the pain complaint, its frequency, precipitating factors, and associated complaints, such as blood or mucus discharge. The character of the pain may suggest its etiology (sharp or stabbing; intermittant or chronic; dull or throbbing; well or poorly localized). A history of anal intercourse or anal receptive sexual practices will help direct the examination and the selection of appropriate culture media and specimens. An immunosuppressed host is an important consideration as physical findings may be obscured. As more than one condition that causes pain may coexist with others, in either a related or unrelated fashion, this anorectal evaluation should serve as a minimum. Select confirmatory studies when the appropriate diagnoses are being considered.
B. Visual inspection of the anal margin will be judged as normal or abnormal.
C. When the anal margin is normal to inspection in a patient complaining of anorectal pain, the cause will either be proximal within the anal canal, rectum, or perianal or perirectal spaces or of functional or idiopathic causes. The latter etiologies are considered to be depression, proctalgia fugax, and levator syndrome.
D. Common causes of acute anal pain are frequently suspected by gently separating the buttocks and carefully inspecting for fissures, abscesses or fistulae, thrombosed external hemorrhoids, or prolapsed internal hemorrhoids. Erythema associated with perianal abscesses and anal margin tumors will suggest further investigations. A patulous anal orifice suggests either anoreceptive intercourse or a degenerative neuromuscular process.
E. Anoscopy may be unremarkable.
F. In patients complaining of anorectal pain when the cause is either more proximal than can be seen with this instrument or when secondary to extrinsic disease processes.

Evaluation of the complaint of anorectal pain

Directed[A] history → Anorectal examination

Anorectal examination → Endoscopy

Endoscopy → Inspection[B]

Inspection[B] → Normal[C] → IBD, anal canal/pelvic tumors, deep perianal abscess, functional/idiopathic causes, levator syndrome

Inspection[B] → Abnormal[D] → Anal margin tumors, descending perineum syndrome, thrombosed external hemorrhage, acute hemorrhagic prolapse, perianal abscess, anal fissure, anal fistula

Anal ultrasound[P]

Anoscopy[E] → Normal[F] → Perianal abscess, degenerative neurologic disease, functional/idiopathic causes, levator syndrome → Treatment[Q]

Anoscopy[E] → Abnormal[G] → Fissures, tumors anal canal, inflammatory processes of the anorectum, prolapsing internal hemorrhoids

Endoscopy → Proctoscopy[H]

Proctoscopy[H] → Normal[I] → Hemorrhoids, fissure, fistula, extraintestinal pelvic tumors or abscesses, functional idiopathic cause, degenerative neurologic diseases

Proctoscopy[H] → Abnormal[J] → Inflammatory conditions of the rectum, incomplete rectal prolapse, tumor distal rectum

Anorectal examination → Palpation[K]

Palpation[K] → External[L]

External[L] → Normal → Anal canal tumors, IBD, functional/idiopathic causes, degenerative neurologic disease

External[L] → Abnormal → Ischiorectal abscess, fissure, anal margin tumors, thrombosed external hemorrhoid

Palpation[K] → Internal[M]

Internal[M] → Normal[N] → Depression

Internal[M] → Abnormal[O] → Pelvic abscess, prostatitis, pelvic inflammatory disease, intersphincter abscess, deep posterior anal abscess, tumors anal canal/distal rectum, tumors (extracolonic) pelvis, IBD, degenerative neurologic disease, levator syndrome, incomplete rectal prolapse

ALGORITHM 6–1

IBD = inflammatory bowel disease

34

TABLE 6–1 CLASSIFICATION OF CAUSES OF ANORECTAL PAIN

Organic causes
Inflammatory conditions
Anorectal abscesses
Anal fistula
Proctitis
Crohn's
Ulcerative
Idiopathic
Radiation
Infectious
Other
Pararectal inflammation
Prostatitis
Tubular ovarian abscess
Endometritis
Diverticular abscess
Pelvic appendicitis
Other
Mechanical causes
Anal fissure
External hemorrhoidal thrombosis
Acute hemorrhoidal prolapse
Incomplete rectal prolapse (retroanal intussusception)
Descending perineum syndrome
Pelvic surgery
Pudendal neuropathy
Neoplastic causes
Benign tumors
Peripheral nerve
Muscle: anal sphincter or pelvis

Peripheral nerve muscle: anal sphincter or pelvis
Bone endometriosis: sacrum or pelvis
Malignant tumors: primary and metastatic
Rectum
Anus
Prostate
Cervix
Uterus
Ovary
Nerve: peripheral cauda equina
Bone
Pelvic muscle
Krukenberg tumor
Neurogenic causes
Multiple sclerosis
Peripheral neuropathy
Degenerative lumbosacral disk disease
Orthopedic causes
Coccygeal trauma
Sacropelvic fractures
Osteogenic tumors
Functional/idiopathic causes
Levator syndrome
Proctalgia fugax
Depression
Chronic idiopathic rectal pain

G. More commonly, anoscopy confirms and clarifies, diagnoses suggested by inspection. Inflammatory conditions affecting the mucosa proximal to the dentate line will be noted and will prompt more thorough endoscopic evaluation.

H. Appropriate cultures and biopsies may clarify the etiology of the disease process. Proctoscopy should be performed only after a careful anoscopic assessment since many common causes of anorectal pain will be missed

I. Proctoscopy permits a careful assessment of the various types of inflammatory bowel disease (IBD), including idiopathic, infectious, radiation-induced, Crohn's disease or ulcerative colitis.

J. Additionally, tumors involving the distal rectum will be noted. An incomplete rectal prolapse can be suspected while having the patient attempt defecation while slowly withdrawing the scope. The finding of a solitary rectal ulcer anteriorly between 6 to 10 cm from the anal verge also suggests this condition.

K. Palpation, both externally about the anus, perineum, and vulva and internally, along the anal canal, levator ani, and vagina in females, should be performed prior to any endoscopic assessment. Such palpation will avoid confusion from traumatic endscopic examination and will direct the subsequent endoscopic evaluation based on pertinent findings.

L. Importantly, gentle palpation of the anal margin will suggest common sources of anal pain. Tenderness over the ischiorectal fossa will suggest a deeper abscess. Fissures and thrombosed hemorrhoids will be readily detected with a gentle examining finger.

M. Palpation of the anal canal and distal rectum will frequently be rewarding when an external cause of pain is not detected. In males, a careful digital palpation of the prostate is mandatory to rule out prostatitis and prostatic malignancy. In females, cervical tenderness or adnexal fullness will suggest gynecologic causes for outlet pain. Extrarectal tumors in the presacral area may be noted as well. Commonly, patients who complain of a deep aching or throbbing perianal or perirectal pain made worse by straining or coughing will have an indurated fullness on careful palpation of the muscular canal. These findings suggest an intersphincteric or deep postanal space abscess. Tenderness to palpation of the levator ani muscles with or without spasticity is compatible with the diagnosis of levator syndrome. A weak anal tone without focal defects suggests an underlying neurogenic problem or receptive relaxation associated with receptive anal intercourse.

N. When inspection, palpation, and local endoscopy are all normal, chronic anorectal pain may be due to mental depression or, more rarely, to degenerative disorders of the cauda·equina or peripheral pelvic pain pathways.

O. In the absence of identification of an etiology for the pain, pelvic CAT scan or ultrasound should be undertaken, particularly in women. Ovarian lesions can present as rectal pain. Obviously, gynecologic referral for a pelvic examination should accompany the request for a pelvic ultrasound. Presacral cysts and tumors can also present as rectal pain.

P. Anal ultrasound is a worthwhile exam as occasionally a chronic intramuscular abscess may be localized.

Q. Treatment of idiopathic rectal pain is very difficult. Electrogalvanic stimulation, levator massage, anxiolytics, antidepressants, analgesics, acupuncture, biofeedback, and direct nerve and muscle blocks are only a few of the myriad attempted therapies. Unfortunately, the sheer number of treatment options attests to the poor understanding of both the etiology and the treatment of this condition.

BIBLIOGRAPHY

1. Ger GC, Wexner SD, Jorge JMN, et al: Evaluation and treatment of chronic intractable rectal pain—a frustrating endeavor. *Dis Colon Rectum* 36:139–145, 1993.
2. Henry MM, Swash M (eds): *Coloproctology and the Pelvic Floor. Pathophysiology and Management.* (3rd ed) London: Butterworth Heineman, 1995.
3. Nivatvongs S: Diagnosis-Chapter 3. In Gordon PH, Nivatvongs S (eds): *Principles and Practice of Surgery for the Colon, Rectum and Anus.* St. Louis: Quality Medical Publishing, 1992.
4. Oliver GC: Proctalgia fugax, levator syndrome, and pelvic pain. In Beck DE, Wexner SD (eds): *Fundamentals of Anorectal Surgery.* New York: McGraw-Hill, 1992.
5. Yang YK, Wexner SD, Nogueras JJ, et al: The rule of anal ultrasound in the assessment of benign anorectal diseases. *Coloproctology* 15:260–264, 1993.

See also Chapters 8, 22, 24, 29.

CHAPTER 7

Anal Disease in the Neutropenic Patient

Walter E. Longo, M.D. and Anthony M. Vernava, III, M.D.

Refer to Algorithm 7–1.

A. Abscess, fistula, perirectal infections, hemorrhoids, fissures, ulcers, and tumors are commonly seen in patients who are neutropenic secondary to either acquired immunodeficiency syndromes, hematologic disorders or adjuvant therapy (chemotherapy/bone marrow transplantation).

B. Patients at risk for neutropenia are (1) those with diseases that require long-term steroids such as inflammatory bowel disease or collagen vascular disease; (2) patients undergoing whole-organ transplantation who receive immunosuppressive medications such as Immuran or cyclosporine; (3) patients receiving adjuvant therapy for malignancy, either chemotherapy or bone marrow transplantation; (4) patients who are homosexual or intravenous drug abusers who may harbor HIV; and (5) patients with other systemic illnesses that predispose to poor wound healing and impaired tissue recovery such as diabetes and cirrhosis.

C. The signs and symptoms of anorectal disease are similar to those of patients with normal and impaired immune competence. Anorectal disease will usually present with either pain, swelling, bleeding, fever, discharge, or diarrhea and tenesmus. The key to early diagnosis is a high degree of clinical suspicion, particularly in those high-risk patients listed above.

D. The diagnosis of anal disease in neutropenic patients centers around a thorough history including recent sexual activity and direct visualization and palpation of the anorectum and perineum. This may not be possible in the office setting, and thus examination under anesthesia should be undertaken if there is uncertainty as to diagnosis or the inability to examine the patient adequately. Leukocytosis may be unreliable due to anergy or malnutrition. computerized tomography (CT) scan of the abdomen and pelvis may aid to determine extent of disease. Any ulcers or drainage must be biopsied and cultured.

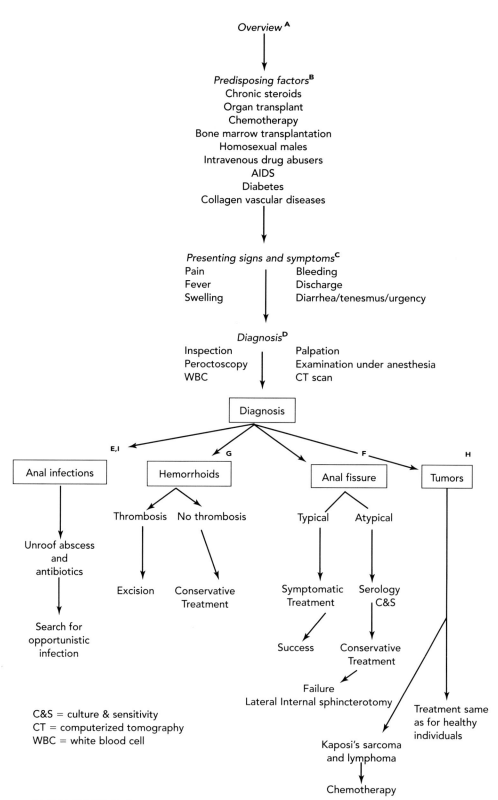

Overview **A**

Predisposing factors**B**
Chronic steroids
Organ transplant
Chemotherapy
Bone marrow transplantation
Homosexual males
Intravenous drug abusers
AIDS
Diabetes
Collagen vascular diseases

Presenting signs and symptoms**C**
Pain   Bleeding
Fever   Discharge
Swelling   Diarrhea/tenesmus/urgency

Diagnosis**D**
Inspection   Palpation
Peroctoscopy   Examination under anesthesia
WBC   CT scan

Diagnosis

E,I   **G**   **F**   **H**

Anal infections   Hemorrhoids   Anal fissure   Tumors

                 Thrombosis   No thrombosis   Typical   Atypical

Unroof abscess
and
antibiotics
                 Excision   Conservative   Symptomatic   Serology
                            Treatment   Treatment   C&S

Search for   Success   Conservative
opportunistic   Treatment
infection

                                            Failure
                                            Lateral Internal sphincterotomy

C&S = culture & sensitivity   Treatment same
CT = computerized tomography   as for healthy
WBC = white blood cell   individuals

                                            Kaposi's sarcoma
                                            and lymphoma

                                            Chemotherapy

ALGORITHM 7–1

40

E. Anal infections (abscess and fistula) are common in neutropenic patients. Suppurative anal disease requires incision and drainage. Perianal sepsis in immunocompromised patients may have little, if any, pus or drainage noted on examination under anesthesia. Any abscess cavity should be unroofed. Intravenous antibiotics are required. Close observation for spread of infection with repeat examination under anesthesia may be necessary. Necrotizing infection requires prompt debridement. A search for opportunistic infections in the anorectal area must be continuous. Fistulas-in-ano are usually treated conservatively.

F. Anal fissures and ulcers are common among male homosexuals as a result of anoreceptive intercourse. In patients with anal fissures and ulcers who are neutropenic, a high index of suspicion for a sexually transmitted disease (chlamydia, syphilis, hemophilus ducreyi, herpes simplex) and neoplasms is necessary, so that all ulcers are biopsied and cultured. All anal fissures are initially treated conservatively; if it is a typical fissure, one can proceed to sphincterotomy for refractory symptoms. If medical management has failed and if the fissure is atypical, then appropriate serologies, cultures, and biopsies are required prior to treatment.

G. Thrombosed external hemorrhoids are treated in a manner similar to that used in nonimmunocompromised patients: excision for pain and conservative therapy are recommended if symptoms are resolving. Otherwise symptomatic hemorrhoids are treated conservatively. Definitive surgical hemorrhoidectomy in the HIV-positive patient is usually contraindicated.

H. Most anal tumors in neutropenic patients (squamous cell, cloacogenic, melanoma) are treated the same as in healthy patients. Epidermoid tumors are found in association with condylomata acuminata. Radical surgery should be avoided in patients with a limited lifespan. In AIDS patients, two types of tumors are commonly encountered: Kaposi's sarcoma and lymphoma. Therapy is mostly palliative employing single or multiple chemotherapeutic drugs.

I. The key to the treatment of proctitis and sexually transmitted diseases is diagnosis. This includes dark-field microscopy, Gram's stain, stool culture, and sigmoidoscopy and biopsy. Sexually transmitted diseases and viral proctocolitidies are treated appropriately.

BIBLIOGRAPHY

1. Barnes SG, Sattler FR, Ballard JO: Perirectal infections in acute leukemia: improved survival after incision and debridement. *Ann Int Med* 100:515–518, 1984.

2. Beck DE, Jaso RG, Zajac RA: Proctologic management of the HIV-positive patient. *South Med J* 83:900–903, 1990.

3. Handler B, Longo WE, Vernava AM, et al: Gastrointestinal disease in neutropenic patients. *Missouri Medicine* 91:637–640, 1944.

4. Safavi A, Gottesman L, Dailey TH: Anorectal surgery in the HIV positive patient: update. *Dis Colon Rectum* 34:299–304, 1991.

5. Schmitt S, Wexner SD, Nougeras JJ, et al: Is aggressive management of perianal ulcers in homosexual HIV-seropositive men justified? *Dis Colon Rectum* 36:240–246, 1993.

See also Chapters 37, 38.

CHAPTER 8

Anal Mass

Juan J. Nogueras, M.D.

Refer to Algorithm 8–1.

A. The evaluation of the perianal mass begins with a detailed history. The patient is questioned about bowel frequency, alterations in bowel habits, and other constitutional symptoms. Specific queries focusing on the anal mass include its onset, the mode of discovery, and the presence of pain, bleeding, drainage, and pruritus. Fluctuations in size suggest a nonneoplastic etiology, as opposed to the more suspicious symptom of progressive, painless growth. Patients are questioned about their sexual histories, including homosexuality, anoreceptive intercourse, the number of sexual partners, and other sexual practices that may place them at risk for sexually transmitted diseases.

B. Visual inspection of the perianal region requires adequate exposure, good illumination, and a calm and reassuring environment. The patient is positioned in the prone jackknife position, which is preferred over the lateral decubitus position. The examiner wears a headlight for enhanced illumination, and the perianal area is inspected as the buttocks are gently spread apart. The general condition of the perianal skin is evaluated, and the location of the mass relative to the anal verge is documented. The presence of erythema, abnormal pigmentation, drainage, and ulceration are noted. A search for satellite lesions should include the perineal body, and the gluteal cleft.

C. Palpation of the anal mass should determine the presence of pain, fluctuance, and drainage, all of which suggest an inflammatory etiology. The characteristics of the mass are documented, including the presence of firmness, ulceration, and fixation to surrounding tissues, which may represent neoplastic invasion. Digital evaluation with a well-lubricated, gloved digit determines the dimensions of the mass relative to the anal canal and rectum.

D. In those situations when the pain is so severe that an office evaluation is inadequate, then an examination under anesthesia is recommended to establish a diagnosis.

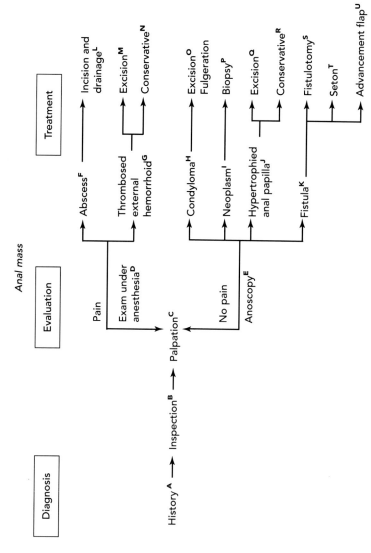

Anal mass

| Diagnosis | Evaluation | Treatment |

History [A] → Inspection [B] → Palpation [C]

Pain → Exam under anesthesia [D]

Abscess [F] → Incision and drainage [L]

Thrombosed external hemorrhoid [G] → Excision [M], Conservative [N]

No pain → Anoscopy [E]

Condyloma [H] → Excision [O] Fulgeration

Neoplasm [I] → Biopsy [P]

Hypertrophied anal papilla [J] → Excision [Q], Conservative [R]

Fistula [K] → Fistulotomy [S], Seton [T], Advancement flap [U]

ALGORITHM 8–1

44

E. The anoscope is gently introduced, and the anal canal is evaluated. The examination should determine the presence of dilated internal hemorrhoids, dilated anal crypts, purulence, proximal extension of the anal mass intranally, satellite lesions, and abnormal mucosa. If the patient complains of severe pain, the examination is aborted and performed under anesthesia.

F. An abscess in the perianal region can present as an expanding, tender mass that may drain spontaneously. The most common locations for an abscess with this presentation include the perianal and ischiorectal spaces. The typical findings in these patients with these abscesses include erythema, swelling, and exquisite tenderness to palpation. Occasionally pus can be visualized from the offending anal crypt with anoscopic examination.

G. A thrombosed external hemorrhoid is a perianal hematoma confined to the anoderm up to the level of the dentate line that presents as a painful perianal swelling. In most cases, there is no obvious etiology for this condition. The natural history of this condition is an acute onset with an increase in the pain corresponding to the degree of swelling, typically peaking by the 3rd or 4th day. The swelling will have a characteristic bluish discoloration, and occasionally the skin overlying the hematoma will develop superficial necrosis, resulting in drainage or spontaneous clot evacuation and bleeding.

H. Condylomata acuminata are sexually transmitted venereal warts caused by certain types of the human papilloma virus. They typically occur in the perianal region and anal canal, but may also be found in other parts of the perineum, vulva, vagina, penis, and oral cavity. These lesions are usually painless, but may result in other symptoms, such as pruritus ani, poor hygiene, drainage, and bleeding. These lesions vary in size from diminutive scattered warts to massive cauliflower-like masses that encircle the anus. They are often friable, and may bleed during the examination. A thorough search for other sexually transmitted diseases, as well as an evaluation of sexual partners, is part of the management of these lesions.

I. Neoplasms of the anal region include squamous cell carcinoma, lymphoma, melanoma, adenocarcinoma, and basal cell carcinoma. Malignancies of the anal canal and anal margin are uncommon, and as a result may be initially undetected. Any chronic, nonhealed ulcer should be biopsied to exclude squamous cell carcinoma. Melanomas are suspected when a pigmented mass lesion is noted, although these tumors may be lightly pigmented or nonpigmented. Lymphomas may present as a perianal mass that may be mistaken for an abscess; however, these tumors are more common in the immunocompromised patient, including AIDS patients. Adenocarcinomas may occur from the anal glands and present as a perianal mass. These adenocarcinomas have also been reported in long-standing fistulas.

J. Hypertrophied anal papillae occur as a result of enlargement of the anal papillae at the level of the dentate line. These may be as a result of an underlying anal disease, such as a chronic fissure, but may also occur without an obvious predisposing factor. The majority of these patients are asymptomatic, but if there is significant enlargement of these papillae, the patient may notice a prolapsing anal mass.

K. The external opening of an anal fistula can present as a perianal mass. The typical history is that of a lump that may fluctuate in size, spontaneously drain, and occasionally hurt. There may be an antecedent history of an anorectal abscess. On physical examination, an obvious external opening can be found anywhere in the perianal region. There may be a palpable tract in the sub-cutaneous tissue extending from the external opening to the anus. The temptation to probe the tract in the office setting should be resisted in order to avoid causing discomfort to the patient and creating false tracts.

L. The management of an anal abscess is incision and drainage. Certain abscesses, such as perianal and superficial ischiorectal space abscesses, may be adequately drained in the office. Complex abscesses should be drained in the operating room.

M. An acutely thrombosed external hemorrhoid of <72-hours duration is usually best managed by complete excision of the perianal hematoma rather than incision and enucleation of the thrombosed pile. This procedure is performed under local anesthesia in the office in the majority of cases.

N. The natural history of a thrombosed external hemorrhoid is dissolution of the clot within 1 week of its occurrence. If the patient is initially evaluated during the phase of the clot when the pain is beginning to diminish, then conservative management with reassurance, nonnarcotic analgesics, and fiber therapy to avoid constipation is an acceptable mode of therapy.

O. The optimal management of symptomatic anal condylomata is excision and fulguration. Topical therapy with podophyllin or bichloroacetic acid is usually inadequate in treating these larger warts.

P. Any suspicious ulcerated, firm, or pigmented mass in the perianal region should be adequately biopsied. In many instances, a punch biopsy performed with local anesthesia will provide adequate tissue for an accurate diagnosis. In other instances, exam under anesthesia is required to allow adequate tissue collection for biopsy. Ancillary studies such as anal ultrasonography may provide detailed information on the consistency, location, and dimension of the mass.

Q. The indications for excision of a hypertrophied anal papilla include inter-ference with perianal hygiene, discomfort, and differentiation from a neo-plasm.

R. The majority of hypertrophied anal papillae can be nonoperatively managed with reassurance of the patient, maintenance of adequate perianal hygiene, and fiber therapy to avoid constipation.

S. The lay-open fistulotomy technique is applicable for fistulas that do not involve a significant portion of the external anal sphincter.

T. Utilization of a seton is reserved for the more complex and recurrent fistulas for which fistulotomy is not feasible. The seton can be of the cutting or the draining variety.

U. The endorectal advancement flap technique is another tool for the manage-ment of complex or recurrent anal fistulas. The internal opening is obliterated utilizing a flap of adjacent rectal wall. This technique has also been successful in the management of rectovaginal fistulas.

BIBLIOGRAPHY

1. Corman ML: *Colon and Rectal Surgery,* 3rd ed. Philadelphia: Lippincott, 1993.
2. Beck DE, Wexner SD (eds): *Fundamentals of Anorectal Surgery.* New York: McGraw-Hill, 1992.
3. Gordon PH, Nivatvongs S: *Principles and Practice of Surgery of the Colon, Rectum and Anus.* St. Louis: Quality Medical Publishing, 1992.

See also Chapters 22, 24, 25, 26, 28, 29, 37.

CHAPTER 9

Pruritus Ani

Terry C. Hicks, M.D. and Frank G. Opelka, M.D.

Refer to Algorithm 9–1.

A. *Pruritus ani* refers to the unpleasant cutaneous sensation that leaves the patient with a nearly uncontrollable desire to scratch. Pruritus ani is not a diagnosis, but a symptom complex that has both medical and surgical implications. The cornerstone to the correct diagnosis and appropriate therapy is a systematic approach with maintenance of appropriate follow-up care. This care ensures that nonresponders are reevaluated, and that their therapy is appropriately adjusted, it also provides a safeguard against the few potentially life-threatening disorders that can present as pruritus ani. Pruritus ani occurs in approximately 1–5% of the population; men are affected more commonly than are women by a ratio of 4:1. This condition is most common in 5th and 6th decades, and usually begins insidiously, but as the area of involvement spreads, the intensity of itching increases and the patient begins to scratch and claw at the skin. This skin trauma leads to further damage, excoriation, and potentially secondary skin infection. This injury unfortunately creates a vicious cycle of itching and scratching that exacerbates the symptoms.

B. A careful history can often aid in identifying the etiology. Attention should be paid to systemic diseases, prior anorectal surgery, perianal medications, and diet. The history should include questions about bowel habits, hygiene practices, antibiotics, topical and oral medications, types of clothing, dietary associations, other pruritus symptoms, menopausal status, history of pelvic radiation, systemic diseases, vaginal discharge, acholic stools, dark urine, anal intercourse, exercise patterns, history of anorectal surgery, and a brief patient stress profile (see Table 9–1).

C. The patient should present to the examining suite without bowel preparation and should be told not to apply any creams or ointments to the perianal area. The examining room should have a bright light source and be well stocked with a magnifying glass, enemas and the clinical equipment necessary to obtain appropriate culture scrapings with evaluation or biopsies. The patient is

49

Pruritus ani^A → **History, physical exam^B** → **Diagnostic evaluations^C**

Diagnostic evaluations^C branches to:
- Systemic diseases
- Diagnosis-specific test
- Anoscopy Sigmoidoscopy

Systemic diseases:
- Diabetes
- Renal failure
- Jaundice
- Lymphoma
- Myeloproliferative disorders

Diagnosis-specific test:
- ^D Culture/O&P exam
- ^E Biopsy
- ^F Serology
- ^G Scrapings/exam by magnification
- ^H Scotch-tape test
- ^I Wood's lamp exam

Anorectal/vaginal infections:
- Viral
- Bacterial
- Parasitic
- Fungal

Diarrheal states:
- IBD

Diet and drugs:
- Coffee
- Topical and oral medications

Anatomic predisposition:
- Deep gluteal cleft
- Obesity
- Hirsutism

Dermatoses:
- Chemical exposure
- Irritant soaps
- Mechanical cleansing
- Psoriasis
- Seborrheic dermatitis

Anorectal neoplasms:
- Bowens
- Paget's
- Cloacogenic
- Squamous

Anorectal diseases:
- Fistula
- Fissure
- Hemorrhoids
- Sphincter incompetence

Other: radiation or psychogenic

Idiopathic → Treatment^J

IBD = inflammatory bowel disease
O&P = Ova & parasites

ALGORITHM 9–1

50

TABLE 9–1 MAJOR CAUSES OF PRURITUS ANI

Personal hygiene	Poor cleansing habits resulting in chronic exposure to residual irritating feces; conversely, overmeticulous cleansing with excessive rubbing and soap use
Diet	Consumption of large volumes of liquids: coffee (caffeinated and decaffeinated, coffee-containing products), chocolate, citrus, spicy foods, tea, beer, and foods high in milk content; vitamin A and D deficiencies
Anatomic compromise	Obesity, deep anal clefts, excessive hair, tight-fitting clothing (tight clothing or clothing that impairs adequate ventilation), fistula, fissure, skin tags, prolapsing papilla, or mucosal prolapse
Systemic disease	Jaundice, diabetes mellitus, chronic renal failure, iron deficiency, thyrotoxicosis, myxedema, Hodgkin's lymphoma, polycythemia vera
Gynecologic conditions	Pruritus vulvae, vaginal discharge (endocervicitis, vaginitis)
Neoplasms	Bowen's disease, extramammary Paget's disease, squamous cell carcinoma, cloacogenic carcinoma, rectal or polypoid lesions
Diarrheal states	Irritable bowel syndrome, Crohn's disease, chronic ulcerative colitis
Radiation	Postirradiation changes
Psychogenic drugs	Anxiety, neuroses, psychoses Quinidine; colchicine; antibiotics (tetracycline); IV hydrocortisone phosphate; ointments or creams that contain "caine" drugs; and nonprescription medications for personal hygiene such as perfumed soaps and ointments that may contain alcohol, witch hazel, or other astringents
Dermatologic conditions	Psoriasis, seborrheic dermatitis, atropic dermatitis, lichen simplex, and lichen sclerosis;
Infections	viruses—herpes simplex, cytomegalovirus, papillomavirus; bacteria—*Staphylococcus aureus*, erythrasma, mixed infections; fungi—*dermatophytosis*, candidiasis; parasites—pinworms, scabies, pediculosis; spirochetes—syphilis
Idiopathic	

placed in a prone jackknife position and after careful inspection of the perianal skin, looking for signs of excessive moisture, swelling, or excoriation, the physician performs a digital examination to evaluate the stool consistency and to obtain a specimen for hemoccult testing. The physician should also document sphincter competency. Furthermore, evaluation of the undergarment may often provide useful clues about hygiene. The patient should then be prepped with a disposable enema so that a sigmoidoscopy and anoscopic exam can be performed to exclude proctitis, infections, or inflammatory bowel disease. The clinician can next complete any cultures, biopsies, scrapings, or Wood's lamp examinations as necessary to make the appropriate clinical diagnosis.

D. Herpes simplex, can be diagnosed by culture.

E. Suspicious skin lesions can be biopsied using a punch biopsy technique.

F. Serology can exclude syphilis and other sexually transmitted diseases.

G. Scrapings are sent for microscopic identification of mycotic infections (Epidermophyton, Tricophyton, and Candida), parasites (sarcoptes, scabiei, pediculosis pubis).

H. Identification of pinworm eggs is done by the scotch tape test.

I. Erythrasma (*Corynebacterium minutissimum*) produces red fluorescence when a Wood's lamp is used for illumination.

J. If primary cause for pruritus ani can be identified, appropriate therapy for that etiology should be instituted. Unfortunately, the majority of patients with pruritus have no identifiable etiology and subsequently fall into the category of idiopathic pruritus ani. This group requires a focused therapeutic approach. The use of a supplemental instruction sheet often leads to a higher degree of patient compliance (see Table 9–2). The goal is to keep the perianal skin dry, clean, and slightly acidic by utilizing appropriate perianal hygiene. Dietary adjustments, as well as efforts to eliminate any further perianal trauma, are undertaken. If symptoms continue in the compliant patient despite aggressive therapy, a second opinion from a dermatologist should be considered.

TABLE 9–2 PATIENT CARE HANDOUT FOR TREATMENT OF PRURITUS ANI

1. Our goal is to keep the skin of the anal area clean, dry, and slightly acidic.

2. During bath or shower, wash the outside of the anal area with water. Do not use soap in the anal area (it is alkaline and will increase discomfort). If a cleansing agent is desired, apply Balneol (Solvay Pharmaceutical, Marietta, GA) with fingertips or wet cotton balls. When drying the anal area, avoid abrasive trauma or vigorous rubbing. This may be accomplished by patting the skin dry with a soft towel or using a hair dryer.

3. Following each bowel movement, make sure the anal area is cleansed of any residual stool or moisture. This may be accomplished with a non-alcoholic towelette. Be sure not to leave pads in contact with the skin for prolonged periods. Avoid the use of toilet paper on irritated skin. If persistent afterdrainage persists even after meticulous hygiene, rectal irrigation with a 4-oz syringe bulb and warm water may be useful.

4. In the morning and at bedtime, apply a thin cotton pledget directly in the anal crease. It should be small enough so that you are not conscious of its presence. You may dust the cotton with baby powder or corn starch if needed. It is important to change the pledget often during the day if it becomes moist.

5. Soaking in a warm sitz bath for 20 minutes can provide relief. Do not add any soaps or skin softeners to the water, and be sure to dry the anal area thoroughly afterward.

6. Maintain a soft, large, and nonirritating stool so that it can pass through the anal canal without causing mechanical or chemical trauma. This may be accomplished by the following:

    a. A bulking agent such as Konsyl (Konsyl Pharmaceutical, Fort Worth, TX), Metamucil (Proctor and Gamble, Cincinatti, OH), or Citrucel (Merrell Dow Pharmaceuticals, Inc., Cincinatti, OH) _____ tablespoons in _____ glasses of water or juice _____ times a day.

    b. Eat a high-fiber diet that includes 8–10 glasses of water or juice a day, plenty of fruits and vegetables, and bran cereal every day.

    c. Avoid foods that cause bowel irritation or are mucus-producing, or aggravate drainage; these include dark colas, spicy foods, citrus fruits and juices, coffee (regular or decaffeinated), beer, nuts, popcorn, milk, and foods known to produce gas or indigestion. Ginger ale, and other light-colored soft drinks may be tolerated.

7. Wearing cotton gloves to bed can be of benefit if you scratch yourself while sleeping.

8. Recurrences are common and to be expected.

9. Don't become despondent over this; just be sure to reconsult your doctor so that appropriate corrections in therapy can be made.

10. You may apply a hydrocortisone cream, but only if it is directed by your physician(s) following a cleaning and drying routine.

BIBLIOGRAPHY

1. Alexander S: Dermatologic aspects of anorectal disease. *Clin Gastroenterol* 4:651–657, 1975.

2. Dailey TH: Pruritus ani. In Shackelford's *Surgery of the Alimentary Tract* (3rd edition) Philadelphia: Saunders, Vol. 4, pp 281–285, 1991.

3. Friend WG: The cause and treatment of idiopathic pruritus ani. *Dis Colon Rectum* 20:40–42, 1977.

4. Hanno R, Murphy P: Pruritus ani: classification and management. *Dermatol Cl* 5:811–816, 1987.

5. Hicks TC, Opelka FG: Pruritus ani: diagnosis and treatment. In Beck DE, Wexner SD (eds): *Fundamentals of Anorectal Surgery*. New York: McGraw-Hill, 1992, pp 157–169.

6. Smith LE: Perianal dermatologic disease. In Gordon P, Nivatvongs S (eds): *Principles and Practice of Surgery for the Colon, Rectum, Anus*. St. Louis (MO): Quality Medical Publishing, 1992, pp 282–299.

7. Sullivan ES, Garnjobst WM: Pruritus ani: a practical approach. *Surg Clin N Am* 58:505–512, 1978.

8. Wexner SD: Pruritis ani and fissure-in-ano. In: Beck DE, Welling DR (eds). *Manual of patient care in colorectal surgery*. Boston: Little, Brown and Co., 1991: 237–254.

9. Wexner S, Smithy W, Milsom J, et al: The surgical management of anorectal diseases in AIDS and pre-AIDS patients. *Dis Colon & Rectum* 29:719–723, 1986.

See also Chapter 1.

CHAPTER 10

Acute Hematochezia

Martti Matikainen, M.D. and Kari-Matti Hiltunen, M.D.

Refer to Algorithm 10–1.

A. *Hematochezia* [Greek haima=blood, chez(ein) to defecate] means the passage of bright red, easily identifiable blood or blood clots from the anus (see also, Chapter 12). Sometimes *hematochezia* and *melena* are used erroneously as synonyms (interchangeably), leading to confusion regarding the proper meaning of these terms.

B. A detailed history is of the utmost importance. If the patient has previously experienced hematochezia and the bleeding is mild (see below), refer to the chapter on chronic hematochezia (Chapter 11). If the patient has experienced prior diarrhea (Chapter 16) or ulcerative (Chapter 52) or Crohn colitis (Chapter 51), the chapters on these topics should be consulted. Liver disease with impaired coagulation, a history of rectal varices, or use of anticoagulant therapy or nonsteroidal antiinflammatory drugs (NSAIDS) are all important clues to the etiology and possible therapeutic options.

C. Along with the standard clinical examination it is mandatory to perform anoscopy. Rigid proctosigmoidoscopy is recommended if the procedure can be performed in the emergency room.

D. It is reasonable to divide acute hematochezia into "severe" and "moderate" bleeding because the management of these patients differs. "Severe" bleeding means that the patient bleeds more than 1500 cc in 24 hours or has signs of shock on admission. These patients have a risk of exsanguination.

E. In case of severe bleeding it is most important to resuscitate the patient to prevent shock. After resuscitation it is possible to continue with diagnostic maneuvers. It may be necessary to proceed with the diagnostic procedures at the same time as the resuscitation if the bleeding continues. Fortunately, colorectal bleeding seldom leads to an uncontrollable situation and will stop spontaneously in about 70–80% of cases, so generally there is time for diagnosis and treatment.

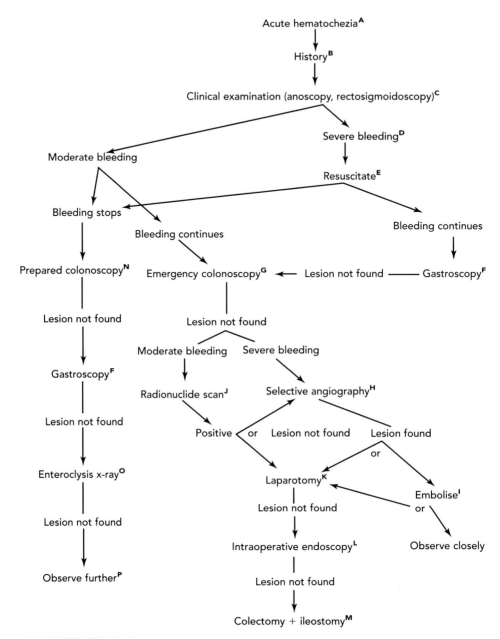

ALGORITHM 10–1

F. In case of severe bleeding it is important to exclude upper gastrointestinal lesions. Massive peptic ulcer bleeding, aortoenteric fistula, and bleeding esophageal varices can cause hematochezia, which is accompanied in these situations with shock. Ten percent of patients with acute severe rectal bleeding, have the lesion proximal to the ligament of Treitz. Thus upper endoscopy should be performed if clinically indicated and technically feasible. At the very least, a nasogastric tube should be inserted and bilious drainage confirmed. If the colonoscopy fails to reveal the site of bleeding and the bleeding has stopped, a lavage type bowel preparation can be given and a more thorough colonoscopy is repeated either later the same day or the next day.

G. If the bleeding continues, emergency colonoscopy should be done as soon as possible. It should be done without bowel preparation to avoid delay. Emergency colonoscopy is difficult with active bleeding, requiring a great deal of experience. If the definitive diagnosis is not reached, often the level of bleeding can be determined; information that may be of help in planning a possible operation. The diagnostic yield of the barium enema is so limited that it should be done only if there are no facilities for endoscopy, radionuclide scanning and/or angiography.

H. If a bleeding lesion is not found, continue with mesenteric angiography. If the bleeding rate is >0.5 mL/min, selective angiography may show the bleeding lesion. The prerequisite for the positive angiography is active bleeding at the moment of contrast injection.

I. If a lesion is found during angiography, it is possible to try to embolize it. The embolization must be as peripheral as possible to prevent bowel wall necrosis. If successful, embolization may stop the bleeding but, at least, it facilitates location of the bleeding lesion during a possible operation.

J. One possibility is to perform a radionuclide scan. It can be done using technetium-99m sulfur colloid or technetium-99m-labeled autologous red cells. A bleeding rate of 0.1–05 mL/min can be demonstrated. The accuracy of these scans varies between 30 and 90%. With a positive scan it is reasonable to continue with angiography. The most sensitive method to detect slow bleeding is to inject technetium through a selectively positioned angiography catheter.

K. If the bleeding continues and no lesions have been found, continue with laparotomy. Intravenous antimicrobial prophylaxis is given during the induction of general anesthesia. Begin with careful exploration of the whole abdominal cavity.

L. Continue with intraoperative upper gastrointestinal endoscopy. A transorally inserted colonoscope can reach the distal small bowel by invaginating the bowel onto the endoscope. Subsequent transrectal passage of the instrument will include intubation of the ileocecal valve and inspection of the distal most ileum. Transilluminate the bowel during intraoperative endoscopy to detect angiodysplasias or telangiectasias.

M. If no lesions are found and bleeding continues, then perform a total abdominal colectomy and ileostomy.

N. If the bleeding has ceased, perform urgent colonoscopy after proper preparation of the bowel. A rapid effective 90 ml phosphosoda prep can be utilized. A single-contrast barium enema is worthless, and a double-contrast barium enema should be used only if there are no facilities for colonoscopy. In these cases a barium enema should be preceded by flexible sigmoidoscopy to exclude colitis.

O. If no lesion is yet found continue with small bowel x-ray by enteroclysis technique.

P. If the diagnosis is still unresolved, it might be reasonable to observe the patient further. In case of rebleeding proceed as in a new case of active bleeding.

Laparotomy and intraoperative endoscopy might be the only way to demonstrate causes for moderate rebleedings.

BIBLIOGRAPHY

1. Cohen SM, Wexner SD, Binderow SR, et al: Prospective randomized endoscopic-blinded trial comparing precolonoscopy bowel cleansing methods. *Dis Colon Rectum* 37:689–696, 1994.
2. Gathright JB Jr., Bozdech JM, Volpe P, et al: Management of lower intestinal bleeding expert exchange. *Perspect colorectal surg* 4:219–232, 1991.
3. Hosking SW, Johnson AG: Bleeding anorectal varices—a misunderstood condition. *Surgery* 104:70–73, 1988.
4. Jensen DM, Machicado GA: Diagnosis and treatment of severe hematochezia. The role of urgent colonoscopy after purge. *Gastroenterology* 95:1569–1574, 1988.
5. Leitman IM, Paull DE, Shires III GT: Evaluation and management of massive lower gastrointestinal hemorrhage. *Ann Surg* 209:175–180, 1989.
6. Lewis BS, Wenger JS, Waye JD: Small bowel enteroscopy and intraoperative enteroscopy for obscure gastrointestinal bleeding. *Am J Gastroenterol* 86:171–174, 1991.
7. Schrock TR: Colonoscopic diagnosis and treatment of lower gastrointestinal bleeding. *Surg Clin N Am* 69:1309–1325, 1989.

See also Chapters 11, 12A, 12B, 13, 15, 16, 51, 52.

CHAPTER 11

Chronic Hematochezia

Stephanie L. Schmitt, M.D. and
Philip F. Caushaj, M. D.

Refer to Algorithm 11-1.

A. Important points of the history and physical exam are the nature of the bleeding ("wipe" bleeding, blood in the toilet bowl, blood mixed with stool), associated symptoms and signs, duration of bleeding, and family history of inflammatory bowel disease (IBD) or colon carcinoma.

B. Anoscopy is a crucial part of the initial evaluation. It is a great disservice to the patient to attribute hematochezia to hemorrhoids or anal fissures without considering the patient's age, nature of the bleeding, any associated symptoms, and family history. If the patient is young with recent onset of hematochezia consisting of "wipe" bleeding or blood in the toilet bowl with bowel movements and symptoms attributable to hemorrhoids or an anal fissure, it is reasonable to begin a trial of conservative therapy appropriate to the diagnosis.

C. If diarrhea is present stool studies should be undertaken. As appropriate for the history and symptoms: culture, ova and parasites, fecal leukocytes, clostridium difficile toxin, and microscopic examination.

D. Conservative therapy consists of high-fiber diet, fiber supplements, increased fluid intake, and sitz baths as appropriate.

E. Nonsurgical management of lateral hemorrhoids includes rubber-band ligation and infrared photocoagulation.

F. Colonoscopy is a superior option for the evaluation of chronic hematochezia. However, if colonoscopy is unavailable then another option for evaluation of the colon is flexible fiberoptic sigmoidoscopy followed by air-contrast barium enema.

G. Medical therapy consists of maintenance of the NPO (nil per os) status, providing adequate intravenous hydration, optimizing cardiac output in "low flow" states, discontinuing any medications that may be contributing to the ischemic state if possible, and implementing close follow-up with regular examinations and follow-up sigmoidoscopy as appropriate.

CHRONIC HEMATOCHEZIA

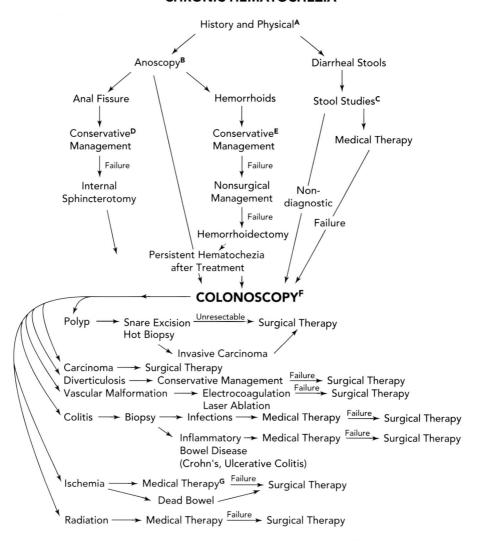

ALGORITHM 11–1

BIBLIOGRAPHY

1. Hutcheon, D: Endoscopic Diagnosis and Management of lower gastrointestinal bleeding. In Cameron JL (ed): *Current Surgical Therapy,* 4th ed. St. Louis: Mosby Yearbook, 1992.
2. Nivatvongs S: Diagnosis. In Gordon PH, Nivatvongs S (eds): *Principles and Practice of Surgery for the Colon, Rectum, and Anus.* St. Louis: Quality Medical Publishers, 1992.

See also Chapters 10, 12A, 12B, 13, 15.

CHAPTER 12A

Melena

Patrick Brillant, M.D. and Heidi Nelson, M.D.

Refer to Algorithm 12A-1.

A. Melena is defined as the passage of black or tarry stools. This finding can occur with the loss of as little as 50 cc of blood and can persist for as long as 5 days after the actual bleeding event. Stool may remain positive for occult blood several weeks after a bleeding episode. Melena can be associated with blood loss anywhere along the gastrointestinal (GI) tract from the mouth to the ascending colon. The black color of melena is a result of the oxidizing effects of the intestinal and bacterial enzymes on heme that produce hematin. Black stools may also result from iron intake, consumption of dyes and food substances, and the use of medicines such as Pepto-Bismol.

B. An initial quick assessment should include vital signs and clinical evaluation of intravascular volume status. The patient should be questioned regarding the presence and amount of associated hematemesis, and the duration of symptoms such as is a useful measure of the severity and source of bleeding. The pace of the ensuing evaluation will depend on the rate of blood loss and the patient's tolerance of the hemodynamic insult.

C. Initial therapy should include establishment of two large-bore peripheral intravenous lines, crystalloid fluid infusion, and obtaining a blood sample for type and cross-matching. Although other tests and procedures may be indicated, (hemoglobin, liver function tests, Prothrombin Time (PT), Partial Thromboplastin Time (PTT), platelet counts, Electrocardiogram (ECG), placement of central venous access), it is of paramount importance to remember that these measures should be sought only after the initial critical steps of resuscitation have been performed.

D. Once the patient is stable, a complete history should now address whether the patient has had previous peptic ulcer disease, bleeding episodes, liver disease, jaundice, bleeding, dyscrasias, systemic illnesses or abdominal surgeries and has been using alcohol, aspirin, nonsteroidal antiinflammatory agents, or anticoagulants. It is also important to evaluate the episode in the context of recent patient activities, such as "binge drinking," violent retching,

61

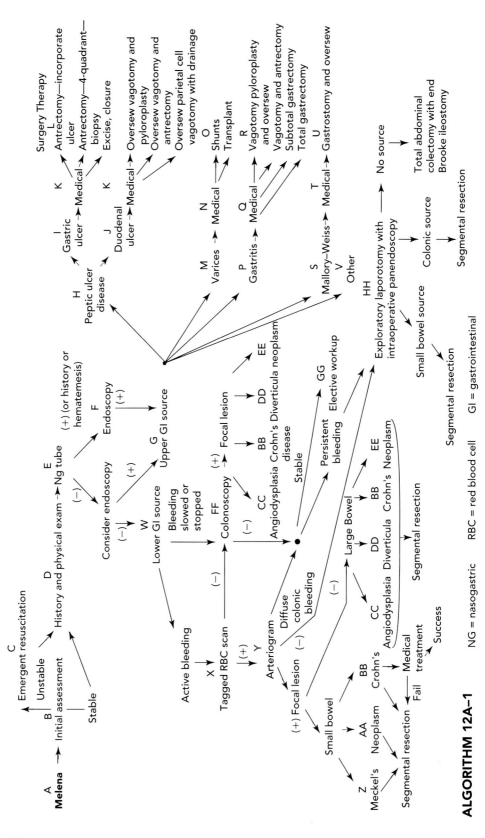

ALGORITHM 12A-1

NG = nasogastric   RBC = red blood cell   GI = gastrointestinal

or mechanical ventilation. The physical examination should include a careful nasooropharyngeal exam for sources of bleeding, and a skin exam to look for changes associated with Osler–Weber–Rendu or Gardner's syndrome. The abdominal exam should focus on detection of an enlarged or tender liver, palpable abdominal masses, adenopathy, an aortic aneurysm, ascites, as well as a careful search for the stigmata of liver disease including jaundice, gynecomastia, Dupytren's contracture, spider angiomata, and testicular atrophy. A digital rectal exam should always be performed.

E. A nasogastric (NG) tube is placed to exclude an upper GI source. As many as 25% of patients with a bleeding duodenal ulcer may not have blood in NG aspirates. It is important to verify the presence of bile in the aspirate to confirm postpyloric aspiration of luminal fluid.

F. Endoscopy should be performed within 24 hours of patient presentation after vascular volume deficits and coagulation abnormalities have been corrected. Esophagogastroduodenoscopy will localize the source of bleeding in about 85% of patients and will allow therapeutic intervention in patients with peptic ulcer disease or varices.

G. The most common causes of upper GI bleeding are peptic ulcer disease (PUD), 45%; esophageal varices, 20%; gastritis, 20%, Mallory–Weiss tear, 10%; and others, 5%.

H. PUD affects approximately 10 million Americans. It is most common in male smokers between the ages of 20 and 60 years.

I. Gastric ulcers are mostly related to mucosal barrier breakdown. Types: I—normal fundic ulcer; II—gastric and duodenal ulcer; III—prepyloric ulcer; IV—juxtocardiac ulcers. 85% of ulcers will improve with conservative medical treatment; however, although it is important to obtain biopsies and washings as well as to consider reendoscopy to confirm healing in any questionable lesions, since 10% of ulcers are malignant. Medical management should also include treatment for *H. pylori.*

J. Endoscopic treatment should control 90% of these lesions.

K. Medical treatment includes H_2 (histamine) blockers, volume resuscitation, correction of coagulation defects, and careful hemodynamic monitoring. Patients who should be *considered* for surgical intervention include those whose initial bleeding episode lead to syncope or hypotension, persistent slow bleeding lasting >24 hours while on appropriate treatments, loss of >1500 cc of blood during an 8-hour period, requirement of ≥6 units of blood, a second acute episode while in the hospital or the endoscopic presence of predictors of high-risk rebleeding. Within this latter category are a giant duodenal ulcer (>2 cm), a visible vessel with a clot, or active bleeding not amenable to endoscopic control.

L. Vagotomy should be added to treatment of type II and III gastric ulcers.

M. Massive hematemesis due to esophageal varices is, perhaps, the most dreaded sequla of portal hypertension; 90% present with hematemesis. This problem most commonly occurs secondary to hepatic cirrhosis, although it may also be due to pre- and posthepatic obstructive phenomenon. As always, initial stabilization of the patient is the first goal. Patient mortality with an acute bleed from esophageal varices approaches 50%. This high fatality is related not only to the severity of the bleeding but also to the underlying nutritional, hepatic and pulmonary dysfunction encountered in these patients.

N. Therapy is guided by endoscopic identification of bleeding varices since as many as half of the patients with known cirrhosis and active GI bleeding have sources of hemmorhage other than their varices at the time of acute gastrointestinal bleeding. Control of the hemorrhage can be accomplished using endoscopic techniques, systemic pitressin therapy, propanalol, placement of a Sengstaken–Blakemore tube, or utilization of a transjugular intrahepatic portosystemic shunt (TIPS).

O. Surgical options include a nonselective end-to-side portocaval shunt, which is technically simpler but has a high incidence of encephalopathy, or a side-to-side portocaval or mesocaval shunt. Options to be considered in the more elective setting include distal splenorenal shunts with total pancreatic disconnection in patients with adequate liver reserve, and liver transplantation in carefully selected patients with poor liver function.

P. Gastritis is commonly associated with shock, sepsis, burns (Curling's ulcers), and central nervous system (CNS) problems (Cushing's ulcers).

Q. Although gastritis was once a common and often lethal problem in the ICU setting, its incidence decreased due to the prophylactic use of H_2 blockers, antacids, Sucralfate, and nutritional support.

R. Although rarely indicated, the surgical options after medical failure include vagotomy and pyloroplasty with oversewing of the bleeding points, vagotomy and antrectomy, subtotal gastrectomy, gastric devascularization, and in rare cases total gastrectomy.

S. Mallory–Weiss tears are longitudinal tears in the gastric mucosa at the level of the gastroesophageal junction most often related to forceful emesis. Average length of the tear is 2 cm, and 15% of patients may have two or more tears. These lesions most often stop spontaneously, and the associated mortality in noncirrhotic patients is essentially 0%.

T. Most patients require only supportive therapy with intravenous (IV) fluids, H_2 blockers, and correction of clotting abnormalities. Occasionally these measures may not be sufficient, in which case endoscopic sclerosant injection, laser therapy, epinephrine injection, or angiographic embolization may be required.

U. In the rare patient who fails the above therapeutic options, it may be necessary to perform a gastrotomy and oversewing of the laceration. If the laceration extends into the proximal esophagus then traction sutures or a left thoracotomy may be required.

V. Other upper GI that can lead to melena include oropharyngeal, esophageal, gastric, hepatic, or pancreatic malignancies; esophagitis; hemobilia; duodenal diverticula; Crohn's disease; trauma; arteriovenous malformations; and aortoduodenal fistulas.

W. Due to the location and nature of lower gastrointestinal bleeding an extensive evaluation may be needed to find these relatively uncommon sources of bleeding. Ninety percent stop spontaneously, which makes diagnosis challenging and renders useless many of the tests that rely on active bleeding.

X. ^{99m}Tc (technetium)-labeled red blood cell (RBC) scan is generally inaccurate as far as locating a site of bleeding, yet it may allow confirmation of the presence or absence of continued bleeding since it may be positive with a bleeding rate as low as 0.1 cc/min. This information improves the yield from arteriography.

Y. Arteriography may identify a bleeding source in up to 70% of patients, but it is invasive, requires active blood loss of at least 0.5 cc/min, carries the risk of dye load, and is operator-dependent. Therapy using intraarterial injection of vasopressin can be used as a temporizing measure.

Z. Meckel's is a true diverticulum located in the terminal ileum 45-90 cm from the ileocecal valve, which is a remnant of omphalomesenteric duct present in about 2% of the population. Of symptomatic diverticulae 40% present as bleeding that arises from ulceration of heterotopic gastric mucosa.

AA. Small bowel neoplasms are uncommon causes for GI bleeding. Hemangiomas and leiomyomas are the most common lesions responsible for bleeding. Other less likely etiologies include lipomas, fibroadenomas, harmartomas, sarcomas, and adenocarcinomas.

BB. Crohn's disease is a nonspecific inflammation of the GI tract that can occur anywhere along its length from mouth to anus. It rarely (<5%) presents with melena as the initial sign.

CC. Angiodysplasia, which is synonymous with arteriovenous malformation and vascular ectasia, can be found in 2% of individuals older than 50. The bleeding, which comes from venule dilation, is responsible for 30% of all colon bleeds. Almost 80% of these vascular malformations are found in the right colon, but they can also be found in the small bowel in younger patients. There is an association with aortic stenosis and Von Willebrand disease.

DD. Diverticulosis is a syndrome in which there is a herniation of mucosa through the site of arteriolar penetration of the bowel wall. These saccular protrusions of colon wall often erode into blood vessels and lead to 30-50% of cases of massive colonic bleeding. They rarely bleed more than 1500 cc and more than 70% stop bleeding spontaneously. Although diverticulae most commonly occur in the sigmoid colon, 75-90% of bleeding lesions are found in the right colon, and 20% rebleed if they are seen during an arteriogram.

EE. Although the most common source of lower GI bleeding, it rarely presents as melena but rather as occult GI blood loss with a positive hemoccult or as hematochezia.

FF. Colonscopy can be done emergently in a nonprepared colon as blood acts as a cathartic or in a prepared colon in the more elective setting. Success rates are as high as 90%. Using current bowel regimens the colon can be prepared in as quickly as 4-8 hours.

GG. Further options include small bowel endoscopy, enteroclysis, intraoperative endoscopy, upper GI studies, and air-contrast barium enema. Elective exploration is usually used as a last resort in the patient who is not actively bleeding but who has had multiple bleeding episodes without having a source identified.

HH. It cannot be overemphasized that in the patient with continued lower GI bleeding without an obvious source it is reasonable to proceed with a total abdominal colectomy. The operation avoids the complication of continued postoperative bleeding after a lesser operation. However prior to blind colectomy, intraoperative panendoscopy with transillumination can be performed. Localization of a segmented source will allow segmental resection. If a subtotal colectomy is performed, an anastomisis should generally be avoided.

BIBLIOGRAPHY

1. Cameron JL: *Current Surgical Therapy.* St. Louis: Mosby Year Book, 1992.
2. Gastout CJ, Wang KK, Ahlquist DA, et al. Acute gastrointestinal bleeding experience of a specialized management team. *J Clin Gastroenterol*; 14:260–267, 1992.
3. Potter GD, Sellin JH: Lower gastrointestinal bleeding. *Gastroenterol Clin N Am* 17:341–355, 1988.
4. Way LW (ed): *Current Surgical Diagnosis and Treatment.* Norwalk (CT): Appleton Lange, 1991.

See also Chapters 10, 11, 12B, 13, 15.

CHAPTER 12B

Melena

David H. Gibbs, M.D. and David E. Beck, M.D.

Refer to Algorithm 12B-1.

A. Melena is a black, tarry, maloderous stool that results from intestinal, bacterial degradation of hemoglobin. It is usually caused by an upper gastrointestinal source or a proximal colonic source. Blood loss in quantities greater than 200-300 mL represents significant, recent bleeding.

B. The rapidity and extensiveness of evaluation depends on the patient's condition. It is important to differentiate between patients who are actively bleeding and those with chronic losses. The acutely bleeding patient needs active resuscitation, while the patient with a slower blood loss may undergo evaluation. The initial assessment includes a basic hemodynamic evaluation including pulse, blood pressure, and orthostatic pressure determinations. The history seeks information to guide the examiner toward an upper or lower gastrointestinal source. Important areas include previous ulcer disease, aspirin or nonsteroidal antiinflammatory drug (NSAID) use, anticoagulation, alcohol abuse, liver disease, and a personal or family history of colon cancer. Physical examination includes a thorough abdominal, genitourinary and rectal examination. Laboratory evaluation includes hemoglobin, hematocrit, platelet counts, BUN (evaluation for azotemia), coagulation studies, type and screen/hold (which can later be changed to type and cross as needed). A chest x-ray and acute abdominal series are obtained to evaluate for free air, ileus, or obstruction.

C. A nasogastric tube is used to exclude major active upper intestinal bleeding.

D. A digital rectal exam excludes anal masses or lesions.

E. A proctoscopic exam that includes a rigid proctoscopic or flexible fiberoptic sigmoidoscopy (FFS) is performed in the clinic or emergency room to exclude a distal source of melena. Sources include inflammatory conditions (proctitis, diverticulitis), hemorrhoids, fissures, fistulas, ulcers, arteriovenous malformations (AVMs), or masses (polyps, cancers). Management of these conditions is described in the appropriate chapters.

67

68

Melena

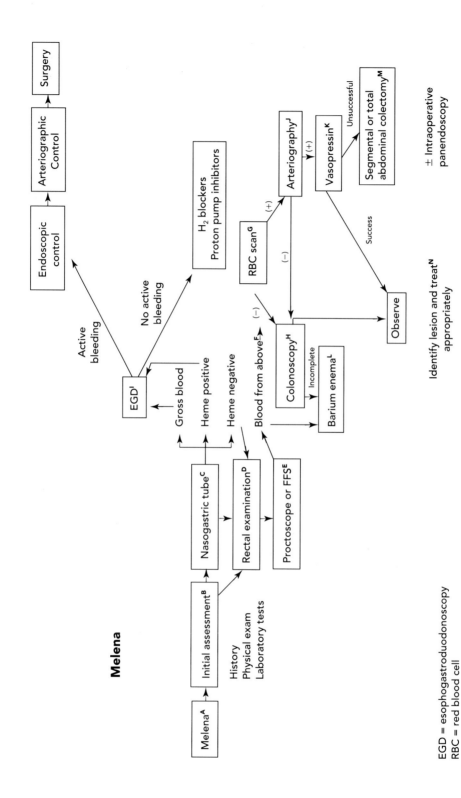

Melena[A] → Initial assessment[B] → Nasogastric tube[C]

History
Physical exam
Laboratory tests

Nasogastric tube[C] → Gross blood / Heme positive → EGD[I]

Rectal examination[D]
Heme negative

Blood from above[F] (−)

Proctoscope or FFS[E] → Barium enema[L]

EGD[I]:
- Active bleeding → Endoscopic control → Arteriographic Control → Surgery
- No active bleeding → H₂ blockers / Proton pump inhibitors

Colonoscopy[H]:
- (−) → RBC scan[G]
- Incomplete → Barium enema[L]

RBC scan[G]:
- (+) → Arteriography[J]
- (−) → Colonoscopy[H]

Arteriography[J]:
- (+) → Vasopressin[K]

Vasopressin[K]:
- Unsuccessful → Segmental or total abdominal colectomy[M]
- Success → Observe

Observe → Identify lesion and treat[N] appropriately
± Intraoperative panendoscopy

EGD = esophogastroduodonoscopy
RBC = red blood cell

ALGORITHM 12B–1

F. Identification of blood proximal to the scope suggests a proximal lesion. If the patient is felt to be actively bleeding, an red blood cell (RBC) scan is indicated. If proximal bleeding is not identified, a barium enema may be indicated to complete the patient's evaluation.

G. A 99m-technetium (^{99m}Tc) pertechnetate-labeled RBC scan requires hemorrhage of at least 0.5 cc/min for a positive scan. In experienced hands, this scan has been reported to have a sensitivity of 91% and a specificity of 95%. A positive scan should be followed by angiography.

H. Colonoscopy requires a clean colon. Stable patients can be prepared with a polyethylene glycol electrolyte lavage solution or a small dose sodium phosphate oral prep. Urgent colonoscopy is successful in 75% of patients with severe hematochezia. Lesions such as arteriovenous malformations (AVMs) or polyps are treated with endoscopic methods. Other lesions such as cancers are biopsied and the appropriate operation is recommended.

I. Esophogastroduodenoscopy (EGD) is used to exclude an upper intestinal source of bleeding. A gastric lavage may be required to empty the stomach of blood permitting an adequate examination. Lesions are managed as described in Algorithm 12B-1.

J. Arteriography of the mesenteric (and celiac if necessary) vessels is indicated after a positive nuclear medicine scan. Hemorrhage of >1-2 mL/min is required for a positive angiographic exam. If the RBC scan is positive and the angiogram is negative, the patient is admitted to the intensive care unit for observation and the percutaneous arterial sheath is left in place for approximately 24 hours. If the patient develops recurrent signs or symptoms of active bleeding, repeat angiography and possible therapeutic interventions are performed with minimal lost time.

K. Vasopressin can be administered in a regional or systemic method. Using selective arterial infusion with a dosage of 2-4 μg/min, hemorrhage may be acutely stopped in 90% of patients. However, rebleeding after cessation of the vasopressin is reported to be as high as 50%. Furthermore, its use is contraindicated in many patients in whom nonoperative methods would otherwise be preferable. Specifically, patients with coronary artery disease or angina pectoris are not candidates for vasopressin therapy.

L. An air contrast barium enema is obtained if the colonoscopic examination is incomplete. It may also be done to assess the remainder of the colon following identification of a distal lesion such as hemorrhoids.

M. If nonoperative measures fail and a bleeding source is localized to the right or left colon, a segmental colectomy is indicated. If a bleeding site cannot be localized, a total abdominal colectomy is the preferred operation. Intraoperative endoscopy is used by some surgeons in this uncommon situation.

N. Colonoscopy, or if incomplete, barium enema, will reveal sources of lower GI bleeding. Small pedunculated and some sessile polyps can be endoscopically removed. Larger benign and malignant neoplastic lesions should be treated by resection. Arteriovenous malformations can usually be treated by endoscopic coagulation.

BIBLIOGRAPHY

1. Cohen SM, Wexner SD, Binderow SR, Nogueras JJ, Daniel N, Ehrenpreis, ED, Jensen J, Bonner GF, Ruderman WB: Prospective, randomized endoscopic-blinded trial comparing precolonoscopy bowel cleansing methods. *Dis Colon Rectum* 37:689–696, 1994.

2. Dent TL: Evaluation of the bleeding patient. *Surg Gynecol Obstet* 151:817, 1980.

3. Gibbs DH, Opelka FG, Beck DE, et al: Post polypectomy lower gastrointestinal hemorrhage. *Dis Colon Rectum* (in press).

4. Hunt PS, Hansky J, Korman MG: Mortality in patients with haematemesis and melaena: a prospective study. *Br Med J* 1:1238, 1979.

5. Jensen DM, Machicado GA: Diagnosis and treatment of severe hematochezia. The role of urgent colonoscopy after purge. *Gastroenterology* 95:1569–1574, 1988.

6. Lieberman DA, Melnyk CS: Gastrontestinal hemorrhage. In Gitnick G, Hollander D, Kaplowitz N, et al (eds): *Principles and Practice of Gastroenterology and Hepatology.* Elsevier: New York. 1988, pp1542–1563.

7. Peterson WL, Laine L. Gastrointestinal bleeding. In Sleisenger MH, Fordtran JS, Scharschmidt BF, et al (eds): *Gastrointestinal Diseases: Pathophysiology. Diagnosis and Management.* Philadelphia: W.B. Saunders. 1993, vol. 1, pp162–192.

8. Schiller, KRF, Cotton PB: Acute upper gastrointestinal hemorrhage. *Clin Gastroenterol* 7:595, 1978.

See also Chapters 10, 11, 12A, 13, 15.

CHAPTER 13

Chronic Rectal Bleeding

James M. Church, M.D.

Refer to Algorithm 13–1.

A. Rectal bleeding is an alarming symptom; it is definitely abnormal, and although the most common causes are benign, there is always the possibility of a life-threatening illness. Investigation of rectal bleeding, therefore, has two aims: to exclude a neoplasm, and to find the cause of the bleeding. Not all rectal bleeding has the same level of risk for an associated neoplasm. Patients are triaged on the basis of risk factors and are offered different approaches to the problem according to the results of the triage. *Hematochezia* means passage of blood in the stools: "suspicious" rectal bleeding in the algorithm supplied in this chapter. A consideration of chronic rectal bleeding needs to include chronic hematochezia as well as those situations where blood is passed separately from stool. Classification of lower gastrointestinal blood loss.

B. Outlet Bleeding

   - Bright red blood on the toilet paper or in the bowl
   - Bleeding associated with defecation
   - No change in bowel habit
   - No risk factors* for colorectal cancer

C. Suspicious Bleeding

   - Dark blood, blood mixed with or streaked on stool
   - Change in bowel habit or passage of mucus
   - Positive risk factor* for colorectal cancer

Hemorrhage: acute rectal bleeding sufficient to warrant admission to hospital. Occult: invisible blood loss though the gastrointestinal tract, detectable by fecal occult blood test.

---

*Risk factors are a personal history of colorectal cancer or polyps, and a family history of colorectal cancer or polyps.

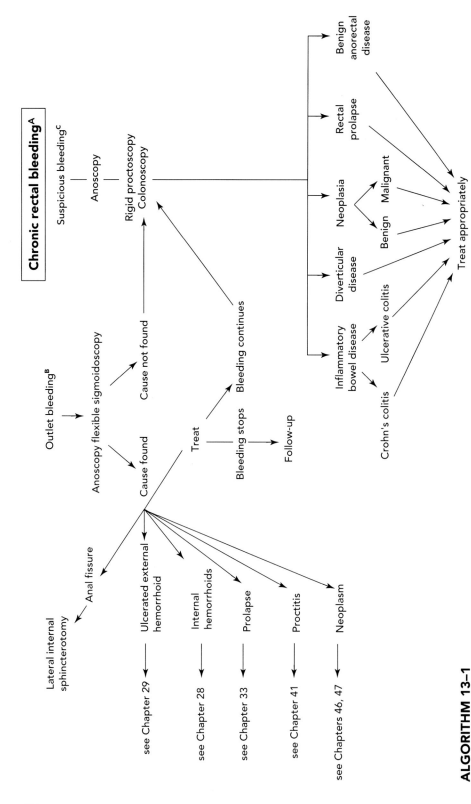

ALGORITHM 13–1

TABLE 13-1 CAUSE FOR BLEEDING

Bleeding Pattern	Cause			
	Colonic	Anal	Possibly Diverticulosis	Not Obvious
Outlet (n = 235)	58 (25%)	139 (59%)	3 (1%)	36 (15%)
Suspicious (n = 199)	96 (48%)[a]	53 (27%)[a]	6 (3%)	44 (22%)

[a] Differences are significant by chi-square (χ^2) analysis.

TABLE 13-2 FINDINGS AT COLONOSCOPY

Bleeding Pattern	Exam Normal?	Cancer	Polyp (>1 cm)	Crohn's Disease	Ulcerative Colitis	AVM	Ischemia
Outlet	124 (53%)	7	29	4	6	6	0
Suspicious	76 (38%)[a]	23[a]	51[a]	2	16[a]	4	4

[a] Significantly different ($p < .05$, χ^2)

In this chapter, only outlet and suspicious bleeding are discussed. Results of colonoscopy in patients with chronic rectal bleeding, categorized as "outlet" or "suspicious," are shown in Tables 13-1 and 13-2. These results confirm the value of differentiating rectal bleeding in this way, according to the definitions presented above. There is some overlap of diagnoses, which is to be expected. In my experience in the patients with outlet bleeding, all except one neoplasm (a 1-cm polyp) has been within reach of the flexible sigmoidoscope. This pattern has not changed with the updated information presented here in Tables 13-1 and 13-2.

EVALUATING THE PATIENT WITH CHRONIC RECTAL BLEEDING: PLAYING "TWENTY QUESTIONS"

When a patient presents with chronic rectal bleeding, take a thorough history. Important questions include the following:

1. How long has the bleeding been going on?
2. How often does it happen?
3. Is the blood with the stool, independent of it, or both?
4. What color is the blood?
5. Where do you see it (paper, bowl, stool)?
6. How much is there?
7. Has it been getting worse?
8. Is there pain with defecation?

   9. If so, is this when the bleeding happens?

 10. Have you noticed a lump near your anus?

 11. If so, is it always there, or does it come and go?

 12. If so, is it painful?

 13. What is your bowel habit like?

 14. Has there been a recent change?

 15. Do you need to strain at stool? How often?

 16. Is this when the bleeding occurs?

 17. Have you had problems in this area in the past?

 18. Have you ever had a polyp or cancer in your bowel?

 19. Has anyone in your family had a polyp or a cancer?

 20. How is your general health?

After asking the patient these questions, you should be able to classify the bleeding as typical outlet bleeding, or as suspicious (not typical outlet bleeding). If it is outlet, plan on a rectal examination, anoscopy, and flexible sigmoidoscopy. If it is suspicious, do a rectal exam and an anoscopy, but also book the patient for colonoscopy.

The questions should also provide enough information for you to make a provisional diagnosis, even before you examine the patient. Confirm the provisional diagnosis with your examination and treat along the lines described or as outlined in other chapters in this book.

BIBLIOGRAPHY

1. Church JM: Analysis of the colonoscopic findings in patients presenting with rectal bleeding according to the pattern of their presenting symptoms. *Dis Colon Rectum* 34:391–395, 1991.
2. Church JM: Colonoscopy for rectal bleeding. *Seminars Colon Rectal Surg* 3:42–47, 1992.
See also Chapters 10, 11, 12A, 12B, 15.

SECTION 3

Symptoms, Systemic

CHAPTER 14

Abdominal Pain

Gregory Weiner, M.D. and Theodore J. Saclarides, M.D.

Refer to Algorithm 14–1.

A. The differential diagnosis in a patient who presents with sudden severe epigastric or upper abdominal pain includes perforation of a hollow viscus, rapid expansion of a solid organ, and rapid bleeding from a major blood vessel. Examples are perforated gastric or duodenal ulcer, perforated upper gastrointestinal neoplasm, ruptured aortic or visceral artery aneurysm, splenic infarction or abscess, and ruptured hepatic adenoma or abscess. Pancreatitis may present in a similar fashion.

B. Excluding pancreatitis, other intraabdominal causes of hyperamylasemia include necrosis of the gallbladder, ischemic bowel, ruptured aortic or visceral artery aneurysm, and torsion of the ovary.

C. Possible sonographic abnormalities include a ruptured or bleeding hepatic adenoma, hepatic abscess, splenic abscess, or aortic aneurysm.

D. Initial treatment of pancreatitis is supportive with intravenous hydration, maintenance of an adequate urine output and normal electrolyte balance, and ventilatory assistance if necessary. If computerized dynamic pancreatography shows necrotic areas within the pancreas, subsequent management is controversial; in the presence of sepsis, some surgeons advocate computerized tomography (CT)-guided aspiration for culture and sensitivity. Pancreatic sterile necrosis may still be managed nonoperatively, provided response to medical management is seen over 3–5 days. Infected necrosis, however, requires operative debridement and drainage.

E. Percutaneous drainage of liver abscesses with ultrasound or CT guidance has proven safe and efficious. If the abscess is secondary to an intraabdominal source, such as choledocholithiasis, diverticulitis, or appendicitis, these entities should be addressed as well. Contraindications to percutaneous drainage include multiple hepatic abscesses, the lack of an appropriate access window, a multiloculated abscess, or ascites. Splenic abscesses are usually due to secondary infection of the spleen from endocarditis or urinary tract infections. The spleen may also be infected by contiguous spread from adjacent organs. In

Epigastric and Upper Abdominal Pain

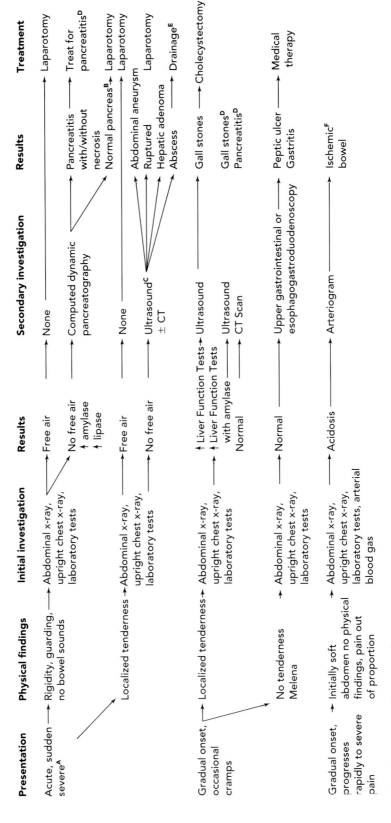

Presentation	Physical findings	Initial investigation	Results	Secondary investigation	Results	Treatment
Acute, sudden severe[A]	Rigidity, guarding, no bowel sounds	Abdominal x-ray, upright chest x-ray, laboratory tests	Free air	None		Laparotomy
			No free air, ↑ amylase, ↑ lipase	Computed dynamic pancreatography	Pancreatitis with/without necrosis	Treat for pancreatitis[D]
					Normal pancreas[B]	Laparotomy
	Localized tenderness	Abdominal x-ray, upright chest x-ray, laboratory tests	Free air	None		Laparotomy
			No free air	Ultrasound[C] ± CT	Abdominal aneurysm	Laparotomy
					Ruptured Hepatic adenoma	Laparotomy
					Abscess	Drainage[E]
Gradual onset, occasional cramps	Localized tenderness	Abdominal x-ray, upright chest x-ray, laboratory tests	↑ Liver Function Tests	Ultrasound	Gall stones	Cholecystectomy
			↑ Liver Function Tests with amylase	Ultrasound	Gall stones[D]	
			Normal	CT Scan	Pancreatitis[D]	
	No tenderness Melena	Abdominal x-ray, upright chest x-ray, laboratory tests	Normal	Upper gastrointestinal or esophagogastroduodenoscopy	Peptic ulcer Gastritis	Medical therapy
Gradual onset, progresses rapidly to severe pain	Initially soft abdomen no physical findings, pain out of proportion	Abdominal x-ray, upright chest x-ray, laboratory tests, arterial blood gas	Acidosis	Arteriogram	Ischemic[F] bowel	

CT = Computerized tomography
SBO = Small bowel obstruction

Midabdominal, lower quadrant pain

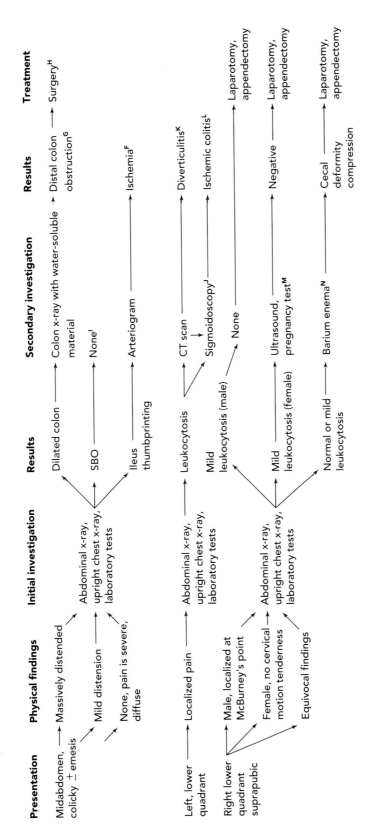

Presentation	Physical findings	Initial investigation	Results	Secondary investigation	Results	Treatment
Midabdomen, colicky ± emesis	Massively distended		Dilated colon	Colon x-ray with water-soluble material	Distal colon obstruction[G]	Surgery[H]
	Mild distension	Abdominal x-ray, upright chest x-ray, laboratory tests	SBO	None[I]		
	None, pain is severe, diffuse		Ileus thumbprinting	Arteriogram	Ischemia[F]	
Left, lower quadrant	Localized pain	Abdominal x-ray, upright chest x-ray, laboratory tests	Leukocytosis	CT scan	Diverticulitis[K]	
			Mild leukocytosis (male)	Sigmoidoscopy[J]	Ischemic colitis[L]	
Right lower quadrant suprapubic	Male, localized at McBurney's point	Abdominal x-ray, upright chest x-ray, laboratory tests		None		Laparotomy, appendectomy
	Female, no cervical motion tenderness		Mild leukocytosis (female)	Ultrasound, pregnancy test[M]	Negative	Laparotomy, appendectomy
	Equivocal findings		Normal or mild leukocytosis	Barium enema[N]	Cecal deformity compression	Laparotomy, appendectomy

ALGORITHM 14–1

79

the absence of severe coexisting medical illnesses, splenectomy should be performed. An intraabdominal abscess secondary to perforation of a viscus should be treated with laparotomy, and the underlying problem—whether due to ulcer disease or cancer—should be corrected.

F. Clear signs of peritonitis mandate laparotomy, and in such instances arteriography is not indicated. If ischemia is suspected in a stable patient with equivocal physical findings, arteriography may be therapeutic as well as diagnostic. Selective injection of vasodilators such as papaverine, phenoxybenzamine, or prostaglandin E_1 may be performed. Fibrinolytic agents may be infused if a clot has been demonstrated in the superior mesenteric artery. Once the patient is stabilized and metabolic defects corrected, the decision to proceed with surgery must be individualized. Operative choices include resection of the involved bowel with exteriorization, revascularization, or embolectomy.

G. In order of decreasing frequency, the differential diagnosis of acute complete colon obstruction includes cancer, diverticular disease, and sigmoid volvulus. Other causes include a stricture from inflammatory bowel disease or a prior ischemic event.

H. For an obstructing right colon cancer, resection, and primary anastomosis is the preferred operation. For an obstructing cancer of the left or sigmoid colon, surgical options are multiple. A primary anastomosis could still be done; however, a subtotal resection with ileosigmoidostomy or ileorectostomy would probably be required because of the dilated, stool-laden proximal colon. Alternatives include hemicolectomy and Hartmann's pouch or mucous fistula. In selected cases resection and intraoperative colonic lavage followed by primary anastomosis can be performed. Finally, fecal diversion followed by resection 7--10 days later can be done in poor-risk patients. If the obstruction is due to a sigmoid volvulus and the bowel is nonviable, resection with end colostomy and Hartmann's pouch or mucous fistula must be performed. If nonoperative detorsion is successful, the bowel may be electively cleansed and resected with primary anastomosis. If the bowel has not been prepared, but is viable at laparotomy, colopexy alone is not acceptable and resection must be performed.

I. Indications for prompt surgery for a small bowel obstruction (SBO) are signs of intestinal strangulation, specifically, pain and guarding on palpation. In the absence of pain, a 24--48-hour observation period may be used to resuscitate and hydrate the patient and correct any metabolic disturbances. If no improvement has been seen after 48 hours, surgery is indicated.

J. In the absence of radiographic signs of diverticulitis (bowel wall and mesenteric thickening, extraluminal air or fluid collections and diverticulae), flexible sigmoidoscopy may be performed. Entities that may be diagnosed include ischemic colitis, pseudomembranous colitis, and inflammatory bowel disease. The examination should be performed gently and with minimal insufflation of air.

K. Unless diffuse abdominal rigidity or pneumoperitoneum is present, acute diverticulitis may be managed initially with nonoperative measures. This course should include bowel rest, intravenous antibiotics specific for Gram-negative and anaerobic bacteria, and close observation. Indications for surgery in patients older than 55 years of age include two or more hospital admissions for diverticulitis associated with pain, fever, leukocytosis, obstruction, or urinary tract symptoms. Inability to exclude cancer is also an indication for surgery. Patients younger than 55 years of age should undergo surgery after only a single attack.

L. Ischemic colitis may follow three patterns: transient mucosal ischemia that is treated nonsurgically; gangrenous and stricturing. Colonic gangrene resembles other intraabdominal catastrophies; patients manifest signs of circulatory collapse, sepsis, and peritonitis. Laparotomy is required. If the ischemic event does not progress to gangrene, the local inflammatory response may produce strictures that can cause obstruction.

M. Nonappendiceal pathology identifiable on ultrasonography include an ectopic pregnancy, tubal ovarian abscess, ovarian cyst, ruptured ovarian follicle, or hydronephrosis.

N. If one suspects appendicitis but the history and physical examination are atypical, a barium enema may be helpful. Indirect signs of appendicitis include nonfilling of the appendix and extrinsic compression on the cecum.

BIBLIOGRAPHY

1. Cameron: *Current Surgical Therapy.* Mosby: St. Louis, 1984.
2. Sabiston DC: *Textbook of General Surgery:* the biological basis of modern surgical practice. WB Saunders: Philadelphia, 1991.
3. Schwartz SI: *Principles of Surgery.* (VI Ed) McGraw-Hill: New York, 1994.
4. Silen W: *Copes Early Diagnosis of Acute Abdomen,* (18th Ed) Oxford University Press, New York, 1991.
See also Chapters 55, 56, 58, 62, 64, 74, 76.

CHAPTER 15

Occult Rectal Bleeding

W. Douglas Wong, M.D. and Douglas D. Berglund, M.D.

Refer to Algorithm 15–1.

A. Fecal occult blood testing (FOBT) has been used for some years as a screening tool for early diagnosis of colorectal neoplasm. A recent report from the Minnesota Colon Cancer Control Study demonstrated a 33% reduction in mortality from colorectal cancer utilizing annual stool examinations with rehydrated hemoccult slides.

B. A thorough history includes questions regarding change in bowel habits, weight loss or gain, abdominal pain, gross rectal bleeding, family history of cancer, prior history of cancer surgery, and other medical diseases.

C. Digital rectal examination and anoscopy should be performed to exclude anorectal causes of bleeding such as anal fissure, fistula, hemorrhoids, proctitis, and anal cancer.

D. Treatment of anal fissure, fistula, hemorrhoids, proctitis, and anal cancer are outlined in Chapters 22, 25, 26, 28, 29, 40 and 43.

E. For young patients with no risk factors for colorectal cancer who are found to have an obvious anorectal source for the bleeding, and a clinical history consistent with this anorectal source, a flexible sigmoidoscopy should be an adequate investigation. However, all other patients should undergo total colonoscopy.

F. Colonoscopy is now considered the best means of evaluating the colon after a positive FOBT. Colonoscoy is both diagnostic and potentially therapeutic. Air-contrast barium enema is a reasonable alternative when colonoscopy is unavailable or not technically possible.

G. Appropriate treatment of the underlying etiology should be performed: excision and retrieval of polyps, notation and photography of vascular malformations, and biopsy of cancers, inflamed areas, and suspicious lesions are followed by appropriate therapy.

H. Patients with a negative colonoscopy that have any upper gastrointestinal symptoms should undergo esophagogastroduodenoscopy.

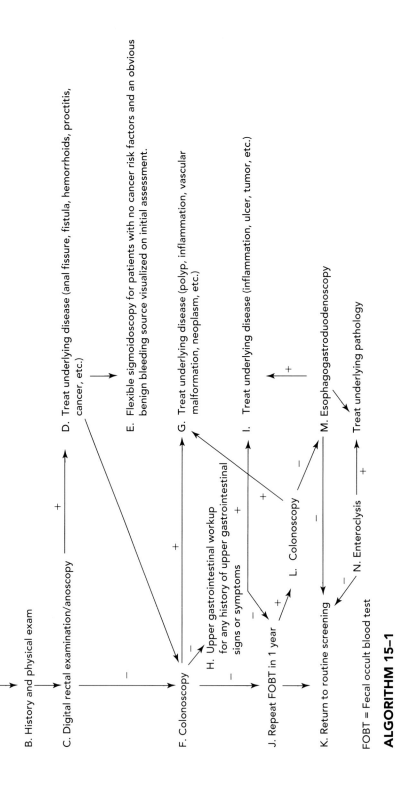

A. + Fecal occult blood test

B. History and physical exam

C. Digital rectal examination/anoscopy

D. Treat underlying disease (anal fissure, fistula, hemorrhoids, proctitis, cancer, etc.)

E. Flexible sigmoidoscopy for patients with no cancer risk factors and an obvious benign bleeding source visualized on initial assessment.

F. Colonoscopy

G. Treat underlying disease (polyp, inflammation, vascular malformation, neoplasm, etc.)

H. Upper gastrointestinal workup for any history of upper gastrointestinal signs or symptoms

I. Treat underlying disease (inflammation, ulcer, tumor, etc.)

J. Repeat FOBT in 1 year

K. Return to routine screening

L. Colonoscopy

M. Esophagogastroduodenoscopy

N. Enteroclysis

Treat underlying pathology

FOBT = Fecal occult blood test

ALGORITHM 15–1

84

I. Most of the upper gastrointestinal etiologies of positive FOBT are benign but should be properly treated. Causes include esophagitis, gastritis, duodenitis, Barret's esophagus, gastric and duodenal ulcers, esophageal varices, and vascular malformation.

J. If colonoscopy is negative, the patient should have a repeat FOBT in 1 year.

K. If repeat FOBT is negative, the patient should be returned to routine screening.

L. If this repeat FOBT is positive, the patient should have repeat colonoscopy and possibly an air contrast barium enema as well as esophagogastroduodenoscopy.

M. If colonoscopy is negative in the presence of two consecutively positive annual FOBT then the patient should undergo esophagogastrododenoscopy. Chen et al. (see Bibliography) have documented that 42% of patients will have an upper gastrointestinal source for their positive FOBT.

N. Small bowel enteroclysis may reveal the source of bleeding as a small bowel lesion.

BIBLIOGRAPHY

1. Chen YK, Gladden DR. Kestenbaum DJ, et al: Is there a role for upper gastrointestinal endoscopy in the evaluation of patients with occult blood-positive stool and negative colonoscopy? *Am J Gastroenterol* 88:2026–2029, 1993.

2. Lieberman DA: Colon cancer screening: the dilemma of positive screening tests. *Arch Int Med,* 150:740–744, 1990.

3. Mandell JS, Bond JH, Church TR, et al: Reducing mortality from colorectal cancer be screening for fecal occult blood. *N Engl J Med* 328:1365–1371, 1993.

4. Matzen RN: Fecal occult blood testing, guidelines for follow-up after positive findings. *Postgrad Med.* 90:181, 1991.

See also Chapters 22, 25, 26, 28, 29, 40 and 43.

CHAPTER 16

Diarrhea

Gregory F. Bonner, M.D.

Refer to Algorithm 16–1.

A. Acute diarrheal attacks are generally due to infectious agents.
B. Symptoms which suggest toxicity include fever, bleeding, and more than minor abdominal pain.
C. Culture should be undertaken for salmonella, shigella, campylobacter, yersinia, and an ova and parasite (O & P) exam for amoeba is recommended.
D. Sigmoidoscopy should search for evidence of inflammatory, infectious, ischemic, or pseudomembranous colitis. Consider gastrograffin enema if symptoms or exam suggest ischemic colitis such as in an elderly patient with other vascular disease, diabetes or hypertension.
E. Check stool for *Clostridium difficile* toxin if the patient recounts a history of recent hospitalization and/or antibiotic exposure.
F. Benign causes include lactose intolerance, antibiotics (*C. difficile* negative), magnesium containing antacids or mineral supplements, sorbitol, drugs (quinidine, quinine, cytotec, chemotherapy), or postoperative conditions (postgastrectomy, cholecystectomy, or ileocecal valve resection).
G. Colonoscopy should include random biopsies for microscopic or collagenous colitis.
H. Medical therapy includes oral or topical azulfidine/mesalamine or steroids.
I. Secretory diarrhea is defined as: stool $[NA^+ + K^+] \times 2$ within 50 of osmolality (stool osmolality should be approximately equal to serum).
J. Osmotic diarrhea is defined as: stool $[NA^+ + K^+] \times 2$ less than 50 below osmolality.

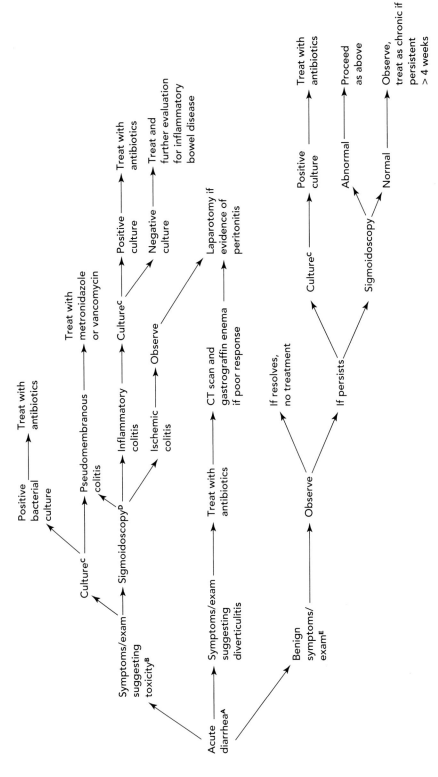

Acute diarrhea[A]

- Symptoms/exam suggesting toxicity[B]
  - Culture[C] → Positive bacterial culture → Treat with antibiotics
  - Sigmoidoscopy[D]
    - Pseudomembranous colitis → Treat with metronidazole or vancomycin
    - Inflammatory colitis → Culture[C]
      - Positive culture → Treat with antibiotics
      - Negative culture → Treat and further evaluation for inflammatory bowel disease
    - Ischemic colitis → Observe

- Symptoms/exam suggesting diverticulitis → Treat with antibiotics → CT scan and gastrograffin enema if poor response → Laparotomy if evidence of peritonitis

- Benign symptoms/exam[E] → Observe
  - If resolves, no treatment
  - If persists
    - Culture[C] → Positive culture → Treat with antibiotics
    - Sigmoidoscopy
      - Abnormal → Proceed as above
      - Normal → Observe, treat as chronic if persistent > 4 weeks

88

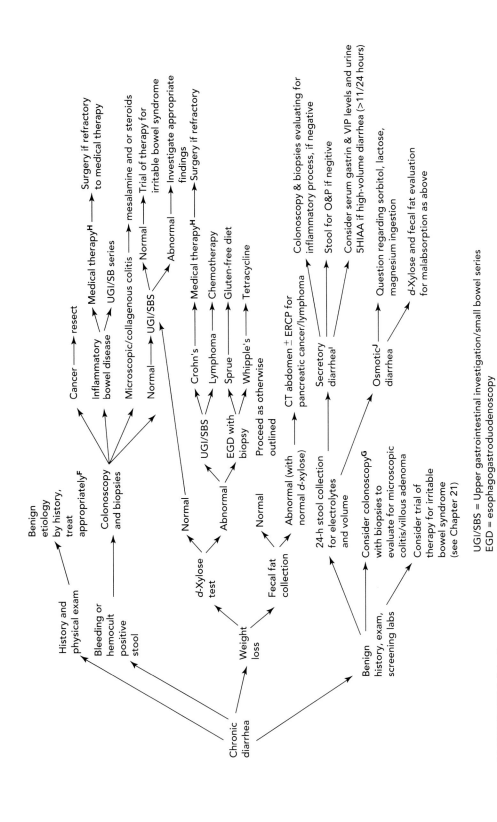

ALGORITHM 16–1

UGI/SBS = Upper gastrointestinal investigation/small bowel series
EGD = esophagogastroduodenoscopy
CT = Computerized tomography

BIBLIOGRAPHY

1. Brandt LJ: Colitis in the elderly. *Am J Gastroenterol* 76:239, 1981.

2. Fine KD, Santa Ana CA, Fordtran JS: Diagnosis of mangesium-induced diarrhea. *N Engl J Med* 324:1012–1017, 1991.

3. Kirsch M: Bacterial overgrowth. *Am J Gastroenterol* 85:231–237, 1990.

4. Rams H, Rogers AI, Ghandur-Mnaymneh L: Collagenous colitis. *Ann Int Med* 106:108–113, 1987.

5. Read NW, Krejs GJ, Read MG, et al: Chronic diarrhea of unknown origin. *Gastroenterology* 78:264–271, 1980.

6. Rickert RR: The important "imposters" in the differential diagnosis of inflammatory bowel disease. *J Clin Gastroenterol* 6:153–163, 1984.

See also Chapters 51, 52, 55.

CHAPTER 17

Diagnosis and Management Approach of Chronic Constipation

Marcelo F. Piccirillo, M.D. and Steven D. Wexner, M.D.

Refer to Algorithm 17-1.

A. To achieve predictable success in the management of chronically constipated patients, it is crucial to objectively identify underlying pathophysiology. The treatment of constipation will not be successful unless extracolonic conditions are accurately identified and corrected. These conditions are listed in Table 17-1. A careful history should reveal many years of hypothyroidism, diabetes, porphyria, amyloidosis, or other endocrine or metabolic pathologies.
B. It is very important to query the patient about consumption of the numerous potentially constipating drugs, including anticholinergics, antidepressants, antacids, and psychotherapeutics; when possible, all such agents should be discontinued or decreased in dosage (Table 17-2).
C. Stool consistency plays an important role in bowel function. The normal colon absorbs over 1300 mL of the 1500 mL of ileal effluent presented to it each day resulting in a stool that is about 70% water. Therefore, poor ingestion of water or the use of diuretics or hypotensives may result in harder stools that are difficult to evacuate. The treatment should be based on common sense: a high-fiber diet (25-35 g/day) with adequate hydration is a crucial facet of initial management. In general, a 6-month supervised trial should be undertaken. The fiber should be slowly added to the diet to prevent gas bloating and discomfort.
D. Hypothyroidism and other endocrine or metabolic disorders as listed in Table 17-1 should be identified by serum testing. In general, a thyroid panel, urine analysis, and routine chemistry profile will uncover such causes. Treatment is undertaken as indicated by the test results.

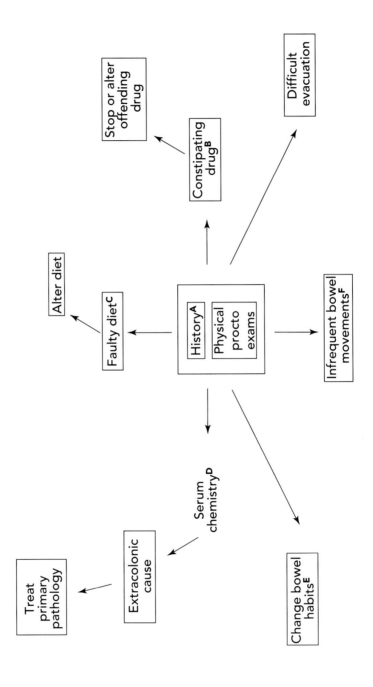

Stop or alter offending drug

Constituting drug**B**

Difficult evacuation

Alter diet

Faulty diet**C**

History**A**
Physical procto exams

Infrequent bowel movements**F**

Serum chemistry**D**

Extracolonic cause

Change bowel habits**E**

Treat primary pathology

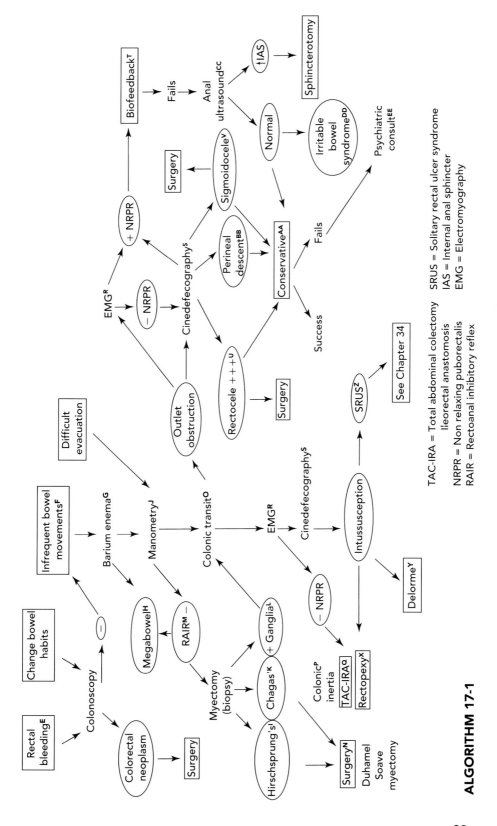

ALGORITHM 17-1

TAC-IRA = Total abdominal colectomy
           Ileorectal anastomosis
NRPR = Non relaxing puborectalis
RAIR = Rectoanal inhibitory reflex

SRUS = Solitary rectal ulcer syndrome
IAS = Internal anal sphincter
EMG = Electromyography

93

TABLE 17-1 ETIOLOGY

Extracolonic constipation
Diet
Drugs
  Anticholinergics
  Anticonvulsants
  Antiparkinsonians
  Anesthetics
  Diuretics
  Hematinics (iron)
  Opiates
  Barium sulfate
  Monoamine oxidase inhibitors
  Antidepressants
  Antacids
  Hypotensives
  Ganglionic blockers
  Metals (arsenic, mercury)
  Psychotherapeutics
  Paralytic agents
Neurological
  Iatrogenic: resection of nervi
Spinal
  Cauda equina meningocele
  Trauma (to spinal cord or cauda equina)
  Paraplegia
  Tabes dorsalis
  Multiple sclerosis

Cerebral
  Parkinson's disease
  Stroke
  Tumors
Peripheral
  Multiple endocrine neoplasia (II B)
  Autonomic neuropathy
  Chagas' disease
  Hirschsprung's disease
  Von Recklinghausen's disease
  Systemic sclerosis
Endocrine/metabolic
  Hypothyroidism
  Hypopituitarism
  Diabetes mellitus
  Pheochromocytoma
  Amyloidosis
  Hyperparathyroidism
  Hypercalcemia
  Porphyria
  Hypokalemia
  Uremia
  Pregnancy
Psychological
  Depression
  Anorexia nervosa

Primary colonic origin constipation
Structural
  Anatomic colonic etiology
    Tumors
    Megabowel
    Hirschsprung's disease
    Chagas' disease
  Anatomic pelvic outlet etiology
    rectocele
    intussusception/rectal prolapse
    Descending perineum syndrome
    Sigmoidocele
    Anal stenosis
    Anal tumors
Physiologic
  Colonic dismotility: colonic inertia
  Physiologic pelvic outlet obstruction
    Paradoxical puborectalis contraction
    PPC, anismus, nonrelaxing puborectalis syndrome; NRPR, spastic pelvic floor syndrome
Others
  Old age
  Lack of exercise

TABLE 17–2 HISTORY

List of current medications
Diet
Differentiate: infrequent bowel movements and difficulty in evacuation
Use of laxatives, suppositories, enemas
Perineal support, anal/vaginal digitation
Abdominal pain, bloating
Change in bowel habits/rectal bleeding
Dorsal trauma

TABLE 17–3 SIGNS AND SYMPTOMS

Infrequent Defecation		Difficult Evacuation
−	Rectal pain	+++
−	Rectal pressure	+++
−	Sensation of incomplete evacuation	+++
++	Discomfort between defecations	++
++	Hard stool consistency	++
+++	Abdominal pain	−
+++	Bloating	−
+++	Laxative dependence	+
+	Enemas, suppositories	+++
−	Anal/vaginal digitation	+++

E. Many patients do not have "chronic" constipation but may experience only a transient change in bowel habits. This condition can be accompanied by sporadic rectal bleeding. Colonoscopy is mandatory in these cases in order to exclude the presence of a colorectal neoplasm.

F. Patients with infrequent evacuation will generally have a history somewhat different from that of patients with difficult evacuation (Table 17–3). Physical exam will usually be unremarkable or may reveal abdominal distention with a palpable full colon.

G. Barium enema may reveal an elongated or redundant colon with retained feces.

H. Megabowel can be considered as megarectum, megasigmoid, megacolon, or a combination of these entities. It also may be indicative of Hirschsprung's disease.

I. Hirschsprung's disease in its classic form is usually diagnosed in infancy or childhood, occurring in one in 10,000 live births. The myenteric plexus is absent for a variable distance of colon, resulting in an aganglionic area with proximal hypertrophied and dilated bowel. The diagnosis is made by a lateral view of the rectum filled with barium or by a full-thickness biopsy (myectomy) of the affected area. In "short-segment" Hirschsprung's disease, which may not be apparent until adult life, the barium enema can be normal because the aganglionic segment extends only to the anorectal junction. In the "ultra-short-segment" form, even the biopsy will be normal because only the distal anal canal is involved.

J. Anal manometry will fail to show a rectoanal inhibitory reflex (RAIR) in all forms of the disease. Thus absence of the RAIR during manometry suggests the diagnosis of Hirschsprung's disease. A myectomy should be performed to assess for the presence of ganglia.

K. Chagas' disease is an acquired form of terminal argyrophyllic neuron disease in which microscopic and histochemical findings are similar to those of Hirschsprung's disease.

L. If biopsy reveals the presence of ganglia, the most common reason for a false-negative RAIR is megarectum. In these instances the rectum is too large to permit rapid balloon insufflation during attempted reflex elicitation.

M. In patients with non-Hirschsprung's megabowel, biopsy shows normal ganglia and the RAIR is present or abnormal but not absent.

N. Treatment for Hirschsprung's disease is either Duhamel's or Soave's operation or a coloanal anastomosis. In the ultra-short segment form an anal myectomy is generally curative.

O. After excluding Hirschsprung's disease the next study to be performed is the pancolonic transit study (PTS). Three possible marker patterns are normal, diffuse slow transit, or rectosigmoid delay (outlet obstruction).

P. A diagnosis of colonic inertia requires that transit-time study demonstrates retention of at least 20% of the markers in the colon on the 5th day after ingestion. The etiology of this syndrome is still poorly understood, especially because no abnormalities can be found by routine examination. However, there is growing evidence that colonic inertia (CI) may be the result of a neuropathy in the colonic wall.

Q. The patients whose symptoms persist despite adequate evaluation and medical therapy may benefit from surgery. A cecorectal anastomosis following subtotal colectomy may result in residual postoperative constipation because the same mitigating factors that were present preoperatively in the colon remain postoperatively in the capacious, readily distensable retained cecum. Therefore, total abdominal colectomy (TAC) and ileorectal anastomosis (IRA) is the best surgical alternative for CI. In order to ensure optimal postoperative results after TAC and IRA, nonrelaxing puborectalis syndrome (NRPR) (paradoxical puborectalis contraction, anismus) must be excluded. Appropriate relaxation of the pelvic floor muscle is best demonstrated by both electromyography (EMG) and cinedefecography (CD).

R. Anal EMG can be performed with either a concentric or single fiber needle. Alternatively, cutaneous patch electrodes or an intraanal plug can be used. Normally, the external anal sphincter and puborectalis should demonstrate decreased electrical activity during attempted evacuation. In patients with NRPR the neuromuscular activity fails to decrease or paradoxically increases.

S. NRPR can also be objectively demonstrated with CD. This lack of coordination between puborectalis and anal sphincters makes defecation exceedingly difficult and prolonged. During CD patients with NRPR will show one or more of the following problems: failure to empty, failure of the anal canal to open or to shorten, maintenance of the puborectalis length, or elevation of the pelvis. There are many causes of structural pelvic outlet obstruction, including descending perineum syndrome, rectal prolapse, rectocele, and sigmoidocele, all of which are well demonstrated by CD.

T. If a rectoanal intussusception is found during CD, a Frykman–Goldberg (sutured) rectopexy can be undertaken during the same surgical act; NRPR may respond to biofeedback. In this method, the patient views the recording with the physician while trying to readjust sphincteric responses, thereby learning to relax the internal anal sphincter (IAS) and contract the external anal sphincter (EAS). Although initially used for incontinence, this method is associated with a 90% success rate in the treatment of constipation. Surgery has no role in the treatment of NRPR.

U. Rectocele is a weakness of the anterior rectal wall, the rectovaginal septum, and the posterior vaginal wall. The patient usually has a variety of anorectal symptoms, the most common being constipation. In those patients who admit to the use of manual pressure adjacent to the anal opening or against the posterior vaginal wall to aid rectal emptying, and after excluding NRPR as the primary pathology, a surgical approach can be considered. Transrectal, transperineal, or transvaginal repair may be performed in these cases, with good results. However, although most females have a small anterior rectocele (< 2 cm), these defects rarely require surgical repair. For a rectocele to be repaired it must be > 2 cm, nonemptying during CD, and the only identifiable cause of constipation.

V. Sigmoidocele is a redundant loop of sigmoid that obstructs anorectal evacuation during CD. These patients will often complain of pelvic or lower abdominal fullness and the need for manual abdominopelvic pressure or positional changes to complete evacuation. In essence, they note a double evacuation syndrome similar to that described in patients with cystocoeles. The overall incidence of sigmoidoceles in constipated patients is 5%. They are classified by the position of the lowest loop of sigmoid during maximal evacuatory effort:

- 1°: above the pubococcygeal line
- 2°: below the pubococcygeal line but above the ischiopubic line
- 3°: below the ischiopubic line

Patients with 1° and 2° sigmoidoceles generally respond to conservative therapy. However, those patients with 3° sigmoidoceles may benefit from sigmoid colectomy. The procedure is ideally suited to laparoscopy.

W. Rectoanal intussusception is the predecessor of rectal prolapse. Early intussusceptions respond to conservative therapy including biofeedback. Advanced intussusceptions can be surgically treated. In general, patients with intussusception complain of incomplete or difficult evacuation with tenesmus. An associated solitary rectal ulcer may also accompany and increases the likelihood of surgery being needed.

X. If the intussusception is noted in a patient with colonic inertia, then a rectopexy can be added to the TAC.

Y. If the intussusception is isolated, a Delorme procedure may be beneficial.

 Z. If the intussusception occurs with solitary rectal ulcer syndrome (SRUS) with normal colonic transit and normal puborectalis function, an anterior resection can be considered.

AA. The vast majority of patients with rectoanal intussusception with normal transit and normal puborectalis function without a solitary rectal ulcer are best treated conservatively. Similarly, most patients with early sigmoidocele and rectocele and all patients with perineal descent are best treated conservatively. Treatment is directed at decreasing straining during evacuation. Options include dietary refinement, laxative, enema and suppository regimes, and biofeedback. Biofeedback has proved successful in 40–70% of patients with non-NRPR outlet obstruction who are not surgical candidates.

BB. Patients with isolated perineal descent (descent > 5 cm at rest or > 5 cm between rest and push) are treated conservatively. Conservative therapy may include a perineal support device to assist in evacuation.

CC. Patients with apparent NRPR who fail biofeedback should undergo anal ultrasonography. Rare cases of isolated internal anal sphincter hypertrophy can be treated by sphincterotomy. Such therapy should be undertaken with caution.

DD. When all evaluations are normal, the patient should be treated for irritable bowel syndrome.

EE. When all conservative measures fail, psychiatric consultation should be considered. Psychological testing of constipated patients has revealed that they are depressed, hypochondriacal, and neurotic. As such, they may greatly benefit from counseling and psychopharmachologic assistance.

SUMMARY

1. The surgeon must exclude dietary and extracolonic causes of constipation.

2. Anorectal physiology investigation is mandatory prior to surgery for constipation.

3. TAC and IRA should only be offered to patients who have colonic inertia.

4. Biofeedback is the treatment of choice for NRPR, early rectocoeles, early rectoanal intussusception, and perineal descent.

5. For patients in whom all diagnostic tests are normal, psychotherapy may be of some benefit.

BIBLIOGRAPHY

1. Beck DE, Jagelman DG, Fazio VN: The surgery of idiopathic constipation. *Gastroenterol Clin N Am* 16:143–156, 1987.

2. Beck DE, Wexner SD (eds) *Fundamentals of Anorectal Surgery,* New York McGraw Hill, 1992.

3. Henry MM, Swash M (eds): *Coloproctology and the Pelvic Floor*, (3rd edition) London: Butterworth-Heineman, 1995.

4. Jorge JMN, Yang YK, Wexner SD: Incidence and clinical significance of sigmoidocoeles as determined by a new classification system. *Dis Colon Rectum* 37:1112–1117, 1994.

5. Lane RHS, Todd IP: Idiopathic megacolon: a review of 42 cases. *Br J Surg* 64:305–310, 1977.

6. Piccirillo MF, Park UC, Nogueras JJ. et al: An objective quantification of the rectoanal inhibitory reflex. *Coloproctology* (in press).

7. Piccirillo MF, Reissman P, Carnavos R, et al: Colectomy for constipation: the best alternative in selected cases. *Br J. Surg* (in press).

8. Schouter W, Tenkate FJ, de Graaf EJ, et al: Visceral neuropathy in slow transit constipation: an immunohistochemical investigation with monoclonal antibodies against neurofilament. *Dis Colon Rectum* 36:1112–1117, 1993.

9. Taylor I. A survey of normal bowel habits. *Br J. Clin Pract* 29:289–291, 1975.

10. Wexner SD, Bartolo DCC. *Constipation: Etiology Evaluation and Treatment.* London: Butterworth-Heineman, 1995.

11. Wexner SD, Cheape JD, Jorge JMN et al: Prospective assessment of biofeedback for the treatment of paradoxical puborectalis contraction. *Dis Colon Rectum* 35:145–150, 1992.

12. Wexner SD, Daniel N, Jagelman DG: Colectomy for constipation: physiologic investigation is the key to success. *Dis Colon Rectum* 34:851–856.

See also Chapters 3, 18, 33 and 34.

CHAPTER 18

Evaluation and Management of Dyschezia

G. Ching Ger, M.D. and Yung Kang Yang, M.D.

Refer to Algorithm 18–1.

A. Difficult defecation includes characteristic symptoms such as prolonged and repeated straining at stool more than 25% of the time, rectal fullness, the sense of incomplete evacuation, and the necessity for manual assistance.

B. A simple history includes the patient's stool frequency, the onset of symptoms, dietary and bowel habits, laxative ingestion, other associated symptoms, and prior abdominal or pelvic surgery.

C. The anal region should be inspected carefully for findings of fissures, hemorrhoids, fistulas, and abscesses. Digital examination might reveal possible neoplasms, fecaloma, anterior rectocele, or prominent puborectalis contraction.

D. Endoscopic examination is mandatory to exclude neoplasia; it will seldom reveal any abnormality in the vast majority of patients. In other patients, melanosis coli means chronic anthracene laxative abuse. A solitary rectal ulcer, which is associated with rectoanal intussusception or digitation, may be found. Occasionally the intussusception itself may be seen. A volvulus can also be endoscopically identified.

E. Barium enema is an excellent tool to demonstrate structural abnormalities in the colon. Colonoscopy is often futile because an unusually redundant and dilated colon or rectum is usually found. The upper limit of the rectosigmoid is 8.5 cm in a lateral view at the pelvic brim.

F. A technique for measuring total and segmental colonic transit time is a useful tool and an important step to establish whether transit is normal, is globally slow, or shows pelvic outlet obstruction. Importantly, it may often demonstrate a normal transit time in patients with bowel neurosis or who deny having bowel actions.

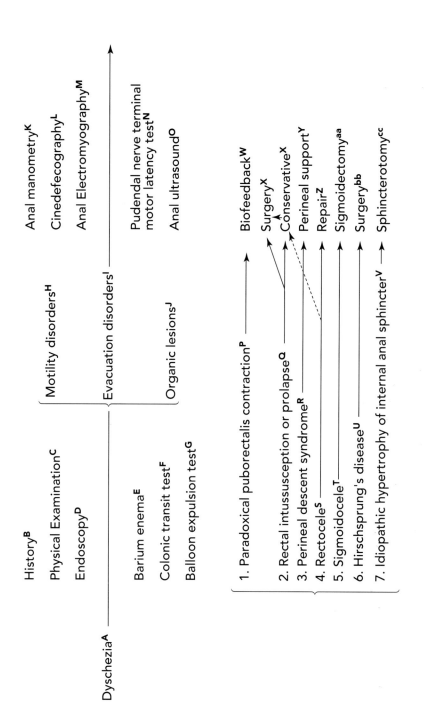

Dyschezia^A

History^B

Physical Examination^C

Endoscopy^D

Motility disorders^H

Anal manometry^K

Cinedefecography^L

Anal Electromyography^M

Evacuation disorders^I

Pudendal nerve terminal motor latency test^N

Anal ultrasound^O

Barium enema^E

Colonic transit test^F

Balloon expulsion test^G

Organic lesions^J

1. Paradoxical puborectalis contraction^P → Biofeedback^W

2. Rectal intussusception or prolapse^Q → Surgery^X

Conservative^X

3. Perineal descent syndrome^R → Perineal support^Y

4. Rectocele^S → Repair^Z

5. Sigmoidocele^T → Sigmoidectomy^{aa}

6. Hirschsprung's disease^U → Surgery^{bb}

7. Idiopathic hypertrophy of internal anal sphincter^V → Sphincterotomy^{cc}

ALGORITHM 18–1

G. A 50-cc balloon is filled within the rectum, and the patient is asked to evacuate it. Failure to achieve evacuation suggests a disorder.

H. To select patients for appropriate treatment, it is necessary to distinguish patients with various slow transit constipation from those with evacuation disorders. The reported results of total colectomy in patients with slow transit constipation are good with a success rate of more than 80%.

I. Patients with pelvic outlet obstruction have a normal colonic transit time, but the radiopaque markers will accumulate in the rectum. If slow transit and pelvic outlet obstruction coexist, the pelvic problem should be addressed either first or simultaneously with the transit problem.

J. Structural abnormalities of the rectum and anus such as neoplasms, anal fissures, fistulas, and hemorrhoids may lead to evacuation difficulty and should be treated on an individual basis. However, correction of pathology such as hemorrhoids or fissures may fail unless the underlying bowel evacuatory pattern is improved first.

K. Absence of the rectoanal inhibitory reflex in anorectal manometry can be used as a reliable test in the diagnosis of Hirschsprung's disease. If the reflex is absent, a myectomy needs to be performed to assess for the presence of the myenteric plexi.

L. Cinedefecography was developed for the dynamic investigation of evacuation. It can assess patients with problems related to defecation such as the perianal descent syndrome, paradoxical puborectalis contraction (PPC), rectoanal intussusception, rectal prolapse, rectocele, and sigmoidocele. The actual anorectal angle is of little importance, although the dynamic changes in the angle during activities such as squeezing and pushing are important.

M. Clinically, anal electromyography (EMG) provides valuable quantitative and objective data in the diagnosis of various pelvic floor disorders and gives an important therapeutic and predictive role following treatment of those various pelvic floor disorders. The EMG diagnosis of PPC is especially important.

N. Transanal pudendal nerve stimulation is the only practical modality of assessing pelvic floor neuropathy. The latent period between pudendal nerve stimulation at the ischial spine and the electromechanical response of anal sphincter muscle is measured. The normal range is 1.6–1.9 ms (milliseconds) for patients < 55 years of age and 1.9–2.2 ms for patients ≥ 55 years.

O. Anal ultrasound is a relatively new technology that can measure the thickness of the internal anal sphincter, external anal sphincter, and puborectalis. It also can evaluate any defects of the anal sphincters and anorectal suppurations.

P. Functional pelvic outlet obstructive constipation is caused by inappropriate contraction of the pelvic floor during attempted evacuation. The pathophysiology is unclear, and the condition may be asymptomatic and therefore found in "normal" individuals. The diagnosis is usually made by a combination of electromyography, manometry, and cinedefecography.

Q. Intussusception of the rectum, or internal procidentia, represents a predecessor to complete rectal procidentia. Women are affected 6 times more commonly than men, with a peak incidence for women in the fifth decade. The most useful diagnostic procedure for identification of internal procidentia is cinedefecography.

R. Perineal descent syndrome may cause obstructed defecation. The etiology is unclear, the relationship to pudendal neuropathy is unproven, and the treatment is elusive.

S. A *rectocele* means a pocket-like weakness of the rectovaginal septum that seldom becomes symptomatic until the 4th or 5th decade of life. A "significant" rectocele is defined as one > 2 cm that requires vaginal or anal digitation for evacuation or perineal support maneuvers and fails to empty during defecography.

T. According to cinedefecography, a sigmoidocele can be Grade I, II, or III as determined by the position of the lowest point during maximal pushing during the evacuatory phase: Grade I—above the pubococcygeal line; Grade II—between the pubococcygeal line and ischiopubic line; Grade III—below the ischiopubic line. Patients with Grade I or Grade II sigmoidoceles respond well to medical management, whereas those individuals with Grade III sigmoidoceles respond well to sigmoid colectomy.

U. Hirschsprung's disease is characterized by an aganglionic colorectal segment with inefficient motility, proximal to which the colon is dilated. Although it usually presents in infancy, it may occasionally present in later life. Anorectal manometry may be helpful in diagnosis because virtually all patients have an absent rectoanal inhibitory reflex. Definitive diagnosis is confirmed by the absence of ganglion cells in a full-thickness rectal biopsy specimen (myectomy). The most common reason for a false-negative reflex is an overly capacious rectum in which the reflex cannot be elicited because the balloon cannot be insufflated rapidly enough.

V. Some patients with symptoms of pelvic outlet obstruction show very high resting pressures, thick internal anal sphincter (IAS) by anal ultrasound, and no paradoxical puborectalis contraction or other abnormalities.

W. One recent study reviewed 18 patients who underwent outpatient treatment of paradoxical puborectalis contraction with intraanal EMG-based sensor biofeedback. A mean of 10-hour-long sessions resulted in an increase in frequency of unassisted bowel movements from 0–7 per week in 89% of patients.

X. The treatment of internal intussusception is similar to that for complete rectal procidentia. The result of various operative therapy that include both abdominal or perineal approaches seem satisfactory in selected patients. However, the vast majority of patients with intussusception respond to conservative means, including high-fiber diet, better bowel regulation, and biofeedback.

Y. The finding of abnormal perineal descent alone is not an indication for surgical intervention. Perineal supportive devices, especially during evacuation, may be helpful to these patients.

Z. A significant rectocele can be corrected by transvaginal, transperineal, or transanal repair.

AA. Sigmoidectomy is the treatment of choice for the symptomatic Grade III sigmoidocele. The operation is well suited to the laparoscopic approach.

BB. In short- or ultra-short segment Hirschsprung's disease, posterior rectal myectomy or anal sphincterotomy may effect a cure. Long-aganglionic-segment disease may benefit by abdominoperineal procedures such as a Duhamel operation, Swanson operation, or Soave operation.

CC. Anal sphincterotomy is the treatment of choice for patients with idiopathic hypertrophy of the internal anal sphincter.

BIBLIOGRAPHY

1. Farouk R, Duthie GS, Bartolo DCC: Functional anorectal disorders and physiological evaluation. In Beck DE, Wexner SD (eds): *Fundamentals of Anorectal Surgery.* New York: McGraw-Hill, 1992.
2. Heymen S, Wexner SD: Biofeedback for constipation. In: Smith L: *Practical Guide to Anorectal Testing.* Igaku-Shoin–New York (in press).
3. Jorge JMN, Wexner SD, Nogueras JJ, et al: Does perineal descent correlate with pudendal neuropathy? *Dis Colon Rectum* 36:475–483, 1993.
4. Pemberton JH: Management of constipation. In Henry MM, Swash M (eds): *Coloproctology and the Pelvic Floor,* 3rd ed. Oxford: Butterworth-Heinemann, 1995.
5. Smith LE: Algorithm for constipation. In Smith LE (ed): *Practical Guide to Anorectal Testing,* 2nd ed. New York: Igaku-Shoin Medical Publishers, 1995.
6. Vaccaro CA, Cheong DMO, Wexner SD, et al: Pudendal neuropathy in evacuatory disorders. *Dis Colon Rectum* 38:166–171, 1995.
7. Vaccaro CA, Cheong DMO, Wexner SD, et al: Role of pudendal nerve terminal motor latency assessment in constipated patients. *Dis Colon Rectum* 37:1250–1254, 1994.
8. Vaccaro CA, Wexner SD, Teoh TA, et al: Pudendal neuropathy is not related to pelvic outlet obstruction. *Dis Colon Rectum* (in press).
9. Wexner SD, Bartolo DCC (eds): *Constipation: Etiology, Evaluation, and Management.* Oxford: Butterworth-Heinemann, 1995.
10. Wexner SD, Marchetti F, Salanga VD, et al: Neurophysiologic assessment of the anal sphincters. *Dis Colon Rectum* 34:606–612, 1991.
11. Yang YK, Wexner SD, Nogueras JJ, et al: The role of anal ultrasound in the assessment of benign anorectal diseases. *Coloproctology* 15:260–264, 1993.

See also Chapters 3, 17, 33, 34.

CHAPTER 19

Fecal Incontinence

Han C. Kuijpers, M.D.

Refer to Algorithm 19-1.

A,B. A thorough history should be obtained focusing on the type and frequency of incontinence. Specifically, an incontinence scoring system should be utilized to classify the frequency and disability caused by incontinence to gas, liquid, or solid stool. An elderly patient who is only rarely incontinent to gas during periods of strenuous activity need not necessarily undergo a thorough physiologic investigation or be a candidate for surgery. Conversely, a young woman incontinent of solid stool on a daily basis who requires the use of a pad and has lifestyle impairment should undergo investigation with a view toward rectification of the problem. The history includes a detailed search for a possible cause of incontinence, including extrasphincteric causes such as diabetes and neurologic disease and sphincteric causes such as trauma from either childbirth, prior surgery, or noniatrogenic trauma.

C. Physical examination should include inspection of the undergarments. Fecal staining is a clue to the severity of the problem. The tone of the anus should be assessed at rest as well as during squeeze. The patient should also be asked to bear down to see whether a prolapse or intussusception occurs. Bidigital examination of the rectovaginal septum and anterior sphincter is particularly helpful, especially if a history of prior trauma has been obtained. Both anoscopy and proctosigmoidoscopy are useful to exclude anatomic causes of staining such as prolapsing hemorrhoids or an advanced rectoanal intussusception or early prolapse.

D. Patients with minor incontinence (incontinence score of 0-5 as noted in Table 19-1) are referred for conservative therapy, including biofeedback, bulking agents such as fiber and cholestyramine, and antidiarrheal agents such as diphenoxylate and loperamide hydrochloride or codeine phosphate.

E. Patients with major incontinence (score of 10-20 or causing disability to lifestyle) are referred for physiologic investigation.

Fecal incontinence

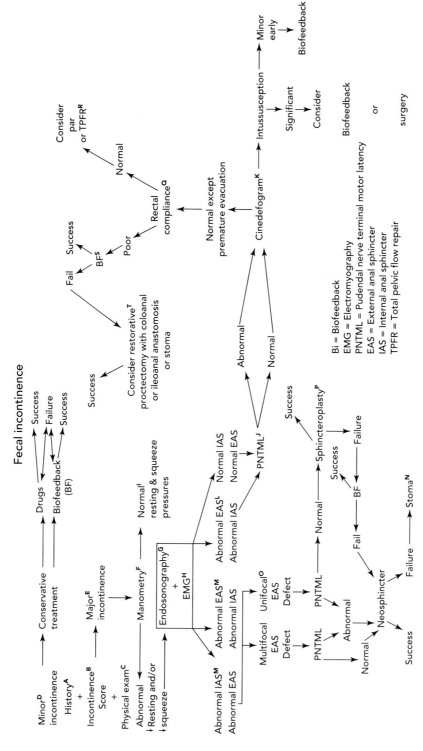

ALGORITHM 19-1

Bi = Biofeedback
EMG = Electromyography
PNTML = Pudendal nerve terminal motor latency
EAS = External anal sphincter
IAS = Internal anal sphincter
TPFR = Total pelvic flow repair

TABLE 19–1 CONTINENCE GRADING SCALE[a]

Type of Incontinence	Frequency[b]				
	Never	**Rarely**	**Sometimes**	**Usually**	**Always**
Solid	0	1	2	3	4
Liquid	0	1	2	3	4
Gas	0	1	2	3	4
Wears pad	0	1	2	3	4
Alteration in lifestyle	0	1	2	3	4

[a] The continence score is determined by adding points from the above grid, which takes into account the type and frequency of incontinence and the extent to which it alters the patient's life.

[b] 0 perfect; 20 complete incontinence; never = 0 (never); rarely = <1 month; sometimes = <1 week, ≥1 month; usually = <1 day, ≥1 week; always = ≥1 day

F. Manometry includes measurement of the resting and squeeze pressures, as well as the length of the high-pressure zone, initial and maximal tolerable sensory volumes, and rectal compliance. Usually 85% of resting pressure is achieved by the internal anal sphincter, and essentially the entire squeeze pressure is contributed by the external anal sphincter and puborectalis. The high-pressure zone length is the functional length of the anal canal. *Initial sensory volume* is the volume at which the patient first senses the presence of a substance in the rectum, and the *volume to fullness* is the volume at which the patient feels full. Maximum tolerable volume is the volume of the sensation to fullness; it is seldom elicited in the laboratory. Rectal compliance is the measure of the distensibility of the rectum. A normally compliant rectum should be able to undergo significant distension with a minimal increase in pressure. A poorly compliant rectum will undergo a significant increase in pressure despite a minor increase in intraluminal volume. Patients with proctitis will have poor compliance and will note tenesmus and leakage.

G. Certain patients confuse staining passage of mucus with fecal incontinence. These patients may display normal resting and squeeze pressures and need not undergo additional physiologic investigation. They can be offered the same conservative treatment as detailed above in D. Alternatively, if clinical suspicion exists, a cinedefogram can be obtained. If the patient displays either perineal descent, premature evacuation of barium, or both, and rectal compliance is poor, then the patient is a candidate for biofeedback therapy. If, however, the patient shows either perineal descent, premature evacuation, or both, and has normal rectal compliance, consideration can be given to either a postanal repair or a total pelvic floor repair. Although these operations were initially thought to improve the anorectal angle, subsequently they have been shown to have little effect on the anorectal angle and, in fact, have poor long-term results. Nonetheless, they are the only alternatives available in these patients with factitious incontinence. On rare occasions, a patient with "incontinence" will have isolated poor compliance due to proctitis but will have normal sphincter pressures. Such individuals may benefit from restorative proctectomy with coloanal anastomosis.

H. If the patient has decreased resting and/or squeeze pressures, then anal endo-sonography and electromyography (EMG) should be obtained. Endosonography allows quantification of the thicknesses of the internal and external anal sphincter and puborectalis as well as the identification of any defects or scars. EMG allows correlation of these findings in a quadrant by quadrant manner.

I. The patient who displays normal internal and external anal sphincter anatomy should undergo pudendal nerve terminal motor latency assessment (PNTML).

J. If latencies are normal, then a cinedefogram should be obtained and inter-preted in the same way as already discussed above.

K. If the cinedefogram reveals an intussusception, then that intussusception should be quantified as to its significance. Patients with early intussusceptions can successfully undergo conservative treatment with biofeedback. Patients with advanced intussusception may, in selected cases, benefit from surgical repair such as either rectopexy or a perineal resection with sphincter plication.

L. A similar approach can be utilized for an isolated abnormality of the internal anal sphincter (IAS). Again, pudendal neuropathy and a rectoanal intussuscep-tion as combined findings may suggest surgical repair of the intussusception. Alternatively, normal nerves and a normal defogram would suggest referral of the patient for biofeedback and conservative therapy.

M. The findings of abnormalities in the external and internal sphincter or in the external anal sphincter alone require quantification as to the defects. If anal endosonography and EMG reveal the defects to be multifocal, then a neo-sphincter should be considered. Failure of a neosphincter can be followed by biofeedback or possibly by a stoma. The varieties of neosphincters available at this time include a stimulated or a nonstimulated gracilis transposition, a bilateral gluteal maximus transposition, or implantation of an artificial sphinc-ter. All of these procedures are associated with success rates ranging from 50 to 85%.

N. As a final option, a stoma should always be considered. It is far better in many cases for the patients to have good control of a well-constructed stoma than no control of a damaged anus. Patients contemplating a stoma for incontinence should be encouraged to speak to other patients with stomas. Moreover, in the age of laparoscopic surgery, stomas can be created without any standard abdominal incision, and hopefully these patients can benefit from rapid recov-ery.

O. If the defect in the external anal sphincter (EAS) is unifocal and pudendal nerves are abnormal, the patients will not do well with sphincter repair. Several studies have shown that the factor of paramount importance in pre-dicting success after overlapping sphincter repair is the status of the pudendal nerves. Therefore, patients with neuropathy should be allowed time to recover from the neuropathy. However, if the injury was remote, then recovery is unlikely and a neosphincter could be considered. If the patient does recover after 6–12 months, as has been shown to happen after childbirth injuries, then a standard sphincter repair may be possible.

P. If the defect is unifocal with either initial or subsequent normal pudendal nerve evaluations, then an overlapping sphincteroplasty can be performed with anticipation of success in approximately 85% of cases. (See continence grading scale in Table 19–1).

Q. If cinedefecography confirms the incontinence, by revealing premature evacuation, and fails to reveal an etiology for the incontinence, rectal compliance studies should be undertaken. Compliance is a measure of the elasticity and accommodative properties of the rectum. It is a measure of the increase in rectal pressure relative to increased volume. The normally compliant rectum (12–15 cc/mmHg) should accommodate up to 200–300 cc with little pressure increase.

R. Patients in whom compliance is normal may benefit from either a postanal repair (PAR) or a total pelvic floor repair (TPFR). Both of these operations entail plication of the striated sphincter muscles.

S. Some patients with poor compliance can improve their control by biofeedback sensory retraining.

T. Some patients, particularly these with radiation proctitis or mucosal ulcerative colitis, will not respond to biofeedback. As medically indicated, appropriate patients may be candidates for restorative proctectomy with either a coloanal or ileoanal anastomosis or a stoma.

BIBLIOGRAPHY

1. Beck DE, Wexner SD (eds): *Fundamentals of Anorectal Surgery*. New York: McGraw-Hill, 1992.

2. Cuesta MA, Meijer S, Derksen EJ: Anal sphincter imaging in fecal incontinence using endosonography. *Dis Colon Rectum* 35:60–65, 1992.

3. Jorge JMN, Wexner SD: Fecal incontinence. *Dis Colon Rectum* 36:77–97, 1993.

4. Kuijpers HC (ed): *Colorectal Physiology: Fecal Incontinence*. Boca Raton: CRC Press, 1994.

5. Kuijpers JHC, Scheuer M: Disorders of fecal incontinence; a clinical and manometric study. *Dis Colon Rectum* 33:207–210, 1990.

6. Laurberg S, Swash M, Henry MM: Effect of postanal repair on progress of neurogenic damage to the pelvic floor. *Br J Surg* 77:519–521, 1990.

7. Oliveira L, Wexner SD, Park UC, et al: Sphincteroplasty for fecal incontinence: is it justifiable in patients over 60 years of age. *Br J Surg* (in press).

8. Vernava AM, Longo WE, Daniel GL: Pudendal neuropathy and the importance of EMG evaluation of fecal incontinence. *Dis Colon Rectum* 36:23–27, 1993.

9. Wexner SD (ed). Practical colorectal physiology: investigation and intervention. *Seminars in Colon and Rectal Surgery*. W.B. Saunders: Philadelphia, 1992.

10. Wexner SD, Marchetti F, Jagelman DG: The role of sphincteroplasty for fecal incontinence re-evaluated: a prospective physiologic and functional review. *Dis Colon Rectum* 34:22–30, 1991.

11. Yang YK, Wexner SD, Nogueras JJ, Jagelman DG: The role of anal ultrasound in the assessment of benign anorectal disease. *Coloproctology*, 5:260–264, 1993.

See also Chapter 3.

CHAPTER 20

Change in Bowel Habits

Philip Huber, Jr., M.D.

Refer to Algorithm 20-1.

A. *Normal bowel function* is a relative term defined as the usual function the patient has experienced over a period of time of good health. The characteristics of defecation, including the timing, consistency and frequency have an established pattern that is normal for that patient. Normal consistency for stool can vary from hard to loose. Similarly frequency can span from 1 stool every 3 days to 3 stools per day. Diet plays an important role in defining normal bowel function as well. The important point is to focus on the patient's usual stool characteristics when the patient felt well or healthy.

B. Onset of changes in bowel habit is usually gradual. The length of time during which the patient has been aware of a change is usually underestimated. Abrupt changes in habit connote acute processes such as infectious or inflammatory conditions.

C. Straining at stool is a frequent complaint gathered under the heading of "constipation." A feeling of incomplete emptying of the rectum is also reported in this subgroup. Both complaints focus on rectal outlet pathology.

D. The most common complaint or symptom in patients with colon cancer is a "change in bowel habit."

E. Fiber and fluid intake are the factors to determine. Even if dietary fiber is high, a poor water intake will cause hard stool. Calorie requirement drops by 30% from age 20 to age 70.

F. Particularly but not exclusively in the elderly, medication can affect bowel habit, usually by slowing stool transit. Supplemental dietary calcium intake generally slows transit, as do calcium channel blockers and antidepressants. All of these compounds are frequently used by older patients.

G. Decreased physical activity is another bowel factor. Aging causes progressive diminution in mobility, but trauma can acutely create similar problems.

H. "Diarrhea" generally connotes increased stool frequency and/or increased water or mucus in the stool.

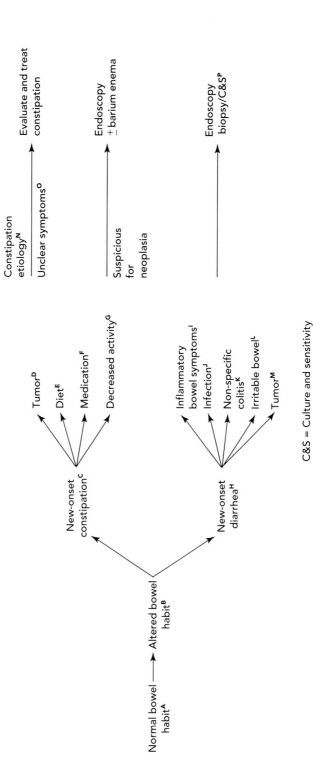

C&S = Culture and sensitivity

ALGORITHM 20–1

I. Systemic symptoms will usually be present with inflammatory bowel disease. Bleeding need not accompany stool, and IBD can present with decreased stool frequency.

J. Dietary and travel history can be very helpful in finding an infectious etiology for new onset of diarrhea. Coexistent systemic symptoms are not always present.

K. What began as "microscopic colitis"—a histologic classification for colitis causing diarrhea—has now been subdivided into multiple new types of colitis that create diarrhea, all based on differing histologic features.

L. One of the most frequent classifications for diarrhea, this syndrome has classically included alternating diarrhea and constipation. It is considered a diagnosis of exclusion if all other colon studies are negative or equivocal.

M. Mucus-secreting villous tumors causing diarrhea and hypokalemia are uncommon (most series report less than 10%). However, both benign and malignant tumors can present with loose stool and increased stool frequency.

N. If there is no suspicion of neoplasia, the evaluation and treatment of constipation can be pursued.

O. If associated symptoms are suspicious for neoplasm, further investigation is warranted. Flexible sigmoidoscopy with air-contrast barium enema remains a more cost-effective, if less accurate, method of surveying the colon than does colonoscopy. An often unstated but compelling point is the quality of the air-contrast barium enema. A detailed study done expertly in a well-prepared patient is often a reliable test.

P. Patients with persistent diarrhea need stool cultures and visualization of the mucosa with biopsy—not only for histology but also for culture and sensitivity (C & S). Particularly with the onset of HIV infections in the colon, the importance of biopsy for viral studies has proved reasonably reliable. Microscopic colitis can only be diagnosed with careful histologic examination.

BIBLIOGRAPHY

1. Sleisenger MH, Fordtran JS (eds): *Gastrointestinal Disease,* (5th ed.). Philadelphia: Saunders, 1993; Vol 1, Chapter 39; Chapter 42, p 917.

2. Yamada T, Alpers D, Owyang C, et al: *Textbook of Gastroenterology.* Philadelphia: Lippincott, 1991, Vol 1, Chapter 38, p 732; Chapter 39, p 779.

See also Chapters 16 and 17.

CHAPTER 21

Irritable Bowel Syndrome

Eli D. Ehrenpreis, M.D.

Refer to Algorithm 21-1.

A. Irritable bowel syndrome (IBS) is defined by the exclusion of structural gastro-intestinal diseases and thus is termed a functional disorder. It is characterized by chronic gastrointestinal symptoms including abdominal pain, altered bowel habits, and abdominal bloating. Predominant symptoms characterizing sub-groups of patients with IBS include pain, constipation, and diarrhea. Anxiety, stress, and depression are frequent findings in patients with IBS who seek medical attention. Symptoms of IBS are common and are found in 15-20% of the adult population.

B. Manning criteria as listed below are useful in separating organic causes of gastrointestinal disease from IBS. Studies indicate that the presence of abdominal pain plus 3 or more Manning criteria are predictive of IBS. The *Manning criteria* are: (1) abdominal distension, (2) pain relieved by defecation, (3) increased stool frequency with pain onset, (4) looser stools with pain onset, (5) mucous discharge from the rectum, (6) incomplete evacuation of the rectum. Other common symptoms of IBS include upper abdominal pain, nausea, flatulence, erudition, thin or pellet-like stools, and alternating diarrhea and constipation.

C. Symptoms suggestive of structural disease should alert the clinician to an alternative diagnosis (rather than IBS). Symptoms not consistent with IBS include weight loss, fever, rectal bleeding, dehydration, and nocturnal awak-ening due to symptoms. Additionally, it should be borne in mind that other organic disorders of the gastrointestinal tract may occur in patients with functional bowel symptoms. Therefore dramatic changes in symptoms should alert the clinician to other disease processes. Experience suggests that incom-plete evacuation in the constipated patient may also result from pelvic floor disorders.

D. No specific physical findings are characteristic of IBS. The examination should be utilized to exclude other causes of IBS-like symptoms (Crohn's disease, hyperthyroidism, Addison's disease, intestinal malabsorptive disorders).

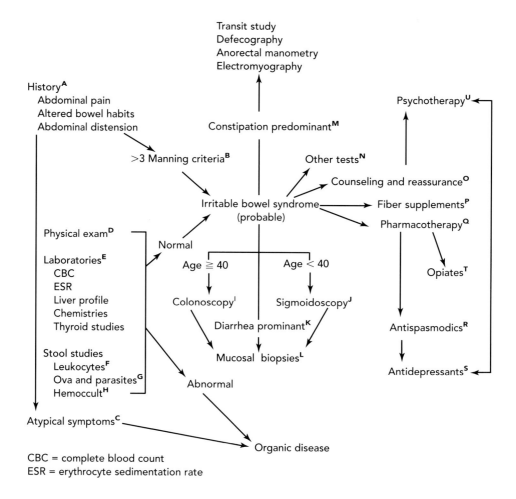

CBC = complete blood count
ESR = erythrocyte sedimentation rate

ALGORITHM 21–1

E. Anemia and elevated erythrocyte sedimentation rate (ESR) are suggestive of inflammatory bowel disease. Hypokalemia and low bicarbonate content may indicate secretory diarrhea.

F. Fecal leukocytes should not be present in IBS. This finding suggests inflammation (ulcerative colitis, Crohn's colitis, infectious colitis).

G. *Giardia lamblia, Entamoeba histolytica,* and *Blastocystis hominis* may cause IBS-like symptoms.

H. Positive hemoccult test should initiate workup for gastrointestinal (GI) blood loss.

I. It is generally recommended that a "low-tech" approach be taken for initial evaluation of patients meeting multiple Manning criteria and having a normal physical examination. Invasive procedures other than sigmoidoscopy, (or colonoscopy if patient is >40 years of age) or advanced radiographic testing should be reserved for those patients' atypical symptoms, abnormal physical findings, or recent change in bowel habits suspicious for colon cancer.

J. The sigmoidoscopic appearance of "colonic spasm" has been utilized in assisting diagnosis, but this finding is very subjective. The main purpose of the sigmoidoscopy is to exclude distal colitis and obstructing lesions of the rectosigmoid. Mucosal biopsies are recommended during sigmoidoscopy or colonoscopy in patients with predominant diarrhea to exclude microscopic colitis or quiescent inflammatory bowel disease.

K. Stool volume >200 mL/day suggests organic causes of diarrhea. Stool may contain phenolphthalein in laxative abusers. Steatorrhea may occur in patients with malabsorption syndromes (pancreatic or small bowel diseases). Fecal electrolytes and osmolality may be useful in characterizing diarrhea.

L. Patients with predominant symptoms of diarrhea may have microscopic colitis diagnosed by mucosal biopsy.

M. Patients with predominant symptoms of constipation may benefit from an evaluation for obstructive anorectal disorders or colonic inertia.

N. Computerized tomography (CT) scan, upper GI x-ray, upper endoscopy, and pancreatobiliary ultrasound may be considered based on the clinical situation. As stated previously, a good history and physical exam should strongly suggest the diagnosis of IBS on initial evaluation. Motility studies (gastric, small bowel and colonic) are generally performed for research purposes.

O. Reassurance regarding the benign clinical course of IBS should be made. Definitions of IBS suggesting that it is a disease (e.g., spastic colitis, mucous colitis) should be avoided. Although some authors chastise clinicians who emphasize the psychogenic aspects of the disorder, evaluation for anxiety disorders and depression is suggested.

P. Although statistically significant benefit from fiber therapy has not been proved, these agents are safe and may relieve constipation or diarrhea associated with IBS. This author prefers a polycarbophil compound for patients with loose stools and psyllium or methylcellulose for firm stools.

Q. It has been suggested that current treatment trials fail to prove the efficacy of any treatment for IBS. The use of pharmacotherapy should therefore be tempered and is at least initially reserved for patients failing counseling, dietary modification, and fiber supplements.

R. Although no firm data exist proving efficacy of antispasmodic medications, these are probably the most commonly prescribed pharmacologic agents for IBS. Contraindications for their use include obstructive uropathy, glaucoma, myasthenia gravis, and gastrointestinal obstruction.

S. Antidepressants may be effective in patients with IBS and overlying depression, insomnia, or fibromyalgia. True proven benefits for the treatment of IBS with antidepressants are lacking, although several studies with positive results have been published.

T. These agents are effective for treatment of diarrhea. No definite effect on IBS has been proved.

U. Several studies have shown beneficial effects of psychotherapy, especially in combination with antidepressant medications.

BIBLIOGRAPHY

1. Creed F, Guthrie E: Psychological treatments of the irritable bowel syndrome: a review. *Gut* 30:1601–1609, 1989.

2. Klein KB: Controlled treatment trials in the irritable bowel syndrome: a critique. *Gastroenterology* 95:232–241, 1988.

3. Lucey MR, Clark ML, Lowndes JO, et al: Is bran effacious in irritable bowel syndrome? A double blind placebo controlled crossover study. *Gut* 28:221–225, 1987.

4. Manning AP, Thompson WG, Heaton KW, et al: Toward positive diagnosis of the irritable bowel. *Br Med J* 2:653–654, 1978.

5. Schuster MM: Irritable bowel syndrome. In Sleisenger MH, Fordtran JS (eds): *Gastrointestinal Disease. Pathophysiology, Diagnosis and Management*. Philadelphia: Saunders, 1993, pp 917–933.

6. Talley NJ, Zinsmeister AR, Van Dyke C, et al: Epidemiology of colonic symptoms and the irritable bowel syndrome. *Gastroenterology* 101:927–934, 1991.

7. Thompson WG, Pigeon-Reesor H: The irritable bowel syndrome. *Seminars Gastroint Dis* 1:57–73, 1990.

See also Chapters 16, 17, and 55.

SECTION 4A

Anorectal Pathology
Nonneoplastic

CHAPTER 22

Anal Fissure

Marco Sorgi, M.D. Mitchell Bernstein, M.D. and
Carlos Sardiñas, M.D.

Anal fissure, a common anorectal disorder that may affect individuals of any age group, usually presents with intense pain that is exacerbated by defecation. The fissure can be acute or chronic in nature. Refer to Algorithm 22-1 (see Table 22-1).

A. The symptoms caused by an acute fissure are intense pain with and after bowel movements. The pain is usually accompanied by a small amount of bright red blood per rectum. Patients can often relate a sensation of "tearing" during defecation to the initial onset of symptoms.

B. Patients with a history suggestive of an acute anal fissure can often have the diagnosis confirmed in the office. While these patients have inordinate perianal tenderness, gentle separation of the buttocks can usually be accomplished to allow sufficient visual inspection of the region, revealing the caudad extent of the open fissure. Some patients may be too tender for this maneuver and an examination under anesthesia may be necessary to confirm the diagnosis. Examination should confirm the usual location of the fissure (posterior midline in 99% of males, 90% of females). A sentinel tag and hypertrophied anal papilla may be seen; however, these are more often associated with chronic anal fissures. Fissures in atypical locations require additional investigation and are addressed below.

C. Following confirmation of the diagnosis, a medical regimen of stool softeners, a high-fiber diet, and sitz baths are usually successful in treating the fissure.

D. Once the fissure is healed, patients should be encouraged to remain on a high-fiber diet.

E. If symptoms persist or recur after conservative therapy, definitive surgical treatment is warrented.

F. Alternatively, some patients are unwilling to undergo medical treatment and opt for surgical intervention after the initial diagnosis is made. A third group of patients who may require surgical intervention are those with fistulas in atypical locations. Such fistulas may have an infectious, inflammatory condi-

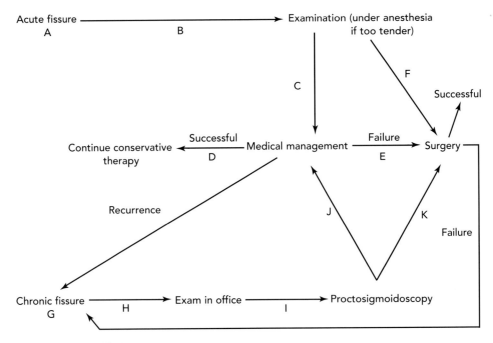

ALGORITHM 22–1

tion of malignant etiology. Bacterial and viral cultures as well as biopsies of the fissure should be performed.

G. Patients with symptoms for more than a few weeks will have a chronic anal fissure. Symptoms of a chronic fissure are slightly different from those of an acute fissure and include pruritis, mucoid or bloody drainage from the wound, and mild pain.

H. The diagnosis of a chronic anal fissure can be made more readily in the office than can the diagnosis of an acute fissure, as pain from the fissure is often mild and does not limit the examination. Visual inspection reveals a well-circumscribed ulcer with indurated edges and a sentinel tag at the fissure's caudad extent. Anoscopy will reveal a hypertrophied anal papilla at the apex of the fissure, and the fibers of the internal anal sphincter should be clearly visible at the fissure's base.

I. Proctosigmoidoscopy should be performed to exclude distal inflammatory bowel disease or concurrent malignancy.

J. Medical regimens of stool softeners, bulking agents, and high-fiber diets may be prescribed for chronic fissures; however, they have not met with the same success as in treating acute anal fissures.

K. The surgical treatment for both acute and chronic anal fissures is a lateral internal sphincterotomy. Sphincterotomy can be performed with the traditional "open" technique (or one of its many modifications) or via the closed lateral subcutaneous sphincterotomy.

TABLE 22-1 ANAL FISSURE/FISSURE-IN-ANO[a]

	Acute					Chronic
	Hours	**Days**	**Weeks**	**Months**	**Year**	**Years**
Symptoms	Acute pain (laceration/acute)	Burning sensation at bowel movement Bleeding [red drops]	Bleeding, contracture, spasm	Bleeding, pressure sensation	Bleeding, pruritus, foreign-body sensation	Spasm and tenesmus, foreign-body sensation
Etiology	Constipation Solid stools or diarrhea Anal trauma (sexual) Iatrogenic	Trauma Sexual Other	Trauma: solid stools Iatrogenic Postpartum Ischemia Herpes	Hypertonic sphincter (i.e., hard and diarrhea) Infectious Radiation therapy	Systemic diseases (i.e., Crohn's)	
Physical Examination	Contracted anus	Difficult anal exploration Intense pain	Fissure, bleeding, pain	Tag or "sentinel tag" chronic fissure	Chronic fissure	Chronic fissure, hypertrophied papilla
Desired exploration	Conversation (talking)	Visualization under anesthesia examination		Digital rectal exam, anoscopy, rigid sigmoidoscopy Laboratory: culture, HIV testing, stools Manometry, colonscopy, biopsy		
Medical treatment	Therapeutics (empirical advice), over-the-counter prescriptions	Analgesics, diet, sitz baths				
Surgical treatment		Fissure bed cleaning, lateral sphincterotomy (partial internal)		Excise hypertrophic papilla + sentinel tag, reconstruction with an anoplasty plus perform a lateral sphincterotomy		

[a] *Definition:* mucosal rupture, longitudinal, from anoderm up to dentate line
Sex and Age: male 60%, female 40%; all ages.
Localization: posterior 75%, anterior 15%, posterior + anterior 8%, lateral 2%.
Time: defined as "Lapse between onset of first symptom and diagnosis"

125

BIBLIOGRAPHY

1. Beck DE, Wexner SD: *Fundamentals of Anorectal Surgery.* New York: McGraw-Hill, 1992.

2. Eiseman B: *Prognosis of Surgical Disease.* Philadelphia: Saunders, 1980.

3. Nicholls J: *Coloproctology.* New York: Springer-Verlag, 1985.

4. Shackelford RT, Zuidema GD: *Surgery of the Alimentary Tract,* 2nd ed. Philadelphia: Saunders, 1991, Vol. 3.

5. Thomson PS, Nicholls RJ, Williams CB: *Colorectal Disease. An Introduction for Surgeons and Physicians.* London: Heinemann Medical Books, 1981.

6. Wexner SD: Pruritis ani and fissure-in-ano. In: Beck DE, Welling DR (eds). *Manual of patient care in colorectal surgery.* Little Brown and Co.: Boston 1991:237–254.

See also Chapters 1, 6, 10, and 13.

CHAPTER 23

Anal Stenosis and Stricture

Mark A. Christensen, M.D. and Richard M. Pitsch, Jr., M.D.

Refer to Algorithm 23–1.

A. The chief complaint is frequently that the anus is "too tight." Associated complaints may also be excessive straining with defecation, pain and associated bleeding or the presence of small caliber stools.

B. Important items in the history are (1) anal operations, especially where tissue was excised or destroyed, such as hemorrhoidectomy, transanal excision of benign or malignant tumors, or coloanal or pouch anal anastomosis; (2) itching, frequently associated with lichen sclerosis; (3) skin diseases, especially involving the perianal and vulvar areas; (4) congenital problems, such as imperforate or ectopic anus; (5) radiation; (6) inflammatory conditions associated with abscesses, fistulas, and strictures such as Crohn's disease; (7) chronic laxative or enema abuse with very thin stools causing the anus to become contracted, and (8) other (noniatrogenic) sources of trauma.

C. Inspection may show the anus to simply be small, and there may be a tag or fissure associated with it. At other times following operations or inflammatory conditions there may be extensive scarring around the anus. Lichen sclerosis presents with thickened skin folds, coarse whitish skin, and often multiple shallow fissures in the anal area. These changes may also be identified on the perineum and the vulva.

D. The digital exam, if possible, calibrates the anal canal and defines the length of the stenosis. It also helps differentiate between tightness in the sphincter muscle and the anoderm. It helps exclude an anal or rectal cancer, other causes of a "stenosis."

E. Anoscopy compliments the digital exam. A small-caliber anoscope and proctoscope are helpful; at times a nasal speculum is necessary. Sometimes the exam must be performed under anesthesia because of pain. Further examinations are indicated if cancer or inflammatory bowel disease are suspected.

F. Anal fissure—see Algorithm 22–1.

G. Lichen sclerosis et atrophicus is of unknown etiology. It is 5 times more common in women; it also affects the vagina, labia, and clitoris. Chronic inflammation leads to sclerosis and narrowing of the anus.

Anal stenosis

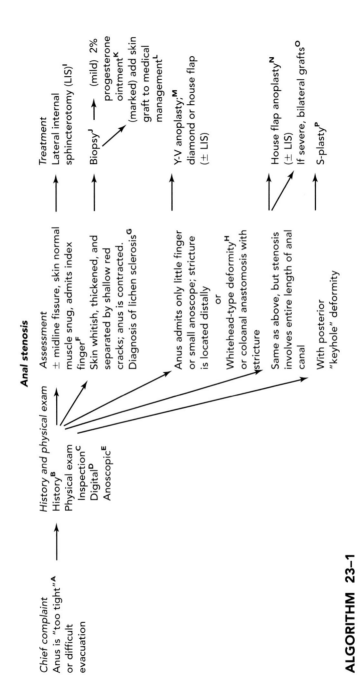

Chief complaint
Anus is "too tight"^A
or difficult
evacuation

→

History and physical exam

History^B
Physical exam
  Inspection^C
  Digital^D
  Anoscopic^E

Assessment

± midline fissure, skin normal muscle snug, admits index finger^F → **Treatment**: Lateral internal sphincterotomy (LIS)^I

Skin whitish, thickened, and separated by shallow red cracks; anus is contracted. Diagnosis of lichen sclerosis^G → Biopsy^J → (mild) 2% progesterone ointment^K / (marked) add skin graft to medical management^L

Anus admits only little finger or small anoscope; stricture is located distally
or
Whitehead-type deformity^H or coloanal anastomosis with stricture → Y-V anoplasty,^M diamond or house flap (± LIS)

Same as above, but stenosis involves entire length of anal canal → House flap anoplasty^N (± LIS) / If severe, bilateral grafts^O

With posterior "keyhole" deformity → S-plasty^P

ALGORITHM 23–1

H. Whitehead hemorrhoidectomy is performed by making an incision at the dentate line and then dissecting the hemorrhoids subdermally and sub-mucosally. Improper technique or poor healing can lead to anal stricture, loss of sensation, or ectropion.

I. Partial lateral internal sphincterotomy (LIS) is the division of the internal sphincter from its outer edge to the dentate line. For details see Algorithm 22–1.

J. Small incisional or punch biopsy confirms the diagnosis. Adequate sampling is needed to exclude dysplasia and malignancy.

K. Lichen sclerosis has no cure; the symptoms may wax and wane. Pruritus can be treated with the usual measures for pruritus ani. The first-line treatment is 2% progesterone cream and hydrophilic ointment 3 times a day for 2 months, then twice weekly. If the patient is poorly responsive to this regimen, then 2% testosterone propionate in stearin lanolin cream may be used. It is applied 3 times a day for 6–8 weeks, then daily for 1 week, and then weekly. However, androgenic side effects can occur, especially if used in the vulvar area as well. Symptomatic relief occurs in 75–90%.

L. If contracted and poorly responsive, skin flap(s) may be required.

M. If an anal stricture is symptomatic, correction can be achieved by performing an anoplasty. This procedure transfers perianal skin into the anal canal. Both the Y-V anoplasty (Fig. 23–1) and diamond flaps (Fig. 23–2) do a satisfactory job of relieving a distal stenosis. Y-V flaps are prone to tip necrosis, a problem relieved by Caplin and Kodner's pedicle flap. Both can be done in more than one area if necessary. LIS is performed if the muscle is tight and appears to contribute to the stenosis.

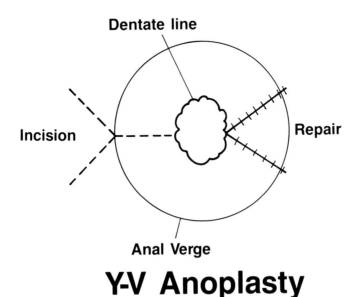

Y-V Anoplasty

FIGURE 23–1 V-Y anoplasty (left—incision, right—repair).

N. The house advancement pedicle flap provides a broad flap of skin for the entire length of the anal canal (Fig. 23–3). Blood supply is always adequate, and there are no small tips prone to necrosis. Extensive rotational flaps have been described. These require more tissue mobilization and have a more tenuous blood supply. These are infrequently used today.

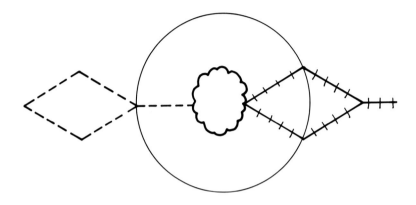

Diamond Flap

FIGURE 23–2 Diamond flap anoplasty (left—incision, right—repair).

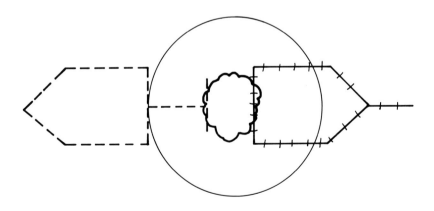

House Flap

FIGURE 23–3 House flap anoplasty (left—incision, right—repair).

O. If, after the first graft, the anus is still smaller than desired, a flap on the opposite side can be created. For conditions like Bowen's disease three or four flaps have been used to reline the anal canal.

P. Associated keyhole deformity is well suited to a unilateral or bilateral S-flap anoplasty (Figs. 23–4 and 23–5).

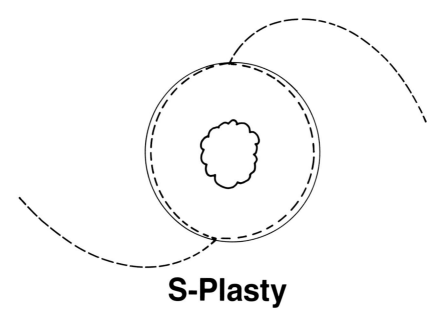

S-Plasty

FIGURE 23–4 S-plasty incision.

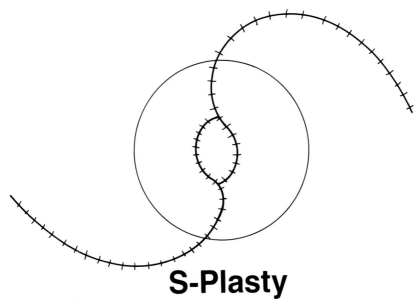

S-Plasty

FIGURE 23–5 S-plasty repair.

BIBLIOGRAPHY

1. Caplin DA, Kodner IJ: Repair of anal stricture and mucosal ectropion by simple flap procedures. *Dis Colon Rectum* 29:92–94, 1986.

2. Christensen MA, Pitsch RM, Cali RL, et al: "House" advancement pedicle flap for anal stenosis. *Dis Colon Rectum* 35:201–203, 1992.

3. Ferguson JA: Repair of "Whitehead" deformity of the anus. *Surg Gynecol Obstet* 108:115–116, 1959.

See also Chapters 6, 18, 20, and 22.

CHAPTER 24

Anorectal Abscess

Steven J. Stryker, M.D.

Refer to Algorithm 24–1.

A. In addition to localized pain and swelling, abscess in the anorectal region may be associated with other local signs and symptoms such as constipation (due to sphincter spasm) and/or purulent discharge (when spontaneous drainage has occurred).

B. Systemic signs and symptoms of fever, chills, and leukocytosis warrant urgent surgical decompression.

C. Abscess is more common in diabetics and immunocompromised patients than in the general population. In these two aforementioned groups, as well as those with valvular heart disease or prosthetic implants, broad-spectrum antibiotics are recommended as an adjunct to surgical drainage.

D. Inspect the perianal area for erythema, induration, or purulent discharge. Determine the anatomic relationship of the process to the anal verge.

E. Superficial and bidigital palpation for induration, localized tenderness, and fluctuance usually reveals the location and extent of abscess.

F. Anoscopy may display pus arising from an anal crypt or the base of a chronic fissure. Proctoscopy may show unsuspected inflammatory bowel disease or tumor. If pain precludes endoscopy at presentation, it can usually be accomplished 1–2 weeks after initial treatment.

G. While radiologic imaging rarely alters treatment of anorectal suppurative conditions, computerized tomography (CT) scan can be extremely helpful if an abscess is suspected but the location and extent remain unclear after physical examination. Similarly, intraanal endosonography can often reveal occult perianal abscesses.

H. A superficial process adjacent to the anal verge, perianal abscess usually arises from an infected anal crypt.

I. Often large, the ischiorectal abscess arises in the ischiorectal space, presenting on the buttock rather than at the anal verge.

J. Occurring in the intersphincteric plane, the intersphincteric abscess arises in the midanal canal and extends proximally. Cutaneous signs of inflammation are often lacking.

Presenting signs and symptoms

Pain

Swelling

Other local signs[A]

Other systemic symptoms[B]

History of associated medical conditions[C]

Evaluation

Inspection[D]

Palpation[E]

Endoscopy[F]

Location and extent unclear

Radiology[G]

Diagnosis

Perianal abscess[H]

Ischiorectal abscess[I]

Intersphincteric abscess[J]

Supralevator abscess[K]

Crohn's associated abscess[L]

Horseshoe abscess[M]

Treatment[N]

Incision and drainage[O]

Incision and drainage[P]

Internal sphincterotomy and drainage[Q]

Internal vs. external vs. percutaneous drainage[R]

Drainage, indwelling catheter or seton, metronidazole[S]

Drainage, counterincisions, bridging drains[T]

Follow-up[U]

Healed at 6 weeks

Persistent discharge[V]

Recurrent abscess[W]

Drain

Evaluate for fistula

ALGORITHM 24–1

K. Relatively rare, a supralevator abscess often presents as occult sepsis. One must look for a pelvic source such as diverticulitis, salpingitis, or Crohn's disease.

L. In patients with multiple or recurrent abscess formation, investigations should be undertaken to exclude Crohn's disease. In patients with established Crohn's disease, optimizing management of the proximal intestinal disease will facilitate healing of the anorectal component.

M. Horseshoe abscess typically refers to bilateral extension into both ischiorectal fossae from a common posterior midline source. Less often, the bilateral extension will be confined to the intersphincteric or supralevator space.

N. The mainstay of treatment for abscess of the anorectal region is prompt and thorough drainage. Anal fistula may be present in 50--70% of patients with abscess. Surgical opinions vary as to the advisability of primary fistulotomy at the time of abscess drainage.

O. Incision and drainage of perianal abscess usually requires only local anesthesia, excision of skin edges facilitates complete drainage and minimizes recurrence.

P. Incision and drainage of ischiorectal abscess more frequently requires regional or general anesthesia, especially for larger abscess or indeterminate extent. The drainage site should be chosen as close to the anal verge as possible to simplify subsequent fistulotomy, should that be required.

Q. Regional or general anesthesia is often required to confirm diagnosis of this extremely painful condition. Intersphincteric abscess is unroofed through the internal sphincter from the anal verge up toward the proximal extent of cavity.

R. If the supralevator abscess is arising from an ischiorectal source, drain externally via ischiorectal fossa. Conversely, if the abscess arises from an intersphincteric source, it should be drained transrectally. Finally, if an underlying pelvic process is responsible for the abscess, percutaneous radiologic drainage can be accomplished with subsequent definitive management of the primary disease.

S. Abscesses associated with anorectal Crohn's disease are often of long-standing duration and, therefore, typically are indurated and fibrotic. Prolonged drainage and symptomatic relief may require placement of an indwelling mushroom catheter or seton. In addition, oral metronidazole is a useful adjunct to lessen discomfort and drainage.

T. A horseshoe abscess usually involves the deep posterior space and requires primary drainage. In addition, anterolateral extensions can be effectively drained by bilateral counterincisions.

U. After surgical drainage of an abscess, the patient should be reexamined until the wound has completely healed and all induration has resolved. If not previously performed, proctosigmoidoscopy is accomplished once the pain has subsided.

V. If drainage persists from the site of original drainage for 6 weeks or more, the likelihood of associated fistula is high.

W. Early recurrence of an abscess may be due to premature healing of the skin edges, unrecognized adjacent areas of abscess, or underlying anal fistula.

BIBLIOGRAPHY

1. Beck DE, Wexner SD (eds): *Fundamentals of anorectal surgery.* New York: McGraw Hill, 1992.
2. Corman ML: *Colon and Rectal Surgery,* 3rd ed. Philadelphia: Lippincott, 1993, pp 133–140.
3. Gordon PH, Nivatvongs S: *Principles and Practice of Surgery for the Colon, Rectum, and Anus.* St. Louis: Quality Medical Publishing, pp 222–234.
4. Wexner SD: Anorectal disease. In: Phillips S, Fazio VW (eds): *Current opinion in gastroenterology,* 1992; 8:70–77.
5. Yang YK, Wexner SD, Nogueras JJ, et al: The role of anal ultrasound in the assessment of benign anorectal diseases. *Coloproctology* 15:260–264, 1993.

See also Chapters 6, 8, 25, and 26.

CHAPTER 25

Fistula-in-Ano

Carol-Ann Vasilevsky, M.D. and Barry L. Stein, M.D.

Refer to Algorithm 25-1.

A. An anal fistula is an abnormal tract communicating with the rectum or anal canal by an identifiable internal opening that results from a preexisting abscess.

B. There may be a history of a surgically or spontaneously drained abscess. Usual complaints include discharge, bleeding, or pain. On physical examination, a secondary opening may be seen and a tract palpated. According to Goodsall's rule, an opening seen posterior to a line drawn transversely across the perineum will originate from an internal opening in the posterior midline of the anal canal. An anterior external opening will originate in a radial fashion from the nearest crypt. The greater the distance from the anal margin, the greater the probability of a complicated fistula.

C. Anoscopy should be done to try to visualize a primary opening in the dentate line, although this opening may not be apparent until the patient is under anesthesia.

D. Sigmoidoscopy should be done to exclude underlying proctitis. Barium enema or colonoscopy and small bowel enema are indicated in patients with inflammatory bowel disease and recurrent multiple fistulas.

E. Manometry is generally not necessary but may be useful in the elderly, or in patients with perianal Crohn's disease or recurrent fistulas because of possible sphincter compromise in these groups.

F. Anal endosonography may be of help with complex fistulas. Hydrogen peroxide injection for fistula tract enhancement is often helpful.

G. Fistulography is generally unreliable but may be helpful in patients with recurrent fistulas or complex fistulas of Crohn's disease.

H. See Figure 25-1 for a classification of fistula-in-ano.

I. An intersphincteric fistula passes in the intersphincteric plane and accounts for about 70% of fistulas.

J. Transsphincteric fistulas account for 23% of fistulas. The tract passes through the internal and external sphincters to the ischiorectal fossa. A high-blind tract

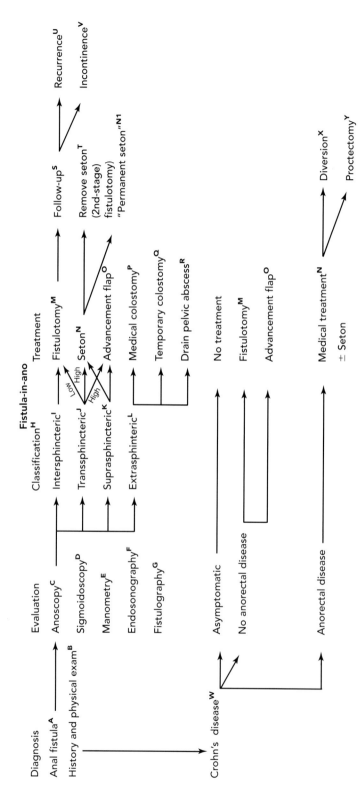

ALGORITHM 25-1

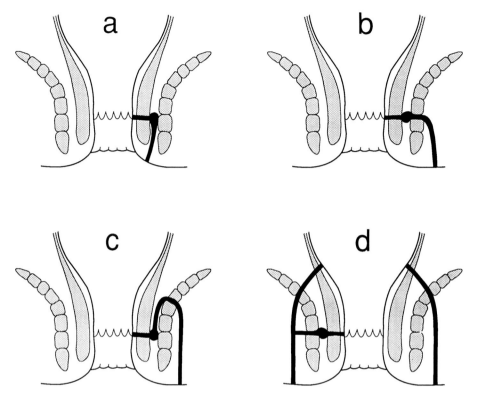

FIGURE 25-1 Classification of fistula in ano: (A) intersphincteric; (B) trans-sphincteric; (C) suprasphincteric; (D) extrasphincteric.

may pass into the levators and even into the pelvis. A rectovaginal fistula is an example of a low transsphincteric fistula.

K. Supralevator fistulas account for 5% of fistulas. The tract passes from the dentate line above the puborectalis, then caudal laterally to the external sphincter in the ischiorectal fossa and to the perianal skin.

L. Extrasphincteric fistulas are the rarest type, accounting for 2% of fistulas. The tract passes from the rectum above the levators to the perianal skin via the ischiorectal fossa. It is important to determine the etiology, which is most commonly due to vigorous probing during abscess or fistula surgery, foreign-body penetration, Crohn's disease, carcinoma, or radiotherapy.

M. Fistulotomy or lay-open technique is preferred to fistulectomy since a smaller wound is created and sphincter injury is minimized. Principles are to eradicate the fistula, prevent recurrence, and preserve continence. The key to successful outcome is identification of the primary opening, which may be accomplished by passage of a probe from the external to internal opening or vice versa, injection of milk or hydrogen peroxide into the external opening, following the granulation tissue or demonstration of puckering at the primary opening. An anterior fistula in a female is best treated with an advancement flap. If multiple fistulas are present, as in Crohn's disease, consideration should be given to seton placement to preserve sphincter function.

N. If the tract crosses the sphincter at a high level, a seton is inserted. A seton may be a nonabsorbable heavy suture or silastic catheter. Its function is to stimulate fibrosis and transect the fistula tract in a slow controlled manner, act as a drain, or delineate the relation of the tract to the sphincter muscles, especially the puborectalis muscle. Its use should be considered in high fistulas, anterior fistulas in women, in the elderly, and in the patient with complex perianal Crohn's, previous fistula surgery, or complex fistulas.

N1. A noncutting seton (such as a vessel loop or silastic) may be used in patients with either Crohn's disease or AIDS. In these latter groups, the seton is generally left in place indefinitely. In these cases wherein incontinence is likely after sphincter division, the purpose of the seton is to provide continuous drainage and prevent abscess reformation.

O. The lay-open technique is inadvisable for anterior fistulas in women or in patients with inflammatory bowel disease with high transsphincteric and suprasphincteric fistulas. An advancement flap of rectal mucosa, submucosa, and partial thickness of the internal sphincter is preferred. Advantages are that no sphincter muscle is divided and the patient experiences less pain.

P. If the extrasphincteric fistula is secondary to iatrogenic probing, the lower part of the internal sphincter is divided and the rectal opening is closed with a nonabsorbable suture. A medical colostomy (mechanical bowel preparation followed by enteral feeding and antidiarrheal agents) will obviate the need for a temporary colostomy.

Q. If the extrasphincteric fistula is due to the presence of a foreign body, the foreign body should be removed, drainage established, and a temporary colostomy constructed.

R. An extrasphincteric fistula may arise from caudad tracking of a pelvic abscess. Drainage of this abscess will allow the fistula to heal.

S. Patients should be seen in frequent follow-up to ensure that the tract heals from the base upward and that no skin bridging has occurred.

T. For complex fistulas, the seton may be removed or the seton-contained muscle may be divided.

U. Recurrence rates range from 0 to 26.5%. The most common cause is failure to identify the primary opening. Other reasons include an unrecognized extension, Crohn's disease, or hidradenitis suppurativa.

V. Incontinence rates range from 0 to 40%. Incontinence may be due to over-zealous division of the sphincter muscle, especially in a patient with Crohn's disease or an elderly patient or may be due to prolonged packing.

W. The presence of Crohn's disease does not obviate the treatment of a fistula. Generally, in the absence of anorectal involvement, fistulas may be treated similarly to cryptoglandular fistulas. The best results have been reported in the absence of anorectal disease.

X. Diversion may be helpful in patients with severe perianal disease with multiple fistulas and sepsis. Diversion may allow resolution of the perineal sepsis or, alternatively, may prepare for eventual proctectomy.

Y. After numerous attempts and unsuccessful medical therapy, intersphincteric proctectomy is indicated.

BIBLIOGRAPHY

1. Cheong DMO, Nogreras JJ, Wexner SD, et al: Anal endosonography for recurrent anal fistulas: Image enhancement with hydrogen peroxide. *Dis Colon Rectum* 536:1158–1160, 1993.
2. Gordon PH: Anorectal abscess and fistula in ano. In Gordon PH, Nivatvongs S (eds): *Principles and Practice of Surgery for the Colon, Rectum and Anus.* St. Louis: Quality Medical Publishers, 1992.
3. Parks AG: Pathogenesis and treatment of fistula in ano. *Br Med J* 1:463–469, 1961.
4. Parks AG, Gordon PH, Hardcastle JD: A classification of fistula-in-ano. *Br J Surg* 63:1–12, 1976.
5. Vasilevsky CA: Fistula in ano and abscess. In Beck DE, Wexner SD (eds): *Fundamentals of Anorectal Surgery.* New York: McGraw-Hill, 1992.

See also Chapters 25, 27, 38, and 51.

CHAPTER 26

Recurrent Fistula-in-Ano

Lester Rosen, M.D.

Refer to Algorithm 26–1.

A. *Inspection* of the perianal region is carried out to demonstrate a secondary opening discharging pus or pouting granulation tissue (transsphincteric fistulas usually have a more laterally placed secondary opening). *Hidradenitis suppurativa* should be considered in the differential diagnosis of recurrent fistula. *Palpation* may disclose a previously overlooked postanal or ischioanal fullness, or a secondary tract or extension that is now the seat of an abscess. Assessment should include anal sphincter tone, presence of unhealed wounds, or significant hemorrhoidal disease.

B. *Anoscopy* is performed to identify a primary opening that is discharging pus or is visibly puckered. *Sigmoidoscopy* may reveal a high rectal opening or the presence of inflammatory bowel disease.

C. The prior *operative report* is reviewed noting the time interval until recurrence, the original description of the abscess–fistula with the presence or absence of a primary opening or secondary tract, and the attempted mode of treatment. The *pathology report* is reviewed to exclude granulomas or other indicators of inflammatory bowel disease that may be supported by previously undisclosed bowel habits.

D. If occult *Crohn's disease* is suspected, lower and upper gastrointestinal (GI) evaluation is indicated when clinically feasible. Negative studies do not reliably exclude the presence of isolated anal Crohn's disease. Anal fistula secondary to other systemic illnesses (e.g., tuberculosis or immunosuppressed states) should be considered. If Crohn's disease is suspected, insertion of a *seton* may be the best option, at least until the proximally active intestinal Crohn's disease is controlled medically or surgically. Metronidazole may be useful for control of anal symptoms, but the side effects of bitter taste, Antabuse (disulfuram) reaction, and possibility of paresthesia should be discussed. Fistulotomy in selected cases is possible but treatment must be individualized.

E. Reoperation is essential for those cases where the primary diagnosis was *correct* but the primary opening was missed, or the wound prematurely closed

Recurrent fistula-in-ano

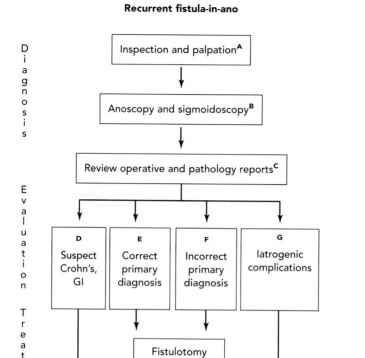

D
i
a
g
n
o
s
i
s

E
v
a
l
u
a
t
i
o
n

T
r
e
a
t
m
e
n
t

ALGORITHM 26–1

GI = gastrointestinal

(bridging or pocketing). Simple unroofing of the entire fistulous track with or without a "backcut" to promote drainage usually suffices.

F. Reoperation is necessary when the previous diagnosis was *incorrect* and an occult horseshoe fistula or secondary tract was overlooked. The etiology of these fistulas must be reclassified in the medical record. The surgeon should be familiar with the anatomic variations of intersphincteric, transsphincteric, extrasphincteric, and suprasphincteric fistulas with awareness that a concomitant extension may have been present (e.g., if a high-blind tract of an intersphincteric fistula is missed, recurrence is expected).

G. Previously created *iatrogenic fistulas* are the most difficult to diagnose and treat. Examples are (1) an original intersphincteric abscess–fistula with an extrarectal extension that was not properly drained into the rectum but was drained through the ischioanal fossa producing a suprasphincteric fistula; or (2) overzealous probing of a high-blind track transsphincteric fistula, creating an extrasphincteric fistula. The former fistula usually requires staged seton fistulotomy, while the latter may require division of the lower half of the internal sphincter, closure of the rectum, and medical or surgical colostomy.

BIBLIOGRAPHY

1. Corman ML: *Colon and Rectal Surgery,* 2nd ed. Philadephia: Lippincott, 1989.
2. Gordon PH, Nivatvongs S: *Principles and Practice of Surgery for the Colon, Rectum, and Anus.* St. Louis: Quality Medical Publishing, 1992.
3. Pearl RK, Andrews JR, Orsay CP, et al: Role of the seton in the management of anorectal fistulas. *Dis Colon Rectum* 36:573–579, 1993.
4. Ustynoski K, Rosen L, Stasik J, et al: Horseshoe abscess fistula: seton treatment. *Dis Colon Rectum* 33:602–605, 1990.

See also Chapters 25, 27 and 51.

CHAPTER 27

Rectovaginal Fistulas

Ann C. Lowry, M.D.

Refer to Algorithm 27–1.

A. Patients with a rectovaginal fistula, a communication between the rectum and the vagina, present with passage of flatus and/or stool through the vagina.

B. The pertinent history and physical includes an obstetrical history, operative history, gastrointestinal symptoms, and history of radiation, neoplasm and inflammatory bowel disease. Low fistulas are generally readily identified during physical exam as a pit in the anterior midline. Higher fistulas may require radiologic evaluation with contrast studies for identification. The rectal mucosa and sphincter muscle should be assessed with digital exam and sigmoidoscopy.

C. From the history and physical exam, the location, size, and etiology of the fistula can usually be ascertained. These facts allow rectovaginal fistulas to be classified into simple or complex. Simple fistulas are low in the rectovaginal septum, are either <2.5 cm in diameter, and result from trauma or infection. The complex fistulas are high in the rectovaginal septum, >2.5 cm in size, and are caused by inflammatory bowel disease, radiation or a neoplasm.

D. Most simple fistulas result from a 4th-degree tear during delivery. The patient's intestinal function and the surrounding tissue are usually normal.

E. Because of the mechanism of injury, it is important to evaluate the patient's sphincter muscle before repair. Identifying an anterior sphincter defect is important for two reasons. The symptoms of a rectovaginal fistula may mask true fecal incontinence that may manifest once the fistula is repaired. In one series, 25% of patients not noted to have true incontinence, were incontinent after a successful endorectal flap repair. Also, the sphincter muscle is the most vascular tissue between the rectum and the vagina. If a sphincter defect coexists anteriorly, then the success of local repair is diminished. At a minimum, every patient should be carefully questioned about symptoms of incontinence and then have sphincter assessment by digital exam. Anal manometry and anal ultrasound are the most specific evaluations of the functional and physical status of the sphincter muscle.

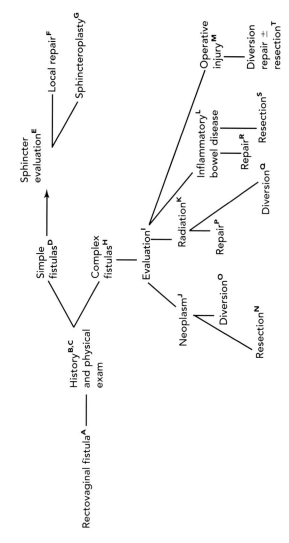

ALGORITHM 27–1

Rectovaginal fistula[A] —— History[B,C] and physical exam

Simple fistulas[D] —— Sphincter evaluation[E] — Local repair[F], Sphincteroplasty[G]

Complex fistulas[H] —— Evaluation[I]

Neoplasm[J] — Diversion[O], Resection[N]

Radiation[K] — Repair[P], Diversion[Q]

Inflammatory bowel disease[L] — Repair[R], Resection[S]

Operative injury[M] — Diversion repair ± resection[T]

F. If the patient is continent and the sphincter muscle is intact, a local repair is used. Endorectal advancement flap involves raising a rectal flap of mucosa, submucosa and circular muscle, approximating the internal sphincter over the fistula site and covering the closure with the flap. Success has been reported in 78 to 100% of patients. Alternatively, a vaginal repair may be utilized. Converting the fistula to a fourth degree tear followed by layered closure is to be discouraged because of unnecessary risk of incontinence.

G. Overlapping sphincteroplasty addresses the sphincter defect and corrects rectovaginal fistula in 95% of patients.

H. Complex fistulas fortunately are uncommon. The etiology of the fistula, the patient's medical condition, and the extent of patient's symptoms are the main determinants of treatment.

I. Complex fistulas require more extensive evaluation because of the higher likelihood of underlying intestinal disease, regional tissue destruction and significant medical illness in those patients. General medical evaluation, endoscopic or radiologic intestinal evaluation, and biopsy of the fistula site may all be necessary.

J. Rectal carcinomas, uterine, vaginal, and cervical carcinomas may all cause rectovaginal fistulas. Frequently, it is recurrent rather than primary disease.

K. Radiation, most frequently for gynecologic malignancies, can lead to rectovaginal fistulas in 0.3–6% of patients. Most fistulas develop 6–24 months after treatment.

L. Patients with Crohn's disease are more likely to develop rectovaginal fistulas than ones with ulcerative colitis. The presence of proctitis or other perianal disease strongly influences treatment decisions. Medical management rarely results in closure.

M. High rectovaginal fistulas may result from pelvic surgery. Hysterectomy for endometriosis is the operation most frequently complicated by rectovaginal fistula. Low anterior resection may also lead to rectovaginal fistulas when an anastomotic leak occurs or the vaginal wall is caught in the stapler.

N. Resection appropriate for the underlying neoplasm is the usual treatment.

O. Diversion is appropriate for high-output fistulas in the presence of extensive pelvis spread.

P. Repair of radiation-induced rectovaginal fistulas is reserved for otherwise healthy, highly symptomatic patients with adequate sphincter function and no evidence of recurrent neoplasm. Biopsy of the area is particularly important in these patients as one-third of fistulas will be a manifestation of recurrent disease. Temporary diversion is generally required. Repair may be done with muscle grafts, such as the bulbocavernous muscle, for low, small fistulas. For others, resection with coloanal anastomosis is appropriate. An alternative is the Bricker onlay patch anastomosis using nonradiated colon as the graft. All choices are reasonably successful in carefully selected patients.

Q. Diversion is the most appropriate treatment for symptomatic, medically frail patients.

R. If the rectal mucosa is normal, local repair of rectovaginal fistulas is possible. Endorectal advancement flap and vaginal flap repairs are the most frequently reported approaches.

S. In patients with proctitis, proctectomy is often required. Rectovaginal fistulas in patients with mucosal ulcerative colitis who require proctocolectomy do not preclude successful ileoanal reservoir construction. The presence of the fistula, however, must raise suspicion that the diagnosis is actually Crohn's disease.

T. Resection with reanastomosis is frequently necessary for high rectovaginal fistulas following pelvic surgery. In some cases, temporary diversion or omental graft interposition results in closure.

BIBLIOGRAPHY

1. Beck DE, Wexner SD (eds): *Fundamentals in Anorectal Surgery.* New York: McGraw-Hill, 1992.
2. Cameron JL (ed): *Current Surgical Therapy,* 3rd ed. Philadelphia: Decker, 1989.
3. Goldberg SM, Gordon PH, Nivatvongs S (eds): *Essentials of Anorectal Surgery.* Philadelphia: Lippincott, 1980.

See also Chapters 25 and 26.

CHAPTER 28

Internal Hemorrhoids

Scott Strong, M.D.

Refer to Algorithm 28–1.

A. Internal hemorrhoids are naturally occurring vascular cushions of the anal canal that typically arise cephalad to the dentate line and contribute to fecal continence. Since hemorrhoids are a normal anatomic finding, their presence does not imply hemorrhoidal disease. Instead, hemorroidal disease is defined as significant symptoms (such as bleeding or prolapse) attributable to hemorrhoid tissue. Symptomatic internal hemorrhoids are classified according to the degree of associated prolapse as follows: first-degree hemorrhoids bulge into the anal canal and bleed with defecation; second-degree hemorrhoids prolapse during defecation and spontaneously reduce when straining ceases; third-degree hemorrhoids prolapse during defecation and require intermittent or persistent manual reduction; fourth-degree hemorrhoids prolapse and cannot be manually reduced.

B. The treatment of problematic internal hemorrhoids depends on the type and degree of associated symptoms. As multiple systemic diseases and local conditions can cause the symptoms of hemorrhoid disease, a thorough patient evaluation is warranted. The patient should be questioned about dietary and bowel habits, bleeding dyscrasias, inflammatory bowel disease, portal hypertension, and immunosuppressive disorders. A regional examination should include anoscopy and rigid or flexible proctosigmoidoscopy with further evaluation dictated by the patient's history and physical findings. If bleeding is present, complete colonic evaluation is recommended for individuals over 40 years of age with a recognized risk for colorectal neoplasia and for all patients 50 years and older.

C. All degrees of internal hemorrhoids may respond to medical treatment. Medical therapy consisting of a high fiber diet, stool modifiers such as psyllium or methylcellulose, warm sitz baths, topical creams, and avoidance of straining will lessen the symptoms in 80–90% of hemorrhoid sufferers.

First- and second-degree hemorrhoids can be treated by medical treatment alone or in combination with various alternative modalities including rubber-band ligation, injection sclerotherapy, infrared coagulation, bipolar diathermy

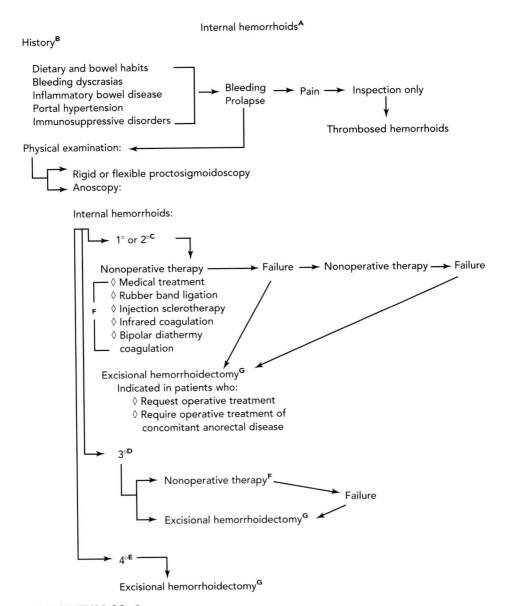

ALGORITHM 28–1

coagulation, and cryotherapy. Should this initial treatment fail to eradicate symptoms, the modality may be repeated or another method can be tried. Excisional hemorrhoidectomy is reserved for patients who have associated external skin tags, patients who fail initial or secondary therapy, and patients who have hemorrhoidal disease and concomitant benign anorectal disease that requires operative treatment such as fistula, fissure, or hypertrophied anal papillae.

D. Third-degree hemorrhoids can be treated by single or combination therapy that includes medical treatment, alternative modalities, and excisional hemorrhoidectomy. If an initial nonoperative treatment fails to eliminate symptoms, excisional hemorrhoidectomy is generally recommended.

E. Fourth-degree hemorrhoids rarely respond to medical therapy, and excisional hemorrhoidectomy is usually indicated.

F. Rubber-band ligation and injection sclerotherapy are the most popular non-surgical techniques. Rubber-band ligation works best for first-, second-, and minor third-degree hemorrhoids with overall patient satisfaction reportedly high (80–91%). Two bands are placed on each of the symptomatic hemorrhoid pedicles in single or multiple sessions scheduled 4 weeks apart. The complication rate is comparable for single and multiple ligations performed with each banding session. Injection sclerotherapy with quinine and urea, tetradecyl sodium, 5% phenol in vegetable oil, carbolic acid, or sodium morrhuate is effective for the treatment of first- and second-degree hemorrhoids with fewer than half of patients with third-degree hemorrhoids significantly improved. Usually, a minimum of 1–2 mL of sclerosant is injected into each symptomatic quadrant with subsequent injections, if necessary, performed at 4-week intervals. The other alternative therapies are used less frequently. Infrared coagulation may not be as efficacious as the previously discussed modalities with repetitive treatments necessary for many first- and second-degree hemorrhoids. If infrared coagulation is to be used for hemorrhoids that are refractory to an initial alternative therapy, local anesthetic may be necessary to lessen the often associated discomfort. Bipolar diathermy coagulation successfully treats 95% of patients with first- or second-degree hemorrhoids. However, nearly 50% of patients experience moderate pain with this modality, and over 30% of individuals require multiple treatments.

G. While excisional hemorrhoidectomy is necessary in only 5–10% of all patients with symptomatic hemorrhoid disease, it is the procedure usually recommended in patients with third- and fourth-degree hemorrhoids. Multiple techniques of excisional hemorrhoidectomy have been described, including open, submucosal, radical, and closed hemorrhoidectomy. Open hemorrhoidectomy is the most widely practiced excisional technique throughout the world; closed hemorrhoidectomy, however, provides a similar outcome with less healing time as the wounds heal by primary, rather than secondary, intention.

BIBLIOGRAPHY

1. ASCRS Standards Task Force: Practice parameters for the treatment of hemorrhoids. *Dis Colon Rectum.* 36:1118–1120, 1993.

2. Mazier WP, Wolkomir AF: Hemorrhoids. *Seminars Colon Rectal Surg.* 1:197–206, 1990.

3. Milsom J: Hemorrhoidal disease. In Beck DE, Wexner SD (eds): *Fundamentals of Anorectal Disease,* New York: McGraw-Hill, 1992, pp 192–214.

See also Chapters 6, 8, 10, 13 and 29.

CHAPTER 29

External Hemorrhoids

Walter R. Peters, M.D.

Refer to Algorithm 29-1.

A. Patients frequently present to the physician with a self-diagnosis of "hemorrhoids." Myriad symptoms are attributed to hemorrhoidal disease, including symptoms of perirectal abscess, fistula, fissure, pilonidal cyst, anal or rectal neoplasm, or inflammatory bowel disease. Therefore, a careful history and physical examination must be done before embarking on treatment of external hemorrhoids. At the very least, an anoscopic exam should be done unless the patient is in such acute pain that this evaluation cannot be accomplished. Further evaluation including a proctosigmoidoscopy, flexible sigmoidoscopy, or colonoscopy may be indicated depending on the nature of the patient's complaints, family history, or physical findings. If other anorectal pathology is found, the associated lesion may well dictate the course of therapy rather than the external hemorrhoids.

B. External hemorrhoids are defined as the dilated inferior hemorrhoidal plexus that are found distal to the dentate line and are therefore covered with a modified squamous epithelium.

C. Simple skin tags are discrete folds of skin arising around the anal verge. These tags usually are the result of a previous thrombosed hemorrhoid. They may also be a finding of inflammatory bowel disease. A solitary skin tag may serve as a sentinel tag in the presence of an anal fissure. Most skin tags are relatively asymptomatic, and the patient requires nothing more than reassurance. Rarely the skin tags are so extensive as to interfere with hygiene. Occasionally, patients will become absolutely obsessed with the abnormality. In either event, simple excision with local anesthesia as an outpatient will provide symptomatic relief.

D. Nonthrombosed external hemorrhoids are usually asymptomatic. Patients may note some degree of swelling in the area as a result of straining. Symptoms, however, are seldom sufficiently severe to prompt the patient to seek care until a thrombosis occurs. Occasionally, patients with large external hemorrhoids and a history of multiple prior thromboses will require excisional hemorrhoidectomy to prevent further episodes of thrombosis.

155

External hemorrhoids

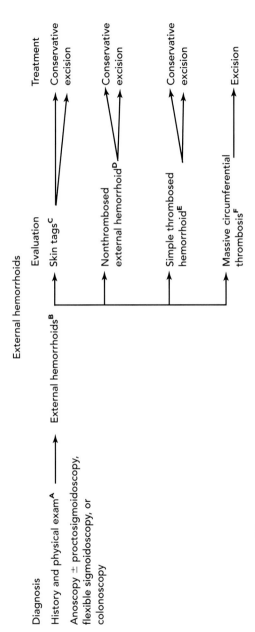

Diagnosis

History and physical exam^A →

Anoscopy ± proctosigmoidoscopy,
flexible sigmoidoscopy, or
colonoscopy

External hemorrhoids^B

Evaluation

Skin tags^C

Nonthrombosed
external hemorrhoid^D

Simple thrombosed
hemorrhoid^E

Massive circumferential
thrombosis^F

Treatment

Conservative
excision

Conservative
excision

Conservative
excision

Excision

ALGORITHM 29–1

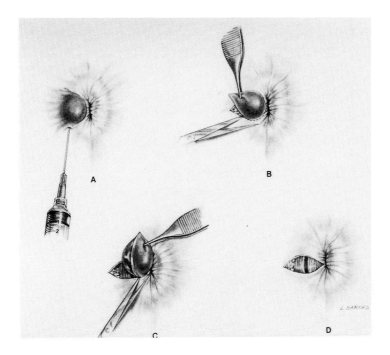

FIGURE 29–1 A: Local anesthetic is injected around, not into, the thrombosed external hemorrhoid. B: The thrombosis is excised, preserving adjacent normal skin. C: Care should be taken to excise the septations and all adjacent small clots. D: After meticulous hemostasis has been secured, the wound can be left open or sutured closed.

E. A single thrombosed hemorrhoid has a distinctive appearance, consisting of a firm nodule within the anal canal or at the anal verge that is usually quite tender. The degree of pain is not necessarily related to the size of the thrombosis, but rather to its position. Even a small thrombosed hemorrhoid can be exquisitely painful if located within the anal canal, whereas a larger thrombosed hemorrhoid on the anal verge may be relatively asymptomatic. The decision to treat the thrombosis conservatively or surgically depends on the severity of the symptoms and the duration of symptoms. If the patient presents within the first 48–72 hours of symptoms, and is very uncomfortable, excision of the lesion often speeds recovery. Excision is recommended because of the high incidence of rethrombosis associated with enucleation alone. (Fig. 29–1) However, once symptoms begin to subside, excision offers little benefit over conservative management with reassurance, analgesics, sitz baths, and stool softeners. Occasionally the thrombosis will cause ulceration of the overlying skin that may lead the patient to present days later with ongoing bleeding. At this time excision of the thrombosis will lead to cessation of the bleeding. If the pain from the thrombosed hemorrhoid is so great that adequate evaluation (as described above) cannot be completed, it is important to have the patient return 6–8 weeks later to complete the evaluation to assure the absence of other anorectal pathology.

F. Massive circumferential thrombosis can be treated conservatively, but the length of disability and the discomfort involved recommends surgical therapy for virtually all patients with this condition. This is often associated with extensive internal hemorrhoids that may also be prolapsed or thrombosed. This condition cannot be adequately dealt with on an outpatient basis. Excisional hemorrhoidectomy with postoperative in-hospital observation is indicated. The surgery is technically more demanding than for an elective hemorrhoidectomy, but can be accomplished with acceptable morbidity. Intraoperative injection of hyaluronidase may be helpful in reduction of swelling.

BIBLIOGRAPHY

1. American Society of Colon and Rectal Surgeons, Standards Task Force: Practice parameters for the treatment of hemorrhoids. *Dis Colon Rectum* 34:992, 1991.

2. Corman ML: *Colon and Rectal Surgery.* Philadelphia: Lippincott, 1993.

3. Goldberg SM, Gordon PH, Nivatvongs S: *Essentials of Anorectal Surgery.* Philadelphia: Lippincott, 1980.

See also Chapters 6, 8 and 28.

CHAPTER 30

Pilonidal Disease

Elliot Prager, M.D. and Sanjiv Bais, M.D.

Refer to Algorithm 30-1.

A. Pilonidal disease (derived from "pilus" meaning hair and "nidus" meaning nest) of the sacrococcygeal area afflicts young adults after puberty and is rare after the age of 40. Other diseases to be excluded are perianal abscess--fistula or hidradenitis suppurativa. The prevalence of this disease in adolescence and in males suggests a hormonal relationship. Increased sweating, buttock friction, and a deep natal cleft can also predispose to pilonidal disease. The incidence of pilonidal disease is higher in whites than in blacks or Asians, suggesting that hair characteristics and growth patterns may also be contributing factors.

B. Pilonidal abscess usually presents with several days' history of pain and swelling in one of the buttocks adjacent to the midline. This exquisitely tender area can be immediately managed with outpatient incision and drainage.

C. Under local anesthesia, a 1-cm cruciate incision is made as close as feasible to the midline and the skin flaps are excised; no drains or packing are indicated, and antibiotics are rarely needed. Patients should note significant improvement almost immediately. About 40% of patients will become asymptomatic, but the remainder will have persistent pilonidal disease.

D. Bascom recommends incision and drainage (I&D) followed by excision of the epithelialized pilonidal pit through a small incision 5 days later when the edema has subsided. According to Bascom this procedure is associated with a recurrence rate of 15% as compared to 60% with I&D alone.

E. About 55--60% of patients with pilonidal disease develop chronic malodorous drainage. The granulation-lined pilonidal cavity drains through a sinus that extends in a cephalad direction in over 90% of cases. The sinus opening is usually located away from the midline, and often there may be more than one opening on the skin. Pain and discharge are the two most common symptoms of pilonidal sinus. Factors to be considered before deciding on a method of treatment are average healing time, recurrence rate, cost of treatment, and the surgeon's experience with a particular procedure.

ALGORITHM 30–1

History and physical exam[A] → Pilonidal disease

Pilonidal disease → Pilonidal[B] abscess

Pilonidal[B] abscess → Incision and drainage only[C]

Incision and drainage only[C] → Asymptomatic (dashed)

Incision and drainage only[C] → Recurrent pilonidal disease

Pilonidal[B] abscess → Incision and drainage followed[D] by pit excision

Incision and drainage followed[D] by pit excision → Recurrent pilonidal disease

Incision and drainage followed[D] by pit excision → Asymptomatic (dashed)

Pilonidal disease → Pilonidal sinus[E] or recurrent sinus

Pilonidal sinus[E] or recurrent sinus → Closed technique[F]

Pilonidal sinus[E] or recurrent sinus → Wide excision[G]

Pilonidal sinus[E] or recurrent sinus → Lay-open[H]

Pilonidal sinus[E] or recurrent sinus → Marsupialization[I]

Pilonidal sinus[E] or recurrent sinus → Excision and[J] primary closure
1. Midline closure
2. Oblique/asymetric closure

Pilonidal sinus[E] or recurrent sinus → Flaps[K]

F. The closed technique could be performed as an outpatient procedure under local anesthesia; the affected, midline epithelial follicles are cored out and hairs within the tract are removed using a small brush. Repeated brushing of the tract is performed in the office. Some authors recommend curetting the tract followed by injection of 50% phenol. The recurrence rate is reported as approximately 18% after 1-year follow-up with a healing time of about 6 weeks.

G. Wide excision involves removing all tissue between skin and presacral fascia. The healing time is prolonged (7 + weeks) and hospital admission and general anesthesia are required. Moreover, this technique carries a recurrence rate of approximately 13% after one year follow-up. This procedure offers no advantage over other techniques.

H. Laying open of the tract can be performed under local anesthesia in the office or in the outpatient surgical facility. It involves sinusotomy with limited excision of the pilonidal tissue, curettage of the sinus tract, side sinuses, and excision of overhanging edges of the skin. The patient is seen in the office on a weekly basis and is instructed to take warm baths twice daily and debride the wound after each bath by using a mechanical spray or a soft toothbrush. Patient discomfort and loss of time from work is minimal. Average healing time is 6 weeks, and this procedure carries a recurrence rate of 5–15% after 1-year follow-up.

I. Marsupialization involves sinusotomy as described above associated with an approximation of the skin edges to the base of the tract. Wound care and follow-up are identical to those for sinusotomy alone. Some authors describe an accelerated healing time and lower recurrence rate than that after laying open alone.

J. Primary closure techniques involve excision of the sinus followed by primary wound closure. Primary healing occurs in over 90% of cases within 2 weeks and avoids the need for frequent dressing changes. This procedure requires hospitalization, restricts activities, and causes loss of time from work. The recurrence rate 1 year after primary midline closure is 15%. Some authors recommend asymmetric or oblique incisions and closure away from the midline. Proponents of this technique report a recurrence rate as low as 3%.

K. Multiple different flap procedures involve wide excision followed by rotation flaps to cover the sacral defect. All of these methods result in flattening of the natal cleft as well as transposition of the scar from the midline. Complications include loss of sensation in the flap, flap necrosis, and infection. Prolonged hospital stay and general anesthesia are required. This procedure carries a recurrence rate of 0–8% after 1-year follow-up and is best employed in patients with complex or multiple recurrent pilonidal disease.

BIBLIOGRAPHY

1. Allen-Mersh TG: Pilonidal sinus: finding the right tract for treatment. *Br J Surg* 77:123–132, 1990.

2. Bascom J: Pilonidal disease: long-term results of follicle removal. *Dis Colon Rectum* 26:800–807, 1983.

3. Fishbein RH: Sacrococcygeal pilonidal sinus. In *Current Surgical Therapy,* 4th ed. St. Louis: Mosby Year Book, 1992.

4. Jones DJ: Pilonidal sinus. *Br Med J* 305:410--412, 1992.

5. Karydakis GE: Easy and successful treatment of pilonidal sinus after explanation of its causative process. *Aust NZ J Surg.* 62:385--389, 1992.

6. Manterola C, Barroso M, Araya JC, et al: Pilonidal disease: 25 cases treated by the Dufourmentel technique. *Dis Colon Rectum* 34:649--652, 1991.

7. Solla JA, Rothenberger DA: Chronic pilonidal disease: an assessment of 150 cases. *Dis Colon Rectum* 33:758--761, 1990.

8. Sondenaa K, Andersen E, Soreide JA: Morbidity and short term results in a randomised trial of open compared with closed treatment of chronic pilonidal sinus. *Eur J Sur* 158:351--355, 1992.

9. Wexner SD. Pilonidal disease. In: Beck DE, Welling DR (eds): *Manual of Patient Care in Colorectal Surgery.* Boston: Little Brown and Co. 1991; 255--265.

10. Wexner SD, Jagelman DG: Pilonidal sinus, pre-sacral cysts and tumors and pelvic pain. In: Zuidema GD, Condon RE (eds): *Surgery of the Alimentary Tract* (3rd ed.). Philadelphia: W.B. Saunders 1991; 390--405.

See also Chapter 31.

CHAPTER 31

Recurrent Pilonidal Disease

John U. Bascom, M.D., Ph.D.

Refer to Algorithm 31–1.

A. Pilonidal problems are a challenge because secondary effects draw attention away from the source: the source is the cleft. Conditions within it are able to create pilonidal disease in any tissue that lies within. Anaerobic bacteria, hair and moisture will perforate normal skin and can perforate all repairs, whether they are full-thickness flaps, split grafts, or scars. Conversely, within clefts that are shallow, dry, and clean, epidermis heals and remains healed. "Epidermis" does not refer to skin, it refers only to the outer layer of the skin. A pinhole in this layer is the initiator of pilonidal disease. The pinhole in pilonidal disease is formed through the epidermis that lines a hair follicle. The pinhole perforates the bottom of a hair follicle that was already distorted and enlarged by strong forces that pull on midline tissue. Only half of all pilonidal abscesses contain hairs, although hairs do sometimes cause and maintain the patency of a hole. Nonetheless, hairs gathered in the cleft foster unclean conditions that nourish anaerobes. Shed body hairs within abscesses become secondary invaders pulled in by the vacuum in fat under the cleft. Scales on the hairs assist the invasion. However, hairs never grow within a pilonidal "cyst" because pilonidals are never "cysts" lined with epidermis that can grow hair. Pilonidal "cysts" are instead actually chronic abscesses lined with granulation tissue. Attempted wide excision of mythical "cysts" often makes for serious recurrent pilonidal disease. Wide excision, marsupialization, Z-plasty, and other operations attack secondary lesions in fat, ignore the source, and aggravate the problem. They often create a sharp, moist fold, place a vulnerable suture line in that fold, and are responsible for most recurrences.
B. An acute pilonidal abscess is either aspirated or incised and drained. If later surgical treatment is chosen for the chronic abscess that may follow, suture lines must be kept away from the deep cleft.
C. *Cleft closure.* For large recurrences, this procedure is best because healthy skin is brought in to repair the midline. The problem is solved using vertical skin from one side of the deep cleft (Fig. 31–1). The skin is incised at the depths and

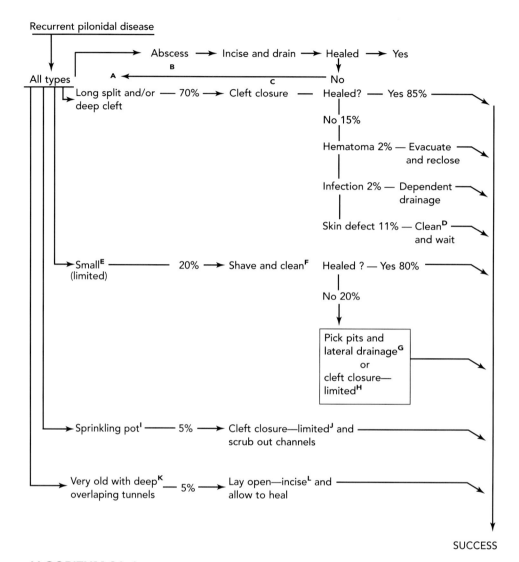

ALGORITHM 31–1

mobilized on the right side as a full-thickness flap hinged at the surface; a large denuded area becomes available. The flap is horizontally drawn across the left buttock until only a shallow groove remains at the upper end of the cleft. A bed is prepared by removing skin from the left side of the cleft wherever the contralateral flap covers it. After the skin is lifted and the fat is either longitudinally incised or the fibrous scar is removed from the old wound in the sides

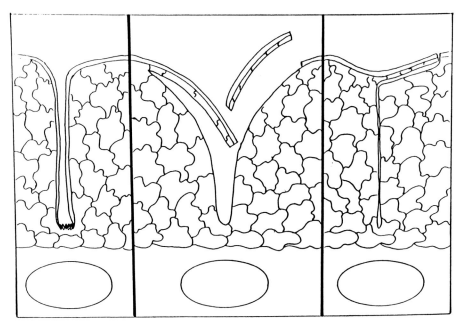

FIGURE 31–1 Cleft closure frees a flap of skin from the vertical side of the cleft and draws it horizontally to a new bed prepared on the opposite buttock. Cleft depth is reduced by half over the sacrococcygeal angle where pilonidal abscesses originate. The suture line lies in a ventilated area that assures drying and healing.

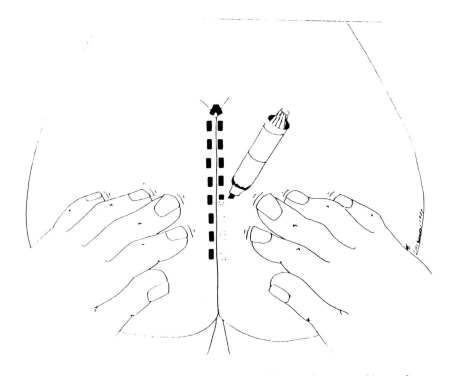

FIGURE 31–2 Cleft closure. The skin is marked along the natural line of contact.

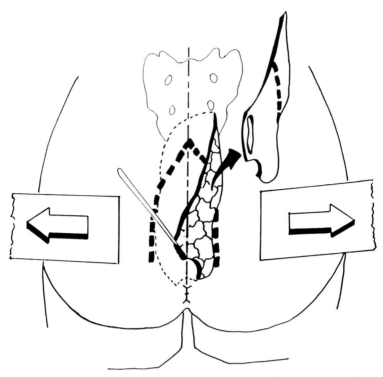

FIGURE 31–3A Skin flap is raised and the infected flap is excised.

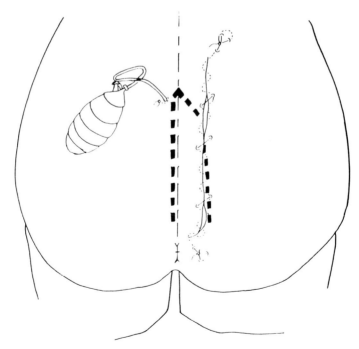

FIGURE 31–4 After contralateral coverage the flap is sutured in place along the previously delineated lines. A suction drain is used to help close the dead space.

and depths of the cleft. Cleft closure moves the suture line away from the cleft where epithelial cells can heal the wound. To permit ease in sitting, 50% of the cleft depth should be retained over the sacrococcygeal angle. Patients can sit at once, and most wounds are healed within 1 week. Such an operation can rapidly heal long-standing wounds.

D. A poorly healed wound in the cleft may heal after thorough cleaning. If surgery becomes necessary, revise the cleft into a shallower, drier, ventilated structure. Fashion a repair so eccentrically shaped as to move suture lines to one side of the cleft. Healing can be assisted with metronidazole and suction drainage.

E. To control limited pilonidal disease, one must limit fresh infusions of anaerobes into fat by cleaning and shaving the cleft. Each week the wound is cleaned of any hairs that perforate the epidermis. Once the hairs are removed, the pinhole or small defect usually closes and the normal vascularity of fat will oxygenate and kill any remaining anaerobes.

F. *Shaving* is the simplest of the treatments. It acts by reducing anaerobic bacteria, bringing the importance of cleanliness to the patients attention, and allowing the surgeon to see and remove tiny hairs crossing epithelium. After three visits the patient and surgeon recognize healing or resistance to healing. At each visit, each option should be reconsidered. Shaving most closely approaches the ideal of a cure that is painless and inexpensive, with no disability or hospitalization; shaving alone can cure some recurrent disease.

G. *Picking pits and lateral drainage* removes the midline holes that started the disease through small laterally placed incisions. Basically the abscess cavity, entered through a separate eccentric incision, is curetted out and left open to heal without packing. The procedure is performed under local anesthesia on an outpatient basis. Half the patients return to work the day after this procedure. This operation may offer a more definitive cure more quickly than shaving.

H. *Cleft closure.* A limited version of the operation described above serves well for small recurrences. It need not reach from the top of the cleft to the anus. Taper each end of the excised elipse to avoid tight folds and sudden changes in cleft depth to avoid recurrences.

I. *Sprinkling pot.* The occasional "sprinkling pot" patient shows 10–20 openings over both buttocks all connected by superficial tunnels. They take origin from an insignificant pore in the midline.

J. *Scrubbing out.* Scrub granulations from the multiple tunnels by pulling gauze through them after excising a 1–2-cm-diameter patch of skin at each drainage opening. Then use a limited cleft closure to heal the midline pore, which is the source of the tunnels. The drainage wounds close in a few weeks.

K. *Deep tunnels.* A rare patient with 20 years of disease may show deep overlapping tunnels. These tunnels must be excised. The differential diagnosis must include hidradenitis suppurativa, which is treated in an identical manner.

L. *Incising.* Disability is minimal after incising to unroof deep tunnels. The incised wounds heal slowly but cease to irritate the patient after a few days.

BIBLIOGRAPHY

1. Bascom JU: Repeat pilonidal operations. *Am J Surg* 154:118–122, 1987.
2. Bascom JU: Pilonidal disease—healing a hole in bottom paint—a review. *Cur Prac Surg* (in press).
3. Crile G Jr: Surgery, in the days of controversy. *JAMA* 262:256–258, 1989.
4. Klass AA: The so-called pilonidal sinus. *Can Med Assoc J* 75:737–742, 1956.
5. Hardaway RM: Pilonidal Cyst—neither pilonidal nor cyst. *AMA Arch Surg* 76:143–147, 1958.

See also Chapters 30 and 32.

CHAPTER 32

Hidradenitis Suppurativa

P. Ronan O'Connell, M.D.

Refer to Algorithm 32–1.

A. Hidradenitis suppurativa (HS) is a chronic, indolent, inflammatory condition of the skin and subcutaneous tissues in areas of the body where apocrine sweat glands are found. The regions most commonly affected are, in order of decreasing frequency, axilla, inguinoperineal, perianal, and inframammary.

B. The etiology of HS is uncertain. It appears that keratinous plugging of apocrine ducts results in glandular dilatation that becomes secondarily infected. Chronic inflammation with gland destruction and fibrosis leads to extension to surrounding tissues, eventually resulting in chronic sinus and rarely fistula formation. No specific microorganism is associated with HS, although *Staphylococci, Streptococci, Escherichia coli, Pseudomonas aeruginosa,* and *Bacteroides* are commonly found.

C. The diagnosis of HS is primarily clinical. In the inguinoperineal region HS is usually easily differentiated from chronic folliculitis, perineal/vulval Crohn's disease, and anorectal fistulas. By contrast, perianal HS is frequently misdiagnosed as pilonidal disease, anorectal fistula, or perirectal abscess.

D. The history is usually of a recurrent and progressive subacute infection in the hair-bearing areas of the perineum and perianal region, which may extend to involve the external surfaces of the labia, base of the scrotum, or the natal cleft. In extreme cases, inflammation and sinus formation may extend to the anal canal with fistula formation, or to the lower back. Examination shows indurated, erythematous, hair-bearing skin with discharging sinuses (Fig. 32–1).

E. Laboratory investigations are rarely helpful except to exclude diabetes and to guide antimicrobial therapy. Histopathology shows chronic inflammation with gland destruction, fibrosis, and sinus formation.

F. HS is associated with diabetes mellitus, Cushing's disease, obesity, and skin diseases that cause pore occlusion. Recently an association with Crohn's disease has been reported.

Hidradenitis suppurativa

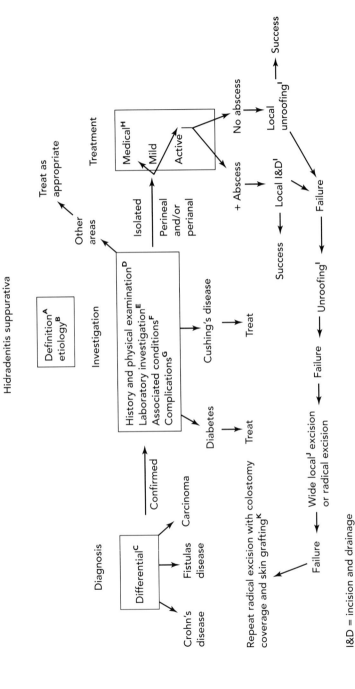

I&D = incision and drainage

ALGORITHM 32–1

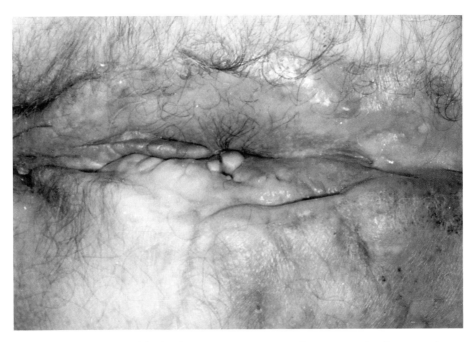

FIGURE 32-1 Perianal hidradentitis suppurativa showing multiple sinus formation and extensive fibrosis.

G. Local long-term complications of HS include marked fibrosis with restriction of mobility, anorectal fistulation, and rarely squamous cell carcinoma. Systemic complications are those of any chronic inflammatory condition, anemia, hypoproteinemia, and amylodosis.

H. While surgical excision is the cornerstone of treatment of HS, medical treatment may suffice in minor cases. A combination of local hygiene with antiseptic solutions systemic antibiotics, particularly erythromycin or tetracycline, will clear up to one-third of mild cases. Topical synthetic retinoids have been reported to be useful.

I. Local excision with primary closure in combination with the medical treatment may be used in acute, localized disease, particularly in the inguinal area. In the presence of abscesses, incision and/or deroofing will give temporary relief.

J. In chronic or recurrent HS only wide surgical excision of all diseased skin and subcutaneous tissue down to deep fascia will control the disease. Skin cover may be obtained with split-thickness graft, rotation, or pedicle grafts. Using these techniques, wound breakdown and recurrence is common (40-50%).

K. Two studies support a more radical approach to severe or recurrent perineal or perianal disease. All affected skin was widely excised with a minimum margin of 1.5 cm. Healing by granulation was controlled with dressings or silastic foam. A colostomy was used only when hygiene or continence could not be maintained. The reported median time for healing was 9 weeks (range 6-14 weeks) for perineal disease and 3 months (range 2-12 months) for perianal disease. Even with these drastic techniques local or distant recurrence was still problematic (at 67%). In general, however, it appears that the more radical the excision, the less likely is local recurrence.

BIBLIOGRAPHY

1. Banerjee AK: Surgical treatment of hidradenitis suppurativa. *Br J Surg* 79:863–866, 1992.
2. Masson JK: Surgical treatment of hidradenitis suppurativa. *Surg Clin N Am* 49:1043–1052, 1969.
3. Morgan WP, Harding KG, Richadson G, et al: The use of silastic foam dressing in the treatment of advanced hidradenitis suppurativa. *Br J Surg* 67:277–280, 1980.
4. Wiltz O, Schoetz DJ, Murray JJ, et al: Perianal hidradenitis suppurativa: the Lahey Clinic experience. *Dis Colon Rectum* 33:731–734, 1990.

See also Chapters 24, 30, 31, 35, 51.

CHAPTER 33

Rectal Prolapse and Rectoanal Intussusception

Stanley M. Goldberg, M.D.

Refer to Algorithm 33–1.

A. Conversion to a reducible rectal prolapse allows preoperative evaluation and preparation and should be attempted when the rectum is viable. Sphincter spasm can be overcome with regional anesthesia, and swelling is markedly reduced by the application of simple table sugar sprinkled over the collapsed rectal mucosa of the rectum.

B. Rectal prolapse is associated with cystic fibrosis (CF) in children. The etiology is due to chronic coughing and associated increases in intraabdominal pressure.

C. Patient and parent education along with establishment of a bowel routine that avoids straining usually allows eventual resolution of rectal prolapse in most children.

D. When conservative efforts fail, additional interventions, such as submucosal sclerosant injection, as in the management of hemorrhoids, are usually successful.

E. A history of incontinence or constipation is sought. Flexible sigmoidoscopy is done to exclude associated pathology. Colonoscopy or barium enema is recommended with a history of rectal bleeding or patient age over 50. Anal manometry and pudendal terminal motor nerve latencies may be indicated to assess sphincter function prior to operation and identification of a nonrelaxing puborectalis may be useful in planning additional therapy such as biofeedback. Colon transit studies in constipated patients will identify those individuals who should be considered for colon resection.

F. Patients with rectal prolapse usually complain of erratic bowel habits, difficult evacuation, and fecal staining of the underclothes. Careful questioning allows

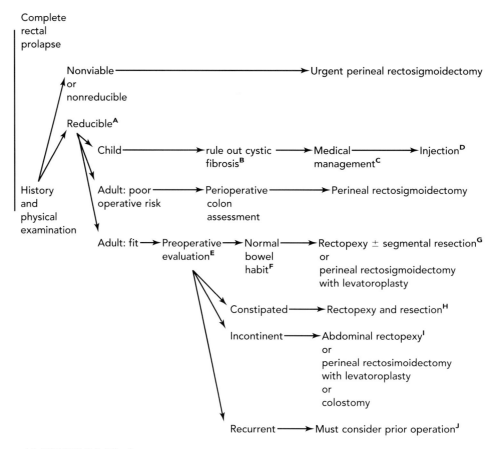

Complete rectal prolapse

Nonviable or nonreducible ──────────────────────────────→ Urgent perineal rectosigmoidectomy

Reducible[A]

Child ──────────→ rule out cystic fibrosis[B] ──────→ Medical management[C] ──────→ Injection[D]

History and physical examination

Adult: poor operative risk ──────→ Perioperative colon assessment ──────→ Perineal rectosigmoidectomy

Adult: fit ──→ Preoperative evaluation[E] ──→ Normal bowel habit[F] ──────→ Rectopexy ± segmental resection[G] or perineal rectosigmoidectomy with levatoroplasty

Constipated ──────→ Rectopexy and resection[H]

Incontinent ──────→ Abdominal rectopexy[I] or perineal rectosimoidectomy with levatoroplasty or colostomy

Recurrent ──────→ Must consider prior operation[J]

ALGORITHM 33–1

identification of those for whom constipation or true fecal incontinence is a predominant clinical feature.

G. An abdominal repair of prolapse in these patients has been the mainstay of treatment in the past because of high recurrence rates with perineal repairs. However, acceptable recurrence rates following perineal rectosigmoidectomy have been reported and may be related to the addition of a routine levatoroplasty to the operation. The risk of impotence after transabdominal rectal mobilization (approximately 1–2%) should be considered in choosing the approach in males. Rectopexy combined with sigmoid resection has been routinely performed with low recurrence rates. Sigmoid resection in all prolapse patients may cause postoperative diarrhea and fecal incontinence and may best be reserved for those patients with documented constipation.

H. Abdominal rectopexy and combined sigmoid resection is the operation of choice for constipated patients. Subtotal colectomy is indicated when colonic transit studies reveal colonic inertia.

I. Rectopexy combined with sigmoid resection is least well tolerated in this group of patients, and rectopexy alone should be considered. Incontinence may continue to improve for up to 1 year following prolapse repair. Patients should be reassured that the results of operation with regard to fecal incontinence will continue to improve over time. Consideration may be given to rectopexy and end colostomy in a fit, elderly patient with severe incontinence.

J. A surgeon planning operation for recurrence must keep in mind the potential for a devascularized segment of rectum if both the initial and subsequent operations include resection. Following abdominal rectopexy with resection, repeat abdominal operation may be the operation of choice, but perineal resection with dissection close to the rectum has been successfully performed. Following perineal resection, repeat perineal resection or abdominal rectopexy can be used.

BIBLIOGRAPHY

1. Goldberg SM, Madoff RD (eds): Rectal prolapse. *Seminars Colon Rectal Surg* 2:169–232, 1991.
2. Johansen OB, Wexner SD, Daniel N, et al: Perineal rectosigmoidectomy in the elderly. *Dis Colon Rectum* 36:767–772, 1993.
3. Madoff RD. Rectal prolapse and intussusception. In Beck DE, Wexner S (eds): *Fundamentals of Anorectal Surgery*. New York: McGraw-Hill, pp89–103, 1992.
4. Wexner SD. Rectal prolapse and intussusception. In: Beck DE, Welling D (eds). Manual of patient care in colorectal surgery. Boston: Little, Brown and Company. 191–192, 1991.
See also Chapters 3, 17 and 19.

CHAPTER 34

Solitary Rectal Ulcer

W. Terence Reilly, M.D. and John H. Pemberton, M.D.

Refer to Algorithm 34–1.

A. Solitary rectal ulcer syndrome (SRU) is a *histologic* diagnosis. Symptoms include: blood per rectum in nearly 100%; straining at stool with difficulty in initiation of bowel movements in over half of patients, passage of mucus in over half, pain on defecation in 50–70%, self-digitation in more than 50%, and the feeling of incomplete evacuation in about 60%.

B. Macroscopically, SRU appears in a spectrum ranging from (1) mucosal erythema to (2) a true, solitary ulcer, often with a white, fibrous base, to (3) multiple areas of erythema, ulceration, and overlying exudate without frank ulceration. These lesions present between 3 and 14 cm from the anal verge. (See photos Figs. 34–1 and 34–2.)

C. Histologic diagnosis is predicated on exclusion of malignancy.

D. Histologically, SRU is defined by thickening of the muscularis mucosa with the finding of fibroblast and smooth muscle infiltrate between the glands of the mucosa. These changes frequently occur in the midst of erosions of the superficial mucosa that may or may not display frank ulceration. (See Figs. 34–3 and 34–4). Histologic findings may also include surrounding localized colitis cystica profunda. This is a name given to changes in the submucosa secondary to some traumatic process and is not specific to SRU. Therefore, when this localized finding is present with SRU, it should be considered part of the same process. Localized colitis cystica profunda, or *proctitis* cystica profunda, may occur from hemorrhage of capillaries that dissects the lamina propria. During repair of this hematoma, the walls of the hematoma become lined with epithelia that migrate from the crypts of the rectal glands when they come into contact with the hematoma. After the hematoma is resorbed, a cystic cavity with a mucin-secreting lining remains. Cystic change may also result from isolation of the deep parts of the glands by inflammation and ingrowth of the fibromuscular cells of SRU. The crypts then become constipated and eventually completely closed off from the enteric lumen. The

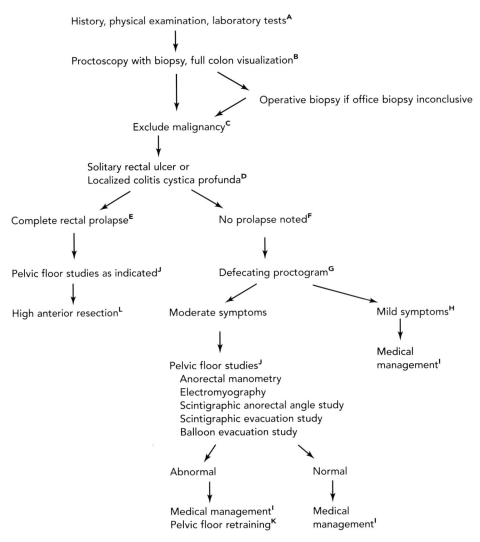

ALGORITHM 34-1

etiology of SRU is still debated, but is probably related to trauma and/or ischemia within the rectal mucosa. These lesions probably occur as a result of some degree of rectal wall prolapse in combination with straining at stool. Prolapse of the rectal wall with tethering of the support structures and microvasculature makes the tissue vulnerable to trauma. Straining submits these tissues to pressures of up to 300 mmHg. Tearing of the microvasculature may occur as a direct result of trauma from squeezing of the prolapsed tissue into the anal canal, yielding microhemorrhage. Alternatively, pressure may cause intermittent ischemia from decreased blood flow through these capillaries, resulting in congestion, fibrosis, and ulceration. Straining may be the result of

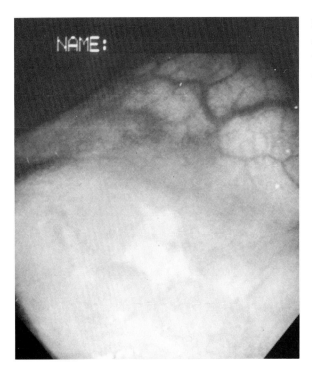

FIGURE 34–1 These colonoscopy photos demonstrate two examples of "nonulcerated" solitary rectal ulcer. In Fig. 34–1, pathology is shown as a focal, superficial area of fibrosis.

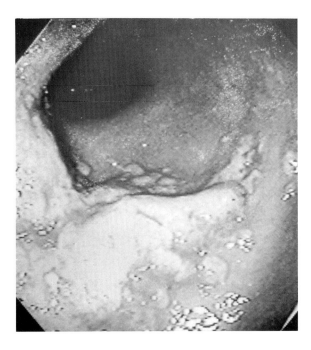

FIGURE 34–2 shows a more diffuse involvement of the mucosa with a raised, polypoid surface and surrounding erythema. Frank ulceration is often absent in these lesions, thus the dependence on histologic confirmation of the disease.

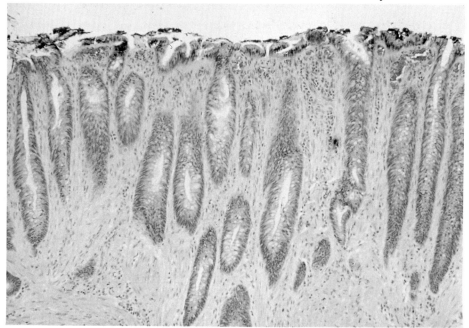

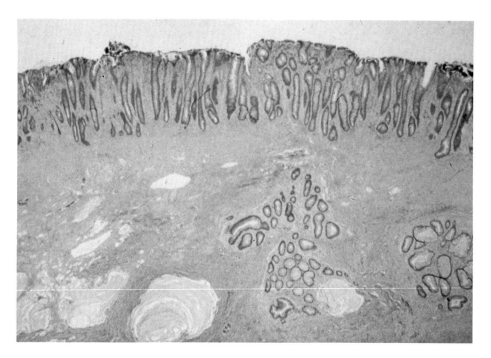

FIGURES 34–3, 34–4 In Fig. 34–3, the histologic features of fibromuscular invasion of the spaces between the mucosal glands can be seen, especially in the lower right part of the photograph. Varying degrees of displacement of the glands to the submucosal areas with the eventual mucous lake formation of colitis cystica profunda are clearly noted. Figure 34–4 gives a higher-power view of the fibromuscular invasion, causing separation and polygonal shaping of the mucus crypts. (Figure 34–3 6× magnification; Fig. 34–4 25× magnification.)

one or more of several associated disorders of pelvic floor physiology. Implicated in the pathophysiology of straining are descending perineum syndrome (with or without subsequent nerve stretch injury) and nonrelaxing puborectalis syndrome.

E. Prolapse may also result from the above factors. Any form of pelvic floor outlet obstruction with straining might result in the posterior displacement of the anterior wall of the rectum, with eventual prolapse. This is, however, speculative.

F. It should be recognized that a small proportion of patients lack any demonstrable prolapse on evaluation. In others, no associated symptoms can be causally related to the lesion encountered. Therefore, definitive etiology is still controversial. Digitation may be both responsible for, and a result of, SRU. Passive anal intercourse has also been associated with the finding of SRU. The clinical context should dictate the evaluation of the patient. Clinical evaluation of SRU begins with the exclusion of malignancy, inflammatory bowel disease, villoadenomatous polyp, or infection. The patient must be examined while straining on a commode to facilitate the finding of frank prolapse, perineal descent, or perineal ballooning. Proctoscopy and colonoscopy or barium enema to exclude proximal lesions are minimal requirements. If definitive diagnosis is not possible on proctoscopic biopsy, operative biopsy should be obtained.

G. In patients with defecatory symptoms, cinedefecography may help identify prolapse.

H. Therapy is directed to the severity of rectal prolapse. Patients without prolapse or with manageable occult prolapse should always be treated conservatively.

I. A diet high in fiber (30–35 g/day) plus added bulking agents such as psyllium products are recommended. Fluid intake should be increased and caffeine and alcohol should be avoided to prevent dehydration of the stool. Counseling on return to a reflex pattern of defecation may improve symptoms. Approximately 60–70% of patients will improve with these conservative measures.

J. Anorectal motility evaluation with colon transit studies, sphincter electromyography, balloon expulsion, anorectal angle evaluation, and anorectal manometry studies should be selectively performed as the clinical presentation demands. Straining and symptoms of outlet obstruction suggest potential benefit from these studies.

K. Pelvic floor retraining may help in those patients demonstrating symptoms and findings of pelvic outlet obstruction or defecation disorder. Biofeedback techniques have been used widely for anismus, which is associated with SRU. Psychological counseling and behavior modification techniques are central to success with this method. Attempted local excision of rectal ulcers has met with a high recurrence rate, and many complications and should not be performed. Patients with complete rectal prolapse (external prolapse) may benefit from repair of the prolapse, but anterior mobilization of the rectum may lead to severe complications such as leakage stricture, and abscess and fistula formation. Elderly or frail patients with significant prolapse may be best treated by a perineal repair or resection. These operations are extremely hazardous, however, because the anterior dissection is performed in the midst of intense fibrosis and scarring.

L. High anterior resection of the rectum, with anastomosis performed in the peritonealized part of the rectum, is associated with relatively low rates of morbidity and recurrence of prolapse. Mortality should be less than 1% in appropriate patients. Technique must include mobilization of the rectum to the coccyx posteriorly and mobilization of the lateral stalks, which are *not* divided. The resection of any redundant sigmoid allows for treatment of the prolapse without any foreign material. Recurrence rates increase with time. One large series resulted in 37% recurrence after 5 years. However, with the technique described above, recurrence over 15–20 years should be less than 13%. Proctectomy with coloanal anastomosis has not been reported as a therapy for SRU. However, one review showed that recurrence rates after low anterior resection of the rectum with anastomosis in the nonperitonealized rectum resulted in a 52% morbidity rate, whereas high anterior resection exhibited only a 19% associated morbidity. This may have a foreboding impact on coloanal anastomosis in this setting. Laparoscopic resection and repair are currently alternative approaches. In the event of failure of the preceding methods, abdominoperineal excision may be considered.

BIBLIOGRAPHY

1. Bogomoletz WV: Solitary rectal ulcer syndrome: mucosal prolapse syndrome. *Pathol Ann* 27(Pt1):75–86, 1992.
2. Ford MJ, Anderson JR, Gilmour HM, et al: Clinical spectrum of "solitary ulcer" of the rectum. *Gastroenterology* 84:1533–1540, 1983.
3. Lam TCF, Lubowski DZ, King DW: Solitary rectal ulcer syndrome. *Bailliere's Clin Gastroenterol* 6:129–143, 1992.
4. Nelson H, Pemberton JH: Solitary rectal ulcer. In Fazio VW (ed): *Current Therapy in Colon and Rectal Surgery*. Philadelphia: Decker, 1990, pp98–102.
5. Nicholls RJ, Simson JNL: Anteroposterior rectopexy in the treatment of solitary rectal ulcer syndrome without overt rectal prolapse. *Br J Surg* 78:222–224, 1986.
6. Rutter KR, Riddell RH: The solitary ulcer syndrome of the rectum. *Clin Gastroenterol* 4:505–530, 1975.
7. Schlinkert RT, Beart RW, Wolff BG, et al: Anterior resection for complete rectal prolapse. *Dis Colon Rectum* 28:409–412, 1985.
8. Stuart M: Proctitis cystica profunda: incidence, etiology, and treatment. *Dis Colon Rectum* 27:153–156, 1984.
9. Wayte DM, Elson BH: Colitis cystica profunda. *Am J Clin Pathol* 48:159–169, 1967.
10. Womack NR, Williams NS, Holmfield JHM, et al: Pressure and prolapse—the cause of solitary rectal ulceration. *Gut* 28:1228–1233, 1987.

See also Chapters 3 and 18.

CHAPTER 35

Anal Margin Lesions

Douglas A. Brewer, M.D. and Patricia L. Roberts, M.D.

Refer to Algorithm 35-1 and Fig. 35-1.

A. The *anal margin* is defined as including the area from the intersphincteric groove to a 5-cm radius around the anal verge. This area includes non-keratinized squamous epithelium, which then changes to keratinized squamous epithelium at the anal verge. Anal margin lesions include premalignant and malignant lesions. Because lesions of the anal canal and anal margin behave differently and are treated differently, it is essential to make a correct diagnosis.

B. Anal margin lesions may be asymptomatic, or patients may have nonspecific signs and symptoms, such as pruritus, burning, bleeding, pain, or a mass, on presentation. A complete history and physical examination are important to exclude other more common causes of these complaints. Examination should include a complete description of all lesions, including size, shape, color, borders, presence or absence of ulceration, and invasion into adjacent structures, including the anal sphincters, rectum, vagina, and scrotum. Examination of the groin is indicated to exclude inguinal lymph node metastases.

C. Anoscopy is necessary to exclude involvement of the anal canal and synchronous lesions.

D. Biopsy of all suspicious lesions should be obtained. Several specimens should be obtained from the periphery and also from the center of the lesion. Biopsy can usually be performed in the office with local anesthesia.

E. Bowen's disease is an intraepithelial squamous cell carcinoma. It tends to spread intraepidermally but may become invasive in 2-6% of patients. It is most common in patients between 40 and 50 years of age, with a female predominance. The lesions appear as erythematous, scaly, and plaque-like with well-defined margins. The cells in Bowen's disease do not take up periodic acid-Schiff (PAS) stain.

F. Paget's disease is an intraepithelial adenocarcinoma. The average age at diagnosis is 65 years; the sex distribution is equal. The lesion appears as well-

ALGORITHM 35-1

Anal margin Lesion[A] → History and physical Examination[B] → Anoscopy[C] → Biopsy[D] →

Anal margin lesions

Premalignant lesions
Bowen's disease[E]
Paget's disease[F] → Pelvic examination[P]
Exclude other malignancies[Q]

Bowenoid papulosis[G]
Leukoplakia[H]
Acanthosis nigricans[I] → Excision/destruction[R]
Symptomatic treatment[S]
Treat underlying malignancy[T]

Malignant lesions
Basal cell carcinoma[J] → Wide local excision[U]
Squamous cell carcinoma[K] → Wide local excision[V]
Groin dissection
Verrucous carcinoma (Buschke–Löwenstein)[L] → Wide local excision[W]
Abdominoperineal resection
? Multimodality therapy

Kaposi's sarcoma[M] → See Chapter 38
Leukemia cutis[N] → Treat perianal complications[X]
Mycosis fungoides[O] → Management of systemic disease[Y]

→ Wide local excision with lesion mapping (Fig. 35–1)[Z] → follow up[AA]

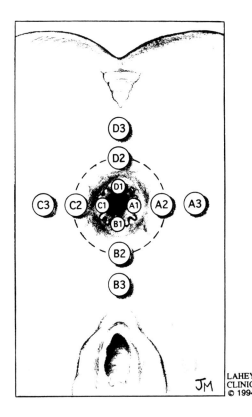

FIGURE 35–1 Lesion mapping has been used to ensure adequacy of excision of Bowen's disease and Paget's disease. Punch biopsies are obtained from the dentate line (1), anal verge (2), and perineum (3). [Adapted from Beck DE, Wexner SD: Anal neoplasms. In Beck DE, Wexner SD (eds): *Fundamentals of Anorectal Surgery*. New York: McGraw-Hill, 1992, pp233; this illustration reproduced with the permission of the Lahey Clinic.]

demarcated, eczematoid, whitish gray plaques that are ulcerated and crusty. Because of the presence of sialomucins, Paget's cells are PAS stain positive. Progression to invasive carcinoma is reported in as many as 40% of untreated patients.

G. Bowenoid papulosis is histologically similar to Bowen's disease; however, the lesions are usually multiple, appearing as numerous raised lesions (2–10 mm in diameter) on the perineum. They occur most commonly in patients in their 20s and 30s, with a male predominance. Bowenoid papulosis is found in association with prior human papillomavirus infection (especially subtypes 16 and 18) and herpes simplex virus.

H. Leukoplakia is a whitish thickening of the mucous membrane epithelium, occurring in patches of diverse size and shape. A male predominance is described. Microscopically, leukoplakia is characterized by hyperkeratosis and squamous metaplasia. It may represent a premalignant condition and, in one series of 27 patients, was associated with synchronous squamous cell carcinoma in 9 patients.

I. Acanthosis nigricans appears as a grayish, velvety thickening of the skin. Microscopic findings include hyperpigmentation, hyperkeratosis, and papillomatosis. It is frequently associated with intraabdominal malignancies, especially gastric adenocarcinoma. The diagnosis of acanthosis nigricans may precede, coincide with, or occur with or after detection of the associated malignancy.

J. Basal cell carcinoma of the anal margin is rare and occurs 3 times more commonly in men than in women. The lesions are similar to basal cell lesions elsewhere on the skin and are characterized by a central ulceration and raised edges.

K. Squamous cell carcinoma of the anal margin is similar in behavior to lesions occurring in other cutaneous areas of the body. The average age at diagnosis is 63 years, with a male predominance. The lesion is usually ulcerated with rolled, everted edges but may be polypoid or fungating. It is a slow-growing, locally invasive carcinoma; however, the rate of synchronous inguinal lymph node metastasis is 8–40%.

L. Although it is still controversial, there is a growing consensus that Buschke–Löwenstein tumor, or giant condyloma acuminatum, probably represents a verrucous carcinoma. Verrucous carcinoma is a well-differentiated squamous cell carcinoma that can be distinguished from large condylomata only by invasion into local tissues. It can arise in the perianal skin, anal canal, or distal rectum. With advanced local disease, multiple sinuses or fistulous tracts may occur although distant metastases are rare.

M. Kaposi's sarcoma (see Chapter 38).

N. Leukemia cutis, infiltration of the perianal area by leukemic cells, is uncommon but may be the first manifestation of leukemia. It is extremely painful and may present as a fistula, abscess, or tender erythematous area with marked cellulitis. It is usually a sign of advanced disease and carries a poor prognosis.

O. Mycosis fungoides is an uncommon, pruritic, usually fatal cutaneous malignancy of the lymphoreticular system (T cells). The cutaneous lesion can occur anywhere, including the anal margin. The overlying skin may have telangiectasia or be violaceous. As the tumor advances, ulcerations occur, and pain is the predominant symptom.

P. Although it was previously believed that Bowen's disease was frequently associated with internal malignancies, this notion has been refuted in several reviews, including a population-based study. Further cohort studies may be needed to settle this controversy. In women with Bowen's disease, careful pelvic examination should be considered because of a possible association with gynecologic (especially cervical) malignancy.

Q. In contrast, the coexistence of visceral malignancies with perianal Paget's disease, most commonly involving the anal canal or rectum, is well established, with an incidence of 50–100% in most reviews. Colonoscopy should be performed.

R. Bowenoid papulosis follows a benign course, and treatment is usually for relief of symptoms. Therapy can be accomplished by excision or destruction, as is done for anal condylomata. Treatment with low-dose recombinant Interferon-2c has also been described.

S. After synchronous squamous cell carcinoma is excluded, treatment should be directed at symptom relief. Operative treatment includes excision with or without skin grafts or flaps. However, the recurrence rate is high. Because of the question of malignant potential, annual surveillance examination is recommended, with biopsy of any suspicious lesion.

T. Treatment for acanthosis nigricans is directed toward the primary malignancy.

U. Local excision with adequate margins is the treatment of choice. The role of radiotherapy has not been determined. Local recurrence after excision is not uncommon (29%) and can be managed by reexcision. The 5-year survival rate exceeds 73%.

V. Local excision with adequate margins is the treatment of choice. For extensive carcinoma that involves the dentate line and deeply invades the underlying sphincter muscles or adjacent organs, abdominoperineal resection offers the best form of local control and best survival. A locoregional recurrent tumor will develop in up to 42% of patients. Local recurrence is treated by local excision or abdominoperineal resection. Groin dissection for synchronous or metachronous inguinal lymph node metastases is indicated. The 5-year survival rate ranges from 35% to 100%.

W. The extent of operation should be individualized. Wide local excision with histologically clear margins is the recommended initial surgical approach. For large lesions or those that involve the anal sphincter, abdominoperineal resection with extended perineal dissection may be required. No substantial experience has been reported in the literature with the use of multimodality (chemoradiation) therapy for patients with anal margin verrucous carcinoma.

X. Treatment is aimed at early recognition and aggressive management of septic perianal complications of the leukemia.

Y. Treatment of mycosis fungoides is aimed at treating the systemic disease.

Z. If evaluation does not demonstrate invasive malignancy, wide local excision is recommended for patients with anal margin Bowen's disease and Paget's disease. "Lesion mapping" is recommended to guide adequate local excision (Fig. 35-1).

AA. Recommendations for follow-up study of patients with anal margin Bowen's disease and Paget's disease include annual complete physical examination, proctosigmoidoscopy, punch biopsy from the edges of the skin graft or scar, and colonoscopy every 2 or 3 years. Recurrent lesions are treated using the same general principles outlined for primary lesions.

BIBLIOGRAPHY

1. Beck DE, Wexner SD: Anal neoplasma. In Beck DE, Wexner SD (eds): *Fundamentals of Anorectal Surgery*. New York: McGraw-Hill, 1992, pp 222–237.

2. Corman ML: Cutaneous conditions. In Corman ML (ed): *Colon and Rectal Surgery*. Philadelphia: Lippincott, 1993, pp420–431, 721–739.

3. Nivatvongs S: Perianal and anal neoplasm. In Gordon PH, Nivatvongs S (eds): *Principles and Practice of Surgery for the Colon, Rectum, and Anus*. St. Louis: Quality Medical Publishers, 1992, pp401–415.

See also Chapters 1, 7, 8, 37, 38, 44 and 46.

CHAPTER 36

Anorectal Trauma

Pedro J. Morgado, M.D. and
Pedro J. Morgado Jr., M.D.

Refer to Algorithm 36–1.

A. Anorectal trauma is less common than is colon trauma and its management is also less controversial. History and physical exam are instrumental in the surgical decision. The primary aim of surgery is to preserve life; secondary aims are maintenance of continence and limiting morbidity and hospital stay. The nature of trauma must be established whenever possible. Sexual assault including foreign-body impalement, insertion injuries, can be labeled as blunt trauma. (Figure 36–1) Conversely stab and gunshot wounds are sharp injuries. Anal and rectal lesions are treated individually according to the standard atomic classifications. (Figure 36–2)

B. Injuries to anal area can be diagnosed by inspection palpation, and instrumentation. Damage to perianal and perineal skin, as well as to adjacent perineal organs (vagina and scrotum), sphincter ani muscles, anal mucosa, and rectal mucosa, must be evaluated.

C. Minor sphincteric and perineal damage may be found.

D. If minor injury is present, wide debridement and primary sphincteroplasty, with tetanus prophylaxis, are generally adequate.

E. However, there may be major sphincteric and/or perineal damage.

F. If major injury is noted, a wide debridement, delayed sphincteroplasty, and a temporary sigmoidostomy are advisable, together with antibiotic prophylaxis.

G. If no mucosal damage is found, a foreign body can be retrieved from the rectum.

H. Using epidural anesthesia, sometimes it is helpful to insufflate air in the rectum above the foreign body to facilitate its extraction. If a perforation is found, it is treated as with any other rectal injury.

I. Rectal injuries can also be diagnosed by inspection, palpation, and instrumentation; it is necessary to locate the site(s) of injury. In addition, plain abdominal and pelvic radiographs, intravenous pyelogram, and a bladder catheter are

Anorectal trauma A

History and physical exam
Nature of trauma

Blunt   Firearm
Stab   Foreign body

Anal → Inspection B
        Digital exam
        Rectosigmoidoscopy

Minor sphincteric C
and perineal damage

Major sphincteric E
and perineal damage

Debridement D
Primary sphincteroplasty

Debridement F
Delayed sphincteroplasty
Temporary sigmoidostomy
Prophylaxis of infection

No mucosal damage G

Remove foreign body H
under epidural anesthesia

Rectal → Inspection I
          Digital exam
          Rectosigmoidoscopy
          Plain abdominal and pelvic x-ray
          Intravenous pyelogram
          Hypaque enema
          Bladder catheter
          Laparoscopy or
          Exploratory laparotomy

Intraperitoneal J
Heavy contamination
Associated pelvic injuries

Proximal end colostomy K
Repair of rectal
and pelvic injuries
Mucous fistula
Rectal washout
Drainage of presacral space
Prophylaxis of infection

Extraperitoneal N

Minimal contamination L
No pelvic injury

Simple closure of wound M
Resection and anastomisis
Rectal washout
Prophylaxis of infection

Rectal washout
Transanal repair
Prophylaxis of
infection

Diagnosis

Evaluation

Treatment

ALGORITHM 36–1

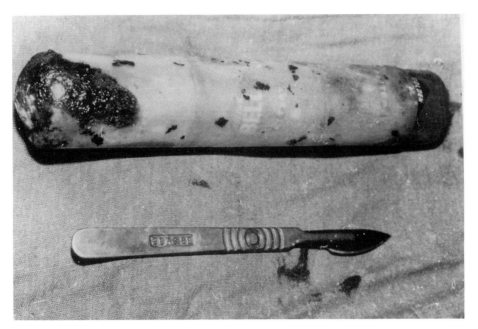

FIGURE 36–1 Three D-size batteries, wrapped in a hard plastic cover, recovered from the rectum. The knife is used for comparison to the size of the foreign body.

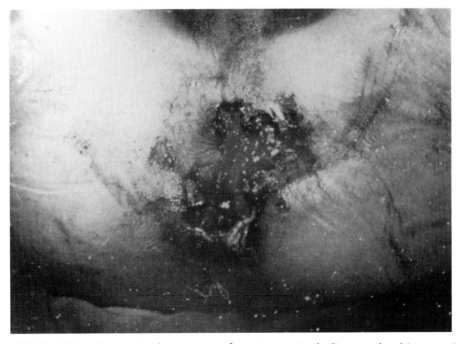

FIGURE 36–2 Extensive laceration of perineum, including anal sphincters, in a man bitten by a Dobermann dog.

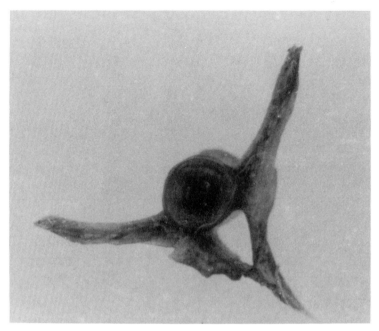

FIGURE 36–3 A fish bone that was impacted in lower third of the rectum.

useful to diagnose any other intraperitoneal injury, particularly to the urinary tract. A water-soluble (Hypaque) enema may be useful to exclude proximal colonic injury. Exploratory laparotomy is mandatory to evaluate whether a rectal lesion is intra- or extraperitoneal. In selected instances laparoscopy may be useful to avoid an exploratory laparotomy.

J. It may be intraperitoneal, with heavy contamination and associated pelvic injuries.

K. A proximal end colostomy must be constructed. Through the distal colonic end, a rectal washout with 5% iodopovidone solution is advisable. After repair of rectal and pelvic injuries drain the presacral space and perform a mucous fistula. An appropriate regime for the prophylaxis of infection is strongly recommended.

L. Contamination may be minimal without an associated pelvic injury.

M. Simple closure of the wound is followed by rectal washout. In these patients, when injury is produced by a firearm, we perform a resection and anastomosis, without a "protective" colostomy. Simple suture in wounds caused by firearms is very risky, due to the damage produced by the expansive wave around the orifice the bullet. The use of the intracolonic bypass (Coloshield™; Davis and Geck, Wayne NJ) may be considered, in order to avoid a "protective" colostomy.

N. Extraperitoneal lesions can be repaired either by the transanal route or through a posterior midline anococcygeal incision, without disturbing the anal sphincter complex, followed by rectal washout and prophylaxis of infection. If the site of the lesion cannot be reached by the transanal route, then a formal exploratory laparotomy should be performed.

BIBLIOGRAPHY

1. Allen-Mersh TG, Sprague DB, Mann CV, et al: Pelvic drainage after anterior resection of the rectum. *Dis Colon Rectum* 32:223–226, 1989.

2. Falcone RE, Wanamaker SR, Santanello SA, et al: Colorectal trauma: primary repair or anastomosis with intracolonic bypass vs. ostomy. *Dis Colon Rectum* 35:957–963, 1992.

3. Fallon WF Jr: The present role of colostomy in the management of trauma. *Dis Colon Rectum* 35:1094–1102, 1992.

4. Morgado PJ, Alfaro GR, Morgado PJ Jr, et al: Colon trauma: clinical staging for surgical decision making: analysis of 119 cases. *Dis Colon Rectum* 35:986–990, 1992.

5. Orsay CP, Merlotti G, Abcarian H, et al: Colorectal trauma. *Dis Colon Rectum* 32:188–190, 1989.

See also Chapters 1, 6, 37 and 59.

CHAPTER 37

Sexually Transmitted Diseases

Victor L. Modesto, M.D. and
Lester Gottesman, M.D.

Refer to Algorithm 37–1.

A. Anorectal complaints range from asymptomatic rectal discharge to associated pain, tenesmus, pruritus, bleeding, or simply the presence of an anal or perianal lesion (mass). Coexisting human immunodeficiency virus (HIV) infection influences the severity, transmission, and host response to a variety of sexually transmitted diseases (STDs). Treatment is often altered in the HIV+/AIDS patient. These patients can present with a different constellation of anorectal disorders than the non-HIV+ individual.

B. In 10–20% of cases of syphilis, a chancre may present as an anal ulcer and may mimic an anal fissure. Although classically solitary, they can present as multiple lesions and appear opposite each other as in a "mirror image" or "kissing" configuration.

C. The Venereal Disease Research Laboratory (VDRL) is a nontreponemal test that detects antibodies to a cholesterol-lecithin-cardiolipin antigen that cross-reacts with antibodies present in syphilitic patients. It is used predominately for screening, but false-positives do occur, especially with rheumatologic disorders. Therefore, it needs to be confirmed by the fluorescent-treponemal-antibody-absorbed test (FTA-ABS). The VDRL does vary according to disease activity; hence titers can reflect persistent disease or responsiveness to treatment. FTA-ABS is a *Treponema pallidum*-specific assay. It becomes positive earlier than does the VDRL and is confirmatory for syphilis. It remains positive throughout the patient's life and does not correlate with disease activity or response to treatment. Biopsy of the chancre will reveal spirochetes on dark-field examination.

D. The treatment for syphilis remains benzathine penicillin 2.4 million units IM (administered intramuscularly) as a single dose. Patients who present with late syphilis or neurosyphilis should be treated with 2.4 million units every 2 weeks for 3 consecutive doses. Those patients allergic to penicillin should be treated with either tetracycline or erythromycin, 500 mg 4 times a day (q.i.d.) for 15 days. Sexual partners during the preceding 12 months should be examined and treated. Follow-up testing with VDRL should be undertaken at 3-month intervals for 1 year or until proved noninfective by low titers.

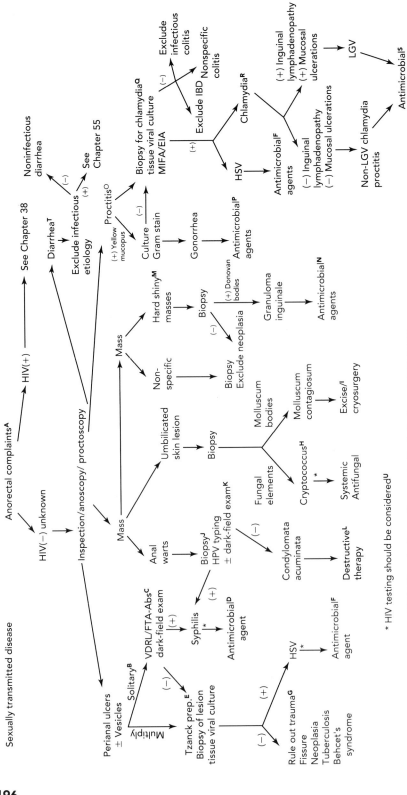

ALGORITHM 37-1

HPV = human papilloma virus
HSV = herpes simplex virus
HIV = human immunodeficiency virus
IBD = inflammatory bowel disease

MIFA/EIA = microimmunofluorescent antibody titre/enzyme immunoassay
VDRI = venereal disease research laboratories test
FTA-ABS = fluorescent treponemal-absorbed test antibodies
LGV = lymphogranuloma venereum

* HIV testing should be considered[U]

E. Scrapings of the ulcerations stained with Giemsa (Tzanck prep.) will reveal multinucleated giant cells typical of herpetic infection. Biopsy of the lesion will also reveal the typical giant cells or intranuclear inclusion bodies. Tissue viral culture will be positive in up to 90% of patients with active herpes infection.

F. No cure exists for herpes; however, antiviral agents, particularly acyclovir (ACV), will shorten the clinical course. The recommended dose of oral ACV is 200–400 mg 5 times daily for 10 days. In severe cases ACV can be intravenously administered at 5 mg/kg over 1 h every 8 h. Once the pain has abated, the patient should be discharged on a 10-day regimen of oral ACV. Recurrence can be a problem, so either early patient-initiated treatment or maintained suppressive dosing of 400 mg twice a day for 1 year is recommended. Acyclovir resistance has been seen not only in HIV+ patients but also in immunocompetent patients. Foscarnet can be used in ACV-resistant herpes; however, it can be administered only intravenously.

G. In the patient whose HIV status is unknown, the presence of perianal ulcerations that have tested negative for herpes or syphilis should suggest AIDS-related ulcers, anorectal malignancy, and tuberculosis. In HIV-negative patients, trauma, benign anal fissures, and Bechet's disease should be considered.

H. Cutaneous cryptococcal infection may mimic molluscum contagiosum in the HIV-positive patient.

I. Although the disease is benign and self-limiting, local destructive treatment with phenol injections, surgical removal, or cryotherapy can be used to prevent spread or for cosmetic purposes.

J. Squamous cell carcinoma (SCCA) of the anus can mimic condylomata acuminata, and both conditions have been known to coexist in the same patient; therefore, biopsy of some of the warts should be performed. Condylomata acuminata is caused by the human papilloma virus (HPV), and certain subtypes of the HPV are known to have oncogenic potential (types 16 and 18). Typing will identify those individuals at risk for subsequent development of SCCA.

K. Condylomata latum is a verrucous lesion of secondary syphilis and can mimic condylomata acuminata; the latter is characteristically more desiccated and keratinized; differentiation can be obtained by dark-field examination.

L. These warts are notorious for recurrence. Warts within the anal canal should be concomitantly treated to prevent recurrence. Treatment options include wart excision, fulguration with either electrocautery or laser, and cytodestruction with either podophyllin or bichloroacetic acid. Immunotherapy with autologous vaccine or interferon injection is usually reserved for recalcitrant or recurrent warts. Recurrence rates vary according to which modality is used. The authors prefer fulguration with electrocautery under either regional or local anesthesia.

M. Red and shiny hard masses located on the genitals or around the anorectum have been classically attributed to infection by a Gram-negative bacillus causing granuloma inguinale. Biopsy reveals Donovan bodies.

N. Effective antibiotic agents against granuloma inguinale include tetracycline 500 mg orally 4 times a day for 7 days or streptomycin 500–1000 mg IM twice a day.

O. A thick yellow mucopurulent discharge with or without proctitis is diagnostic of gonorrhea. Mucopus can be expressed from the anal crypts by gentle external pressure with the anoscope inserted. Gram stain obtained under direct visualization will be positive for gonococcus 79% of the time.

P. Because of the tremendous rise in the prevalence of penicillinase-producing strains of *Neisseria gonorrhea* (PPNG), ceftriaxone, 250 mg IM (single dose) followed by doxycycline 100 mg orally (PO) b.i.d. for 7 days is currently preferred. Alternative treatment includes spectinomycin, 2 g (IM as a single dose) or cefoxitin (IM) or ciprofloxacin (PO). Guidance from regional public health services should dictate therapeutic choices.

Q. Microimmunofluorescent antibody (MIFA) titer is the most sensitive serotyping test available for chlamydia, but is not universally available. The enzyme immunoassay (EIA) is the most commonly used test for diagnosing chlamydia. Antichlamydial antibody titers usually become positive after 1 month or more of active infection.

R. At present, 15 immunotypes of chlamydia are known. Serotypes D through K are responsible for lymphogranuloma venereum non-(LGV) chlamydial proctitis. Serotypes L_1, L_2, and L_3 are responsible for LGV.

S. Treatment of chlamydia is either with oral tetracycline or erythromycin, 500 mg q.i.d., which should extend for 7–14 days for non-LGV infections and for 21 days for LGV infections.

T. Many parasitic infections that were once considered unusual are now seen with increasing regularity in the homosexual and bisexual male population, spread via oral–anal intercourse.

U. Ulcerative perianal Herpes simplex virus (HSV)-2 disease, if present for at least 1 month in a patient with no other identifiable cause of immunodeficency, is diagnostic of AIDS. Several studies have shown a statistically significant association between herpes infection and subsequent HIV infection. The HSV must be recognized, not only as an ulcerative pathogen but also as a harbinger of HIV infection. Patients with STD should be screened for other sexually transmitted pathogens in addition to the HIV virus. Cutaneous cryptococcal infection is not seen in immunocompetent individuals; therefore, its presence should alert the physician to the presence of HIV infection.

BIBLIOGRAPHY

1. Dailey TH: Sexually transmitted diseases. *Seminars Colon Rectal Surg* 3:221–260, 1992.
2. Modesto VL, Gottesman L: Sexually transmitted diseases and anal manifestations of AIDS. *Surg Clin N Am* (in press).
3. Schmitt SL, Wexner SD. Colonic sexually transmitted diseases. *Seminars in Colon and Rectal Surgery*, 1992; 3:247–252.
4. Sim AJW, Wexner SD, Andrews HA. Sexually transmitted diseases in coloproctology. In: Keighley MRB, Williams NS (eds): *Surgery of the Anus, Rectum and Colon*. London: Belliere-Tindell, 1993; 2185–2222.
5. Wexner SD, Beck DE: Sexually transmitted and infectious diseases. In Beck DE, Wexner SD (eds): *Fundamentals of Anorectal Surgery*. New York: McGraw-Hill, 1992.
6. Wexner SD. Sexually transmitted disease of the colon, rectum & anus: the challenge of the nineties. *Dis Colon Rectum* 1990; 33:1048–1062.
7. Wexner SD, Beck DE. Sexually transmitted and infectious diseases. In: Beck DE, Wexner SD (eds): *Fundamentals of Anorectal Surgery*. New York: McGraw-Hill, 1992; 402–422.

See also Chapters 16, 38, 55.

CHAPTER 38

Anorectal Disease in AIDS

Thomas H. Dailey, M.D.

Refer to Algorithm 38–1.

1. Symptoms include pain, bleeding, drainage, diarrhea, mass, and pruritus.
2. Exam includes a digital rectal exam, inspection, anoscopy, and proctoscopy with biopsies.

A. *Neisseria gonorrhea.* Gonococcal proctitis is nonulcerating. The mucopurulent discharge is viscous and watery "mucopus." (See Chapter 37.)

B. *Syphilis.* Primary syphilis of the anal canal or the perianal skin occurs as an ulcer. It is seen almost exclusively in the anoreceptive homosexual male. The primary chancre may be single or multiple, painful or painless. The ulcers have a smooth base with raised borders and may be confused with fissures. Proctitis may occur with or without ulcerations. *Diagnostic test* (see Chapter 37): negative serology does not exclude syphilis. Immunocompromised patients may have a prolonged interval between acute infection and seroconversion. However, with the anal lesions of secondary syphilis, the serologic tests are almost always positive. *Treatment* (see Chapter 37): some experts advise that a treatment appropriate for neurosyphilis be used in HIV-infected patients.

C. *Chlamydia* (see Chapter 37). Lymphogranuloma venereum (LGV) causes a severe proctitis that may ulcerate. Serologic responses may be impaired in HIV disease; therefore, cultures from a rectal swab or from a mucosal biopsy specimen, in addition to the Frei test and complement fixation tests, should be performed.

D. *Shigella* is epidemic in the male homosexual population and in others with AIDS. It is sexually transmitted via the oral–fecal route. *Shigella flexneri* causes inflammation and ulceration of the mucosa of the rectosigmoid and presents with diarrhea. In AIDS patients, the disease may become systemic. All immunocompromised patients with stool cultures positive for shigella should be treated aggressively with antibiotics. *Treatment* is with bactrim/ampicillin/ciprofloxacin. Treatment should continue until the stool cultures are negative.

E. *Granuloma inguinale* is rare (see Chapter 37). The disease shows a cauliflower-like proliferation that may be ulcerated with sinuses and scarring.

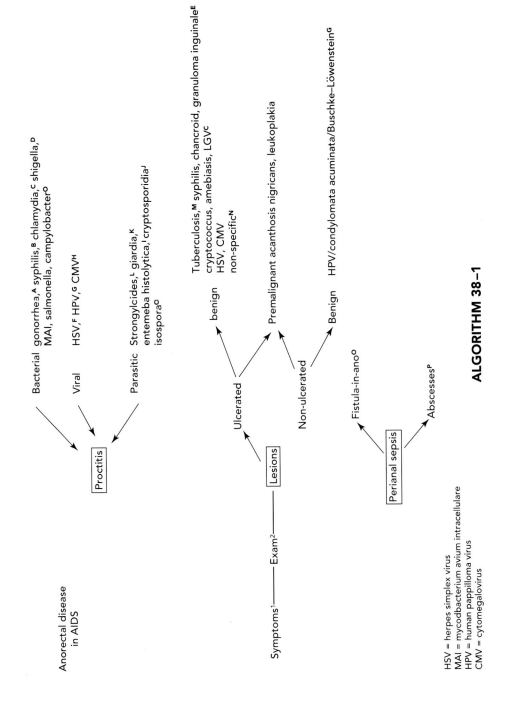

Anorectal disease
in AIDS

Symptoms[1] —— Exam[2]

Lesions

Proctitis

Bacterial gonorrhea,[A] syphilis,[B] chlamydia,[C] shigella,[D]
          MAI, salmonella, campylobacter[O]

Viral   HSV,[F] HPV,[G] CMV[H]

Parasitic Strongylcides,[L] giardia,[K]
          entemeba histolytica,[I] cryptosporidia[J]
          isospora[O]

Ulcerated — benign

Ulcerated — Premalignant acanthosis nigricans, leukoplakia

Tuberculosis,[M] syphilis, chancroid, granuloma inguinale[E]
cryptococcus, amebiasis, LGV[C]
HSV, CMV
non-specific[N]

Non-ulcerated — Benign HPV/condylomata acuminata/Buschke–Löwenstein[G]

Perianal sepsis

Fistula-in-ano[O]

Abscesses[P]

ALGORITHM 38–1

HSV = herpes simplex virus
MAI = mycodbacterium avium intracellulare
HPV = human pappilloma virus
CMV = cytomegalovirus

200

F. *Herpes simplex virus* (HSV) (see Chapter 37) is the most common cause of nongonococcal proctitis in the homosexual population. The perianal clusters of vesicles coalesce and ulcerate. In persons with AIDS, the infection may develop into a persistent ulcerative lesion. Acute infection may cause fever, severe constipation, urinary bladder obstruction, perianal, and/or abdominal pain. *Diagnosis* is made by culture swabs of the vesicle fluid using a viral Tzanck preparation. Biopsy of the ulcer is usually diagnostic. *Treatment:* oral acyclovir for prophylaxis and early symptoms; intravenous for severe local or systemic infections

G. *Human papilloma virus* (HPV) (see Chapter 37). The infection may be condylomatous, papular, or keratotic. Lesions may be small (condyloma acuminatum), or large (giant condyloma acuminatum or Buschke–Löwenstein tumor). HPV rarely causes proctitis. The virus and its lesions are 5–10 times more common in the AIDS patient. HPV types 6, 11, and 42 are more commonly associated with "benign" genital warts, whereas types 16, 18, and 33 are commonly associated with dysplastic lesions and carcinoma of the anus. *Diagnosis:* biopsy and hybridization typing of all lesions is recommended. *Treatment* depends on CDC (Centers for Disease Control, Atlanta, GA) staging: debulking and fulguration for early stages of AIDS. There is a high recurrence rate requiring multiple procedures. Biopsy of suspicious lesions in late stages of AIDS is mandatory. Immunotherapy (interferon) for external lesions shows promise.

H. *Cytomegalovirus* (CMV) causes a pancolitis or isolated ulcerations, erythematous patches, or multiple coalescing ulcers of the rectosigmoid. *Diagnosis:* biopsy reveals diagnostic inclusion bodies, 92% sensitive. Cultures are only 30% sensitive positive. Serologies may not be helpful because of the ubiquitous prevalence of the virus in the homosexual population.

I. *Amebiasis*—is a common STD in the homosexual population. It is common in the carrier state in the homosexual population. On proctoscopy, there are flask-shaped ulcerations of the rectal mucosa. It may cause a severe diffuse proctitis. *Diagnosis* is based on stool test for ova and parasites (O&P). *Treatment:* generic metronidazole. Follow-up is mandatory for patients and their sexual contacts.

J. *Cryptosporidia* is the most frequent pathogen in HIV-positive patients who have chronic diarrhea. It may cause a nonspecific proctitis. *Diagnosis* is based on the demonstration of the oocyte in the stool and/or mucosal histology. *Treatment:* no effective treatment is available.

K. *Giardiasis* causes an ulcerative proctitis. An increased incidence in the homosexual population results from oral–fecal contamination. *Diagnosis:* stool examination or rectal biopsy. *Treatment:* quinacrine hydrochloride/metronidazole.

L. *Strongyloides* may cause a proctitis. *Diagnosis:* stool for O&P. *Treatment:* mebendazole or piperazine.

M. *Tuberculosis.* In addition to the constitutional symptoms associated with the acid-fast bacilli (AFB), it may cause superficial circumferential ulcers of fissures of the anorectum and perianal skin. The disease may reactivate in immunosuppressed patients. *Diagnosis:* tuberculin skin test may yield false-positive reaction from a nontuberculous mycobacterium. The patient may be anergic. Cultures and biopsy of the ulcers are diagnostic. *Treatment:* Isoniazid (INH)/rifampin/pyrazinamide/ethambutol long-term.

N. Non-specific—Anorectal ulcerations that are "idiopathic" respond to intralesional or systemic steroids. The patients should have exam under anesthesia (EUA), biopsies, cultures, and wide debridement and drainage of any deep septic foci. Culture and biopsy of the ulcers are usually nondiagnostic.

O. *Fistula-in-ano.* Because of advanced immunosuppression, AIDS patients may not heal well. Surgery should be carefully tailored to avoid extensive operations. Liberal use of setons and aggressive drainage is encouraged. Abscesses and fistulas usually heal with appropriate conventional operations.

P. *Abscesses.* Drainage in AIDS patients should be done early with adequate drainage through a conservative but adequate incision. Cultures and biopsy are recommended at the time of drainage.

BIBLIOGRAPHY

1. Cohen SM, Schmitt SL, Lucas FV, et al: The diagnosis of anal ulcers in AIDS patients. *Int J Colorect Dis,* 9:169–173, 1994.

2. Connolly MG, Hawkins DA: Proctitis. In Allen-Mersh TG, Gottesman L (eds): *Anorectal Disease in AIDS.* London: Arnold, 1991.

3. Corman LM: Infectious and non-infectious colitides. In Corman LM (ed): *Colon and Rectal Surgery,* 2nd ed. Philadelphia: Lippincott, 1993.

4. Schmitt SL, Wexner SD, Nogueras JJ, et al: Is aggressive management of perianal ulcers in HIV positive patients justifiable? *Dis Colon Rectum,* 36:240–246, 1993.

5. Sim AJW, Wexner SD, Andrews HA. Sexually transmitted disease in coloproctology. In: Keighley MRB, Williams NS (eds): *Surgery of the Anus, Rectum and Colon.* London: Belliere-Tindall 1993; 2185–2222.

6. Soler ME, Gottesman L: Anal and rectal ulceration. In Allen-Mersh TG, Gottesman L (eds): *Anorectal Disease in AIDS.* London: Arnold, 1991.

7. Veidenheimer MC, Dailey TH (eds): Sexually transmitted diseases. *Seminars in Colon Rectal Surg* 3(4):221–259, 1992.

8. Weiss EG, Wexner SD. Surgery for anal lesions in HIV infected patients. *Ann Med* (in press).

See also Chapters 37 and 55.

CHAPTER 39

Necrotizing Infections of the Perineum

Ian G. Finlay, F.R.C.S.

Refer to Algorithm 39–1.

A. Necrotizing infections of soft tissues are uncommon rather than rare. Most surgeons will be required to diagnose and treat such an infection within their working life. Occasionally an "epidemic" will occur after natural disasters such as earthquakes or volcanic eruptions. Although recognized from antiquity, the first clear description of necrotizing soft tissue infection occurred during the United States Civil War when it was named "hospital gangrene." The condition was subsequently described in the male genitalia by Fournier in 1883 and as a more generalized condition by Meleney in 1924. Initially Meleney implicated the β-hemolytic streptococcus as the etiologic agent but later recognized that there may be synergy with anaerobic streptococcus and staphylococcus. Since then, many organisms have been implicated in necrotizing infections, usually in combination. These bacteria include Gram-negative aerobic bacilli, anaerobic streptococci, bacteroides species, coliforms, and clostridia, to name only a few. Although attempts have been made to classify necrotizing infections, according to the infecting agent, many clinicians continue to use either the terms "Meleney's synergistic gangrene" or "necrotizing fasciitis." A clearer and clinically useful classification, however, has recently been proposed comprising three groups:

1. *Necrotizing cellulitis.* These skin lesions are caused by a single organism, usually the group A streptococcus. The subcutaneous tissue is spared.

2. *Necrotizing fasciitis.* Infection is initially of the subcutaneous tissue with relative sparing of the skin until the disease progresses. The muscle and muscle fascia are not involved. Invariably fasciitis is polymocrobial in origin with synergy between aerobic and anaerobic organisms.

3. *Myonecrosis* (gas gangrene). Caused by clostridial species, primarily *Clostridium perfringens.* Involves muscle fascia. Although necrotizing

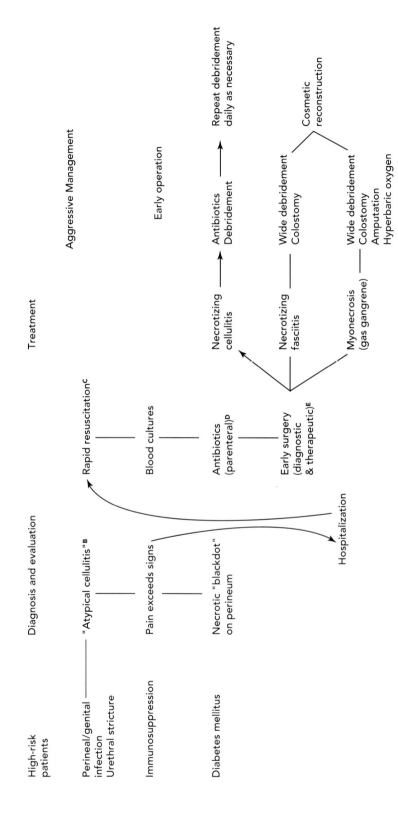

Necrotizing infections of the perineum[A]

High-risk patients — Diagnosis and evaluation — Treatment — Aggressive Management

Perineal/genital infection
Urethral stricture ——— "Atypical cellulitis"[B] ——— Rapid resuscitation[C]

Immunosuppression

Pain exceeds signs ——— Blood cultures

Diabetes mellitus ——— Necrotic "blackdot" on perineum

Hospitalization

Antibiotics (parenteral)[D]

Early surgery (diagnostic & therapeutic)[E]

Early operation

Necrotizing cellulitis ——→ Antibiotics → Debridement → Repeat debridement daily as necessary

Necrotizing fasciitis ——— Wide debridement Colostomy

Myonecrosis (gas gangrene) ——— Wide debridement Colostomy Amputation Hyperbaric oxygen

Cosmetic reconstruction

ALGORITHM 39–1

204

infections may occur at any site in the body, they are particularly common in the perineum, arising from perianal, ischiorectal, supralevator, and labial infections. If infections arising from the lower end of the genitourinary tract are included, then approximately 75% of necrotizing infections occur at this site. Debilitated and immunocompromised patients are particularly at risk, including those with diabetes, alcoholism, leukemia, major burns, AIDS, and prolonged antibiotic therapy.

B. *Clinical features.* The clinical features in necrotizing infections are similar in all patients. In the early stages, skin signs are minimal but pain is disproportionate to these signs. Disease progression brings subcutaneous edema with relative anesthesia related to the underlying necrosis. Only in the late stages is there skin blistering, crepitus, and necrosis. The rate of progression, however, is unpredictable, varying from a few hours to several days. Without treatment the condition progresses, invariably to septicemic shock, multiorgan failure, and death. Histologically, patients have inflammation and necrosis extending from the epidermis to the subcutaneous fat and fascia. There is widespread destruction and liquefaction of the fat. Although gas is present in the subcutaneous tissue, the muscle and skin are spared in necrotizing fasciitis. The severity of the necrotizing process has been positively correlated with the degree of thrombosis. This is the key pathologic event that explains the potential for rapid extension and the failure of the condition to respond to antibiotics. Those patients who exhibit rapid deterioration to death invariably have evidence of disseminated intravascular coagulation (DIC).

C. *Diagnosis and treatment.* The mainstay of diagnosis and treatment is a high degree of clinical suspicion and early radical surgical debridement. Blood cultures are positive in only 50% of patients, while microscopy of subcutaneous aspirates are similarly unreliable. Finding clostridial organisms in the blood does not necessarily indicate myonecrosis, whereas absence of these species does not exclude it. Since shock and multiorgan failure are common, general and rapid resuscitative measures are necessary.

D. Broad-spectrum antibiotics are mandatory, although there is no evidence that they prevent disease progression. The Public Health Laboratory Service suggests benzyl penicillin (2.4 g q.4hour), Clindamycin (0.6–1.2 q.6h) with an aminoglycoside for enterobacter cover. Although hyperbaric oxygen is strongly advocated by some, the benefits have been questioned by others. If a hyperbaric unit is readily available, it may be worth using, but not if interhospital transfer would delay definitive surgery. Both necrotizing fasciitis and myonecrosis are approved for hyperbaric oxygen therapy by the Under Sea and Hyperbaric Medical Society and are recognized for reimbursement by the Federal Health Care Finances Administration.

E. Radical surgery is the key to successful management. Surgical exploration is also the main diagnostic tool when gray edematous fat is found that readily strips off the underlying fascia. Debridement of all the affected subcutaneous fat with overlying skin is required, leading to potentially disfiguring wounds. It is crucial, however, to obtain adequate clearance, irrespective of the area involved. In the presence of myonecrosis, amputation may be required. Where there is extensive debridement of perineal skin, a temporary colostomy may be necessary. Further second-look procedures have been advocated. Meticulous wound care and dressing changes are then required and, when the wound is clean and granulating, skin grafting. Using these principles of aggressive surgery in early disease, death rates are less than 10%. Delay, however, and mortality rises to 30–60% for necrotizing fasciitis and 80% for gas gangrene.

BIBLIOGRAPHY

1. Barker FG, Leppard BJ, Seal BV: Streptococcal necrotizing fasciitis. Comparison between histological and clinical features. *J Clin Path* 40:335–341, 1987.
2. Beck DE, Wexner SD (eds). *Fundamentals of Anorectal Surgery*. New York: McGraw-Hill, 1992.
3. Burge TS: Hyperbaric oxygen—still unproved in necrotizing fasciitis. *BMJ* 307:936, 1993.
4. Clayton MD, Fowler JE, Sharifi R, et al: Causes, presentation and survival of 57 patients with necrotizing fasciitis of the male genitalia. *SGO* 170:49–55, 1990.
5. Fournier JA. Gangrene foudrouant de la verge. *Semaine Med* 3:345, 1883.
6. Giuliano A, Lewis F, Hadley K, Blalsdell FW: Bacteriology of necrotizing fasciitis. *Am J Surg* 134:52, 1977.
7. Jones J: Investigation upon the nature, causes and treatment of hospital gangrene: 1861–65, United States Sanitary Commission, Memoirs: Surgical 2, Hamilton FH (ed). New York Riverside Press 146–170, 1871.
8. Kindwall EP: Hyperbaric oxygen. *BMJ* 307:515–516, 1993.
9. Meleney FL: Hemolytic streptococcus gangrene. *Arch Surg* 9:341, 1924.
10. Meleny FL: A differential diagnosis between certain types of infectious gangrene of the skin. *SGO* 57:847, 1933.
11. Patino JF, Castro D: Nectotizing lesions of soft tissues: a review. *World J Surg* 15:235–239, 1991.
12. Pruitt BA: Burns and soft tissues. In *Infection and the Surgical Patient,* Clinical Surgery International, Vol 4, Polk HC, Jr; Ed Churchill Livingston 113–131, 1982.
13. Risenang A, Samboni WA, Curtis A, et al: Hyperbaric oxygen therapy for necrotizing fasciitis—reduced mortality and the need for debridement. *Surg* 108:847–50, 1990.
14. Simmons RL, Ahrenholz DH: Infections of the skin and soft tissues. In *Surgical Infectious Diseases,* second edition. Ed RJ Howard, Simmons RL: Norwalk, Appleton & Lange, 404–408, 1988.
15. Ward RG, Walsh MS: Necrotizing fasciitis: 10 years' experience in a district general hospital. *Br J Surg* 78:488–489, 1991.
See also Chapter 7.

CHAPTER 40

Idiopathic Proctitis

William B. Ruderman, M.D.

Refer to Algorithm 40-1.

A. One of the typical features of ulcerative proctitis is rectal bleeding. Loose, frequent stools can occur as well, although true diarrhea is uncommon. Fecal urgency and tenesmus are characteristic symptoms of distal colonic inflammation. Since proctitis is a limited process, systemic symptoms such as fever, malaise, and weight loss are usually absent. Attention to historic features such as recent travel, prior broad-spectrum antibiotic use, sexual behavior, and prior radiation therapy is critical in assessing the differential of nonspecific ulcerative proctitis.

B. Laboratory testing is useful in excluding other conditions and should include a routine stool ova and parasite (O&P) testing, and culture. *Clostridium difficile* toxin should be obtained if there has been previous administration of broad spectrum antibiotics. Specialized testing including viral, chlamydia, and *Neisseria* gonorrheal cultures, serology titers, wet prep stool examination, and dark-field examination for syphilis can be obtained on the basis of appropriate historic and endoscopic information.

C. Proctosigmoidoscopy is the diagnostic test of choice. Distal mucosal inflammation is the hallmark feature of proctitis. Endoscopic features of erythema, edema, friability, and granularity should extend proximally from the dentate line, with an abrupt transition between normal proximal and distal involved rectum. Grading can be based on the severity of visible features. Mucosal exudate and ulceration are suggestive of more severe disease. If a transition zone to normal tissue is appreciated, then colonoscopy is generally unnecessary. Pathologic biopsy can suggest specific etiologies such as pseudomembranous colitis, Crohn's disease, radiation, or ischemia.

D. With the appropriate testing, known causes of nonspecific proctitis can be excluded. Once the diagnosis has been established, a treatment plan can be initiated. Idiopathic proctitis usually follows a benign course. About 15% of patients will have only a single disease episode, while about 75% will follow a

Clinical presentation[A]
Rectal bleeding
Urgency, tenesmus
Associated history

Laboratory[B]
Stool ova and parasite, culture
clostridium-difficile toxin

Proctosiqmoidoscopy[C]
Biopsy

→ Idiopathic proctitis[D]

Topical therapy[E]
5-ASA
Hydrocortisone
4-8 weeks

Resolved → Disease-free—Observe[F]

Resolved ← Relapse—retreat
Topical[G]

Refractory

Resolved → Maintenance[I] → Oral
5-ASA
→ Topical
5-ASA

Refractory → Oral 5-ASA[H]

Resolved → Maintenance[I] → Oral
5-ASA
→ Topical
5-ASA

Refractory—oral
steroids
4–8 weeks

Resolved → Maintenance[I]

Refractory → Cyclosporin-A[J]
enema?
→ Proctocolectomy[K]

ALGORITHM 40–1

5-ASA = 5 aminosalicylic acid

course of intermittent symptomatic relapses. Approximately 10–15% will develop extension of their disease beyond the rectum, with extension into the sigmoid or descending colon being more common than the development of pancolitis. Since idiopathic proctitis is usually a benign illness, treatment should be directed towards suppression of local inflammation and control of symptoms.

E. The initial treatment of choice is topical therapy with either a corticosteroid such as hydrocortisone, or a 5-aminosalicylic acid (5-ASA) preparation given either in enema, foam, or suppository form. Treatment for 4–8 weeks will result in symptomatic improvements in 70–90% of patients. Administration of 5-ASA enemas in a prolonged course of up to several months of therapy can result in the induction of remission in 80–90% of patients, even in those previously refractory to topical hydrocortisone. In the future an additional therapeutic option may include newer corticosteroids with less systemic effects such as budesonide, or tixocortol pivalate.

F. For the patient in remission after a first course of therapy, observation alone is reasonable without maintenance therapy. This course of action will be successful in approximately 10–15% of patients with idiopathic proctitis.

G. Intermittent disease exacerbations will occur in two-thirds of patients. However, retreatment with topical therapy usually is quite satisfactory and results in disease remission in the majority of individuals.

H. For those individuals who do not respond to topical therapy, another option is that of the oral 5-ASA preparations. These drugs include either oral sulfasalazine or the newer forms of delayed-release 5-ASA compounds. In limited studies oral agents appear to have an efficacy similar to that of topical 5-ASA.

I. For those patients with relapsing disease, maintenance therapy is beneficial once remission has been reinduced. Effective regimens include both oral and topical 5-ASA preparations. Maintenance regimens with topical 5-ASA have been shown to reduce the 1-year relapse rate from 80% to 20%. Topical 5-ASA can be administered on an every other day, or even on a less frequent basis. Oral 5-ASA maintenance dosages usually are about half of the drug dosage given for active disease. Optimal maintenance regimens have yet to be adequately defined, and empiric dosage adjustment may be needed. Truly refractory idiopathic proctitis is uncommon. However, an oral corticosteroid regimen is useful in those patients with intractable disease. Typical treatment duration with oral corticosteroids is 4–8 weeks with gradual tapering thereafter. There is no documented benefit to a combination regimen of topical and oral corticosteroids.

J. For truly refractory patients, an intriguing experimental regimen has been that of cyclosporin-A enemas. Rectal absorption appears to be limited, and efficacy has been demonstrated in about 50% of patients refractory to other forms of medical therapy.

K. In only a few patients, incapacitating symptoms will persist despite all attempts at medical therapy. In these individuals with prolonged refractory disease, surgical intervention can be curative. Colon-sparing operations have been attempted, but proximal disease extension is quite common after distal resection requiring completion colectomy in the majority of patients. Therefore, if surgery is necessary for refractory proctitis, proctocolectomy should be performed.

BIBLIOGRAPHY

1. Biddle WL, Greenberger NJ, Swan JT, et al: 5-Aminosalicylic acid enemas: effective agent in maintaining remission in left-sided ulcerative colitis. *Gastroenterology* 94:1075, 1988.

2. Biddle WL, Miner PB Jr: Long-term use of mesalamine enemas to induce remission in ulcerative colitis. *Gastroenterology* 99:113, 1990.

3. Cobden I, Al-Mardini H, Zaitoun A, et al: Is topical therapy necessary in acute distal colitis? Double-blind comparison of high-dose oral mesalamine versus steroid enemas in the treatment of active distal ulcerative colitis. *Aliment Pharmacol Ther* 5:513, 1991.

4. Keighley MRB: Ulcerative proctitis. In Keighley MRB and Williams NS (eds): *Surgery of the Anus, Rectum, and Colon.* Philadelphia: Saunders, 1993, Vol 2, p 1324.

5. LaRosa D, Rubin PH, Bodian C, et al: Maintenance oral sulfasalazine prolongs remission in ulcerative proctitis and proctosigmoiditis. *Am J Gastroenterol* 86:1456, 1991.

6. Powell-Tuck J, Ritchie JK, Lennard-Jones JE: The prognosis of idiopathic proctitis. *Scand J Gastroenterol* 12:727, 1977.

7. Thomson ABR: Review article: New developments in the use of 5-aminosalicylic acid in patients with inflammatory bowel disease. *Aliment Pharmacol Ther* 5:449, 1991.

See also Chapters 51, 52 and 55.

CHAPTER 41

Radiation Proctitis

James W. Fleshman, M.D.

Refer to Algorithm 41-1.

A. Radiation injury to the rectum occurs most frequently after radiation therapy for gynecologic (cervical, uterine) or prostate malignancy. The incidence of proctitis after irradiation of the prostate is reported as 4-12%. Proctitis after irradiation of the uterus and cervix occurs in up to 75% of patients. The development of radiation proctitis is dose-dependent [0% < 4000 cGy (centi-gray units of absorbed radiation dose), 20% at 6000 cGy, 18-60% at 7000 cGy]. The proximity of the prostate and the cervix to the anterior rectal wall causes radiation injury to the rectum most commonly in that area. Other factors that predispose a patient to proctitis include diabetes, hypertension, advanced age, previous pelvic surgery, and previous pelvic irradiation.

B. Acute proctitis occurs in virtually all patients during the radiation treatment period and usually resolves within 6 months after completion of the treatments. The proctitis is a direct result of the toxic effect of the radiation on the mucosal cells of the rectum, which are themselves rapidly dividing. The symptoms include diarrhea, mucus production, bleeding, cramps, rectal pain, tenesmus, and incomplete evacuation.

C. Chronic radiation effect to the rectum occurs after a period of several months to years following irradiation of the rectum. Complications of late radiation-induced proctitis include bleeding from telangiectatic vessels or ulceration, stricture, rectovaginal fistula, diarrhea, and incontinence due to a noncompliant rectum and poor anal sphincter function. The frequency of chronic bowel injury is dependent on the radiation dose and occurs in 5-75% of patients.

D. A thorough history and physical examination will usually provide the diagnosis of radiation proctitis. The differential diagnosis includes *Clostridium difficile* colitis, inflammatory bowel disease, rectal neoplasm (villous adenoma or cancer), or other infectious colitides. Proctoscopy reveals mucosal erythema and edema, friable mucosa with easy bleeding, ulceration, and occasionally focal

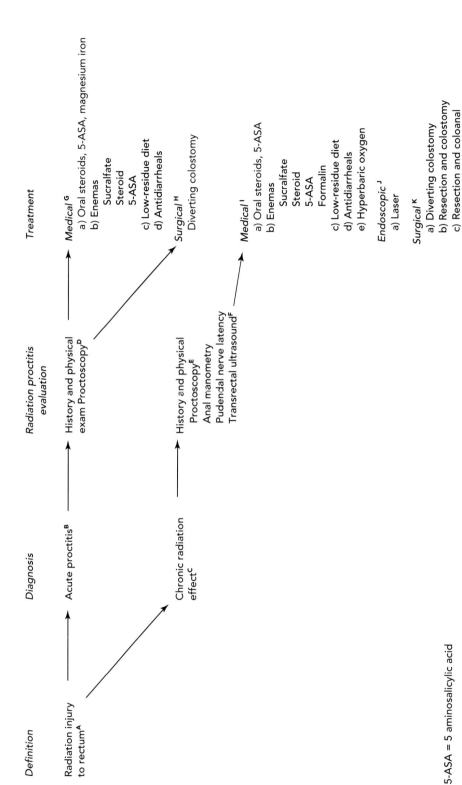

Definition

Radiation injury to rectum[A]

Diagnosis

Acute proctitis[B]

Chronic radiation effect[C]

Radiation proctitis evaluation

History and physical exam Proctoscopy[D]

History and physical
Proctoscopy[E]
Anal manometry
Pudendal nerve latency
Transrectal ultrasound[F]

Treatment

Medical[G]
a) Oral steroids, 5-ASA, magnesium iron
b) Enemas
   Sucralfate
   Steroid
   5-ASA
c) Low-residue diet
d) Antidiarrheals

Surgical[H]
Diverting colostomy

Medical[I]
a) Oral steroids, 5-ASA
b) Enemas
   Sucralfate
   Steroid
   5-ASA
   Formalin
c) Low-residue diet
d) Antidiarrheals
e) Hyperbaric oxygen

Endoscopic[J]
a) Laser

Surgical[K]
a) Diverting colostomy
b) Resection and colostomy
c) Resection and coloanal
   anastomosis

5-ASA = 5 aminosalicylic acid

ALGORITHM 41–1

areas of necrosis. The extent (length of affected rectum) and nature of the proctitis should be documented. A note of rectal distensibility may be helpful in understanding other symptoms. Biopsy of the anterior rectum should be performed with care to avoid the development of an iatrogenic rectovaginal fistula.

E: A history and physical examination should include details of the maximum radiation dose, predominant symptoms, and any previous treatment. The differential diagnosis is the same as for acute proctitis and always includes recurrence of the original cancer. Proctoscopy will reveal findings consistent with the presenting symptom:

1. Bleeding: telangiectatic vessels in the mucosa; ulceration with fibrotic base and friable bleeding edges.

2. Stricture: fibrotic noncompliant rectum with a firm stenotic area. The length of the stricture varies with the length of the most intensely radiated portion of the rectum. An ulcer is usually present on the anterior rectum within or near the stricture.

3. Rectovaginal fistula: an ulcer with a fibrotic base is seen on the anterior rectal wall. An opening extends to the posterior vagina at the level of the cervix. The rectal mucosa is usually thinned and the rectal wall noncompliant and nondistensible. Rectal biopsy often precedes the development of a fistula.

F. Evaluation of the anal sphincter is essential if a rectal resection and reanastomosis is planned. Anal manometry allows objective definition of anal canal pressures. Pudendal nerve terminal motor latency quantitates pudendal nerve injury in the pelvis. Radiation may effect the nerve at the presacral plexus of S2-4 or in the lateral pelvis at Alcock's canal at the level of the ischial spine. Ultrasound of the anal canal provides an anatomic definition of the internal and external anal sphincter. It is useful to distinguish global muscle dysfunction due to radiation from a defined mechanical defect from obstetric trauma, fistulotomy or trauma.

G. Medical therapy for acute radiation proctitis is usually directed toward control of the symptoms of diarrhea, tenesmus, and bleeding. Sucralfate, steroid, and 5-aminosalicylic acid (5-ASA) enemas have all been reported to promote resolution of proctitis, but no single regimen has been shown to be universally successful relative to either no preparation or symptomatic resolution. There may be an advantage to sucralfate enemas since they are inexpensive and result in a good clinical response (Table 41-1).

H. Acute radiation proctitis that is severe enough to cause massive bleeding, intractable diarrhea, or necrosis of the rectum is rare. In these circumstances, a diverting colostomy and continued local therapy is the safest approach. Definitive surgical therapy is extremely dangerous in the acute phase of radiation. Resection and restoration of rectal function should be postponed until the acute changes of radiation resolve, approximately 5-10 weeks to 6 months after treatment. The symptoms of tenesmus and pain and the progression of an ulcer may not be altered by a diverting colostomy.

TABLE 41–1 SUCRALFATE ENEMAS

Enema preparations	Frequency of Administration
Prednisolone 20 mg in 60-cc enema	b.i.d.
Betamethasone 5 mg in 60-cc enema	b.i.d.
5-ASA 4 g in 60-cc enema	b.i.d.
Sucralfate 2 g in 20-cc enema	b.i.d.
Oral preparations	
Prednisone 40 mg PO	q.d.
Sulfasalazine 1 tablet PO	t.i.d.
Dipentum 400 mg PO	t.i.d.

I. Medical therapy for chronic radiation proctitis is similar to therapy for acute proctitis; the results are also similar. The use of 3.6% formalin enemas for treatment of bleeding in chronic radiation proctitis has been reported with good results. However, diffuse destruction of the rectal mucosa should be undertaken with care. Focal "swabbing" of the bleeding mucosa with Formalin may be as effective and safer. Steroid, sucralfate, and 5-ASA enemas should be tried first. Recent reports suggest hyperbaric oxygen treatments may be beneficial in the treatment of both diffuse hemorrhagic chronic proctitis and necrotic or fibrotic bleeding ulcers in chronic proctitis. A treatment regimen of 90 min at 2.5 atmospheres (atm) twice daily has been reported.

J. Bleeding from chronic radiation proctitis may be from telangiectatic vessels or necrotic ulceration. Laser therapy for the control of bleeding is usually successful but may require multiple applications. Laser therapy should be reserved for the treatment of hemorrhage requiring transfusion. The effect of laser ablation may be to create ulceration of the already fragile rectal mucosa. Deep penetration of the laser energy is to be avoided. Nd:YAG (neodymium:yttrium aluminum garnet) lasers have been used more often but reports of the use of more superficially penetrating Argon laser suggest less trauma with equal results (Table 41–2).

K. Only 2–10% of patients with radiation proctitis and complications thereof require operation. The surgical therapy of chronic radiation proctitis should be tailored to address the specific complication(s). Diverting colostomy has been shown to be a temporizing procedure yielding temporary relief of diarrhea, incontinence, and bleeding. Bleeding usually recurs and requires resection if it is unable to be controlled by laser or enema. Stricture and rectovaginal fistula may be amenable to low anterior resection and reanastomosis if the damaged area is more proximal in the rectum. Alternatively a total proctectomy with mucosal stripping to the level of the radiation damage with a coloanal pull-through and hand-sewn anastomosis at the dentate line is required. A protective loop ileostomy is usually recommended. Radiation change in the pelvis makes this procedure a very difficult one with much blood loss, and high likelihood of ureteral and bladder injury. For these reasons, it may be safer to perform a distal Hartmann procedure with a permanent colostomy to remove the bleeding source. If a coloanal anastomosis is performed, the proximal

TABLE 41-2 LASER THERAPY

Nd:YAG	40-W · s pulses up to 4000–5000 in 2–3 s
	Avoid circumferential treatment; destroy vessels in a circle around the telangiectasia rather than "painting" the malformation
Argon	40-W · s pulses up to 1500 in 0.5–5.0 s

bowel component of the anastomosis must be nonirradiated tissue, and the sphincter mechanism must be deemed adequate by preoperative evaluation. The operative morbidity for surgical therapy of radiation proctitis ranges from 20 to 80%. The use of intraoperative ureteric stents is helpful.

BIBLIOGRAPHY

1. Alexander TJ, Dwyer RM: Endoscopic Nd:YAG laser treatment of severe radiation injury of the lower gastrointestinal tract: long-term follow-up. *Gastrointerol Endosc* 34:407–411, 1988.

2. Allen-Mersh TG, Wilson EJ, Hope-Stone HF, et al: The management of late radiation-induced rectal injury after treatment of carcinoma of the uterus. *Surg Gyn Obst* 164:521–524, 1987.

3. Charneau J, Bouachour G, Person B, et al: Severe hemorrhagic radiation proctitis advancing to gradual cessation with hyperbaric oxygen. *Dig Dis Sci* 36:373–357, 1991.

4. Gazet J–C: Parks' coloanal pull-through anastomosis for severe, complicated radiation proctitis. *Dis Colon Rectum* 28:110–114, 1985.

5. Jacobs M: YAG laser treatment for radiation proctitis (letter). *Gastrointerol Endosc* 35:355–356, 1989.

6. Jao S–W, Beart RW Jr, Gunderson LL: Surgical treatment of radiation injuries of the colon and rectum. *Am J Surg* 151:272–227, 1986.

7. Jagelman DG, Rothenberger DA, Wexner SD. Irradiation injuries to the intestine. In: Schrock T (ed): *Perspectives in Colon and Rectal Surgery.* St. Louis: *Quality Medical Publishing* 3:275–296, 1991.

8. Kochhar R, Patel F, Dhar A, et al: Radiation-induced proctosigmoiditis: prospective, randomized, double-blind controlled trial of oral sulfasalazine plus rectal steroids versus rectal sucralfate. *Dig Dis Sci* 36:103–107, 1991.

9. Kochhar R, Sharma SC, Gupta BB, et al: Rectal sucralfate in radiation proctitis (letter). *Lancet* 8607:400,1988.

10. Lucarotti ME, Mountford RA, Bartolo DCC: Surgical management of intestinal radiation injury. *Dis Colon Rectum* 34:865–869, 1991.

11. Rubinstein E, Ibsen T, Rasmussen RB, et al: Formalin treatment of radiation-induced hemorrhagic proctitis. *Am J Gastroenterol* 81:44–45, 1986.

12. Saclarides T, King D, Franklin J, et al: Formalin instillation for refractory radiation-induced hemorrhagic proctitis. *Dis Colon Rectum,* April 1995 (Abstract).

13. Seow-Choen F, Goh HS, Eu KW, et al: A simple and effective treatment for hemorrhagic radiation proctitis using formalin. *Dis Colon Rectum* 36:135–138, 1993.

See also Chapters 51, 52 and 55.

CHAPTER 42

Unhealed Perineal Wounds

Harry K. Moon, M.D. David Caminer, M.D. and
J. Brian Boyd, M.D.

Refer to Algorithm 42–1.

A. *Assessment.* The etiology of most perineal wounds is usually known and the problem is one of reconstruction. History, physical examination, and special investigations are rarely concerned with forming a diagnosis, but rather serve as indicators of the patient's general health, reveal the extent of previous surgery, and allow estimation of the size and position of the defect. The wound is assessed for the size of the skin defect as well as the loss of bulk. The condition of the surrounding skin is noted and the wound bed examined for the presence of necrotic tissue, exposed bone or a fistulous communication with the rectum, vagina, or urinary tract. A rectal examination is undertaken in men and a bimanual examination, in women. Finally, potential donor sites for local or distant tissue are reviewed. Examination under anesthesia may be performed in complex cases but is usually unnecessary. Special investigations of use in deeper complex wounds include a sinogram, fistulogram, computerized tomography (CT), and magnetic resonance imaging (MRI). These investigations will assess depth and extent of the wound and if there is any involvement of adjacent organs. A bone scan may help determine whether there is osteomyelitis involving the pelvic bone.

If adjacent organ involvement is found, appropriate consultations should be sought.

B. *Infective wounds. Fournier's gangrene,* a necrotizing infection of the perineum, groin, and genitalia, was described by Fournier in 1887. The causative agents consist of staphylococcus aureus together with microaerophilic streptococcus or *Klebsiella, E. coli,* enterococci, proteus, or citrobacter. Because of the prevalence of 2 or more species of bacteria, the term "synergistic gangrene" has been used. Necrotizing perineal infection is a life-threatening disease. Treatment is as follows:

1. Provide broad-spectrum antibiotic cover (e.g., metronidazole plus clindamycin)
2. Provide tetanus prophylaxis.

217

Perineal Wounds

No box — reason
[ ] — decision

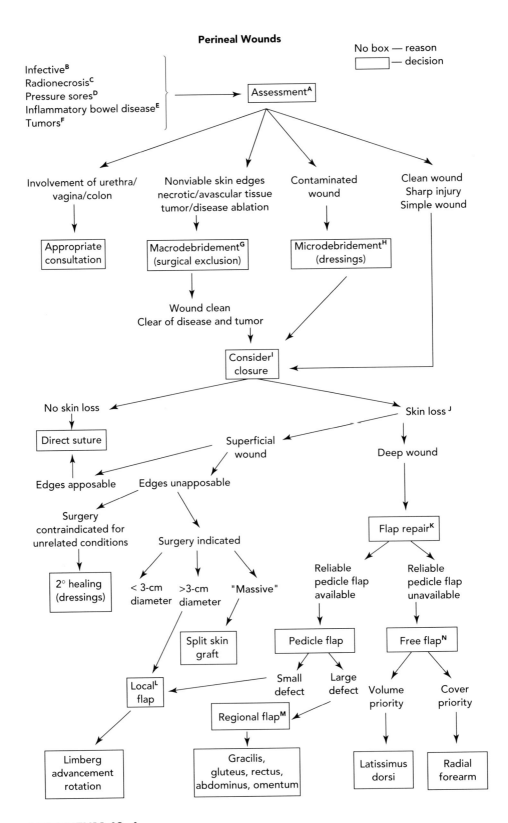

Infective[B]
Radionecrosis[C]
Pressure sores[D]
Inflammatory bowel disease[E]
Tumors[F]

Assessment[A]

Involvement of urethra/vagina/colon

Nonviable skin edges necrotic/avascular tissue tumor/disease ablation

Contaminated wound

Clean wound
Sharp injury
Simple wound

Appropriate consultation

Macrodebridement[G] (surgical exclusion)

Microdebridement[H] (dressings)

Wound clean
Clear of disease and tumor

Consider[I] closure

No skin loss

Skin loss[J]

Direct suture

Superficial wound

Deep wound

Edges apposable

Edges unapposable

Surgery contraindicated for unrelated conditions

Surgery indicated

Flap repair[K]

Reliable pedicle flap available

Reliable pedicle flap unavailable

2° healing (dressings)

< 3-cm diameter

>3-cm diameter

"Massive"

Pedicle flap

Free flap[N]

Split skin graft

Small defect

Large defect

Volume priority

Cover priority

Local[L] flap

Regional flap[M]

Limberg advancement rotation

Gracilis, gluteus, rectus, abdominus, omentum

Latissimus dorsi

Radial forearm

ALGORITHM 42–1

3. Debride the infected area until a point is reached where the fascia is no longer separated from the subcutaneous tissue.

4. Apply betadine or saline dressings 4 times daily until the area is clean.

5. Reconstruct skin and soft tissue loss. If gross fecal contamination of the wound exists, a temporary colostomy must be considered.

Three infectious conditions are described here:

- *Pilonidal sinus.* Various treatment techniques have been described for this condition. They include excision of the area and primary closure: marsupialization, excision, and skin grafting; excision and secondary healing; and excision and local flap repair. These techniques are discussed in greater detail in Chapters 30 and 31.

- *Hidradenitis suppurativa.* (Chapter 32) This is a chronic, recurrent, indolent infection involving the skin and subcutaneous tissue arising in the apocrine glands. The axillae are most frequently involved, but the perineal area can also be affected. Small areas may be conservatively treated with meticulous hygiene, antibiotics, local injections of steroids, incision, and drainage. More extensive or chronic disease usually requires excision after preliminary conservative treatment. The involved area is excised down to unaffected subcutaneous fat or fascia. Closure can be direct only if the area is small or if adjacent tissue it loose. If the area is large, split-thickness skin grafting or planned secondary healing with dressings are both appropriate. Occasionally a local or a regional flap may be employed.

- *Actinomycocis.* Actinomycocis is a chronic infectious disease that usually involves the cervicofacial area, thorax, or abdomen, but can involve the perineal area. The causative organism is a Gram-positive aerobic bacterium, Actinomyces israeli. It produces a suppurative, fibrosing inflammation that forms sinus tracts and discharges sulfur granules. The diagnosis is made by isolating the organism from a culture of the tissue exudate. Sulfur granules are diagnostic. Penicillin, tetracycline, and sulfonamides are all effective agents for infections. Abscesses and chronic scarring may require surgical therapy.

C. *Radionecrosis.* Radiotherapy causes intense fibrosis and decreases the blood supply to the radiotherapy field. This fibrosis and ischemia begins approximately 6 weeks after treatment and worsens over time. The perineum develops a chronic unhealing wound centered on the treated area. The stigmata of radiotherapy should be obvious during examination. These signs are thin atrophic skin (often pigmented), tattoos, dots used to mark the target area, and telangiectasia. Principles of treatment are

1. When debrided, the affected area will not support a skin graft.

2. The entire field is affected, and therefore local flaps are not an option, due to the poor blood supply caused by radiation vasculitis.

3. The most reliable option to reconstruct a radionecrotic ulcer is to use a flap that comes from outside the radiotherapy field, i.e., a regional or free flap. This should be performed after thorough debridement and wide excision of the involved area.

D. *Pressure sores.* Perineal decubitus ulcerations are uncommon. Pressure areas are much more common over bony prominences such as the ischium, trochanter, and sacrum. Paraplegic individuals are particularly affected. Perineal pressure sores tend to occur when the ischia have been surgically removed and no longer bear the weight of the seated patient. As the perineum bears more weight, it becomes more susceptible to ulceration. There is a significant risk of a urethral fistula in perineal pressure ulcers. Treatment includes

1. Prevention: optimal nutrition; meticulous skin, bowel, and urinary-tract care; frequent position changes; weight control; upper body fitness; special wheelchair cushions and air mattresses.
2. Debridement of eschars with wide opening of bursae.
3. Frequent saline dressings (microdebridement).
4. Urinary diversion if a urethrocutaneous fistula is present.
5. Flap repair.

E. *Inflammatory bowel disease.* Unlike mucosal ulcerative colitis, Crohn's disease is a common cause of perianal fistulas. Nevertheless, both disorders can result in perineal wounds that require closure. Only after appropriate treatment of the fistula should the cavity and skin defect be repaired. Total proctocolectomy for ulcerative colitis can result in perineal wound breakdown—as can an abdominal perineal resection for low rectal tumors.

F. *Tumors.* Malignant neoplasms of the skin in this area include basal cell carcinoma, Bowen's disease, malignant melanoma, epidermoid (squamous cell) carcinoma, and extramammary Paget's disease.

G. *Excision (macrodebridement).* Debridement is performed to healthy bleeding tissue (*macrodebridement*). In an outpatient setting or in a hospital bed without anesthesia, this debridement may be subtotal. Frequent wet to dry dressings can be used to remove the remaining necrotic tissue (*microdebridement*) over the subsequent days or weeks.

H. *Dressings and preparation for closure (microdebridement).* Wet to dry dressings are performed to (1) remove contaminated and necrotic tissue in preparation for definitive operative closure (direct suture, skin grafting or flap repair) or (2) keep the wound clean, promote the growth of healthy granulation tissue, facilitate contraction, and encourage reepithelialization from the wound edges. This *healing by secondary intent* is often a lengthy process if the wound is large; but, even then, the final result is often satisfactory. Although there are many different dressings and dressing solutions, there is no evidence that any are superior to saline soaked gauze 4 times daily—*provided the wound has been adequately laid open and debrided.* This dressing removes small amounts of necrotic tissue and keeps the wound clean and moist for optimum healing to occur. Betadine, sodium hypochlorite solutions (eusol, hygoel), or silver sulfadiazine may be used initially in contaminated or infected wounds to decrease the bacterial count and possibly aid sloughing. These solutions, however, have all been shown to be tissue toxic and inhibit reepithelialization.

I. *Wound closure*. Wound closure should only be attempted in a clean wound, free of necrotic tissue, and free of infection. When considering wound closure, one should consider the following questions:

   1. Can the wound be closed safely by direct suture?
   2. If not, will the wound close reasonably quickly on dressings alone?
   3. Can the wound be closed adequately by skin grafting?
   4. If not, can the wound be closed by a local flap?
   5. If not, can the wound be closed by a regional flap.
   6. If not, can the wound be closed by a free tissue transfer?

   This pathway needs to be considered when closing any wound.

J. *Skin loss*. A wound without skin loss, which remains open for some length of time, appears deficient in skin due to retraction of the surrounding skin edges. Such a wound, closed by direct suture, will be under excessive tension and likely to break down. An alternative method of closure is required.

K. *Flap repair*. Large-volume wounds need not only skin but also bulk to obliterate the dead space. Composite tissue such as this can only be obtained by using a flap. Depending on the condition of the surrounding tissue as well as the actual requirements for wound closure, either a local, regional, or free flap might be appropriate.

L. *Local flaps*. Local flaps can be used when the blood supply to the surrounding skin is adequate and has not been damaged by scars or radiotherapy. Local flaps may be transpositional, advancement, or rotational.

M. *Regional flaps*. Regional flaps for defects of the perineum include the gracilis muscle or musculocutaneous flap, the gluteus musculocutaneous flap, the rectus abdominis muscle or musculocutaneous flap, and the omental flap.

   - *Gracilis musculocutaneous flap*. The vessel on which this flap is based is medial branch of the profunda femoris artery. Anatomy of the flap is constant. Both artery and vein diameters are 1–2 mm. The skin paddle is small and unreliable unless placed over the proximal two-thirds of the muscle. This anatomy severely restricts its arc of rotation and limits its use. The donor scar down the medial aspect of the thigh is cosmetically satisfactory, and there is no functional morbidity from sacrificing the muscle. This flap is non innervated.

   - *Gluteus maximus musculocutaneous flap*. This flap is based medially on the inferior gluteal artery. In the context of perineal reconstruction, this flap may be transposed inferiorly to the ischial/lateral perineal region. The flap is reliable, has good donor scar, and has no functional morbidity.

   - *Rectus abdominus muscle or musculocutaneous flap (RAM)*. The rectus flap is based on the (constant) inferior epigastric artery, which is 2–3 mm in diameter. The pedicle length is 9–13 cm. This flap can include a great deal of tissue bulk and may be rotated on its pedicle or transferred as a free flap. For perineal reconstruction, the latter is highly unlikely. Depending on the type of incision, the donor scar is acceptable to very good. With rectus flaps, a portion of the anterior rectus sheath is either sacrificed or devascularized. Its repair should be performed meticulously—probably with the aid of a synthetic mesh—since there is a possibility of an incisional hernia developing.

- *Omental flap.* This flap is based on either the right or left gastroepiploic artery, has constant anatomy, and bears a large amount of soft tissue. The vessel diameters are 2~3.5 mm, giving it an abundant blood supply. Its abdominal function of infection control may be used advantageously in the perineum. The drawbacks of this flap include all the potential complications of a laparotomy, and the fact that there is no skin paddle for surface reconstruction. Its primary roles are therefore as a filler of dead space, and as an interposition between two fistulizing epithelial surfaces.

N. *Free flaps.* Free tissue transfers usually involve much more operating time than does a pedicle flap, and are used only when the previous options are unsuitable. From the many free flaps available, the ones applicable to the closure of perineal defects are the radial forearm flap and the latissimus dorsi muscle (or musculocutaneous) free flap. As mentioned earlier, rectus abdominis and gracilis flaps are generally pedicled for perineal reconstruction.

- *Radial forearm free flap.* The "Chinese" forearm flap is based on the radial artery and is a fasciocutaneous flap. It is reliable, has a constant anatomy and a long pedicle. The vessel diameters are approximately 2.5 mm. The skin is thin and pliable and may be innervated. An Allen test must be performed preoperatively to determine whether the ulnar artery is present and patent. The donor site is poor cosmetically, but there is no functional disability. Healing of the donor site skin graft can be slow, but is rarely a problem. This flap would be used to close a wound only where bulk is undesirable. It is ideal for reconstruction of complex defects involving the male or female genitalia, and is excellent for the resurfacing of radiation ulcers or any perineal deficiency that, if allowed to heal spontaneously, would result in scar contracture with functional limitation.

- *Latissimus dorsi free flap.* This is the workhorse free flap of plastic surgery. It is based on the thorocodorsal artery. The flap has a constant anatomy with vessel diameters of 1.5~4 mm, and is extremely reliable. The pedicle length is about 9 cm. This flap provides a large amount of soft tissue and can be used as a muscle or musculocutaneous flap, the skin paddle not having the potential to be reinnervated. The donor site is satisfactory from a cosmetic standpoint; however, there is a residual functional loss: it should be avoided in patients who require crutches and in certain athletes—swimmers, mountain climbers, and weight lifters.

BIBLIOGRAPHY

1. Beck DA, Wexner SD (eds): *Fundamentals of Anorectal Surgery*. New York: McGraw-Hill, 1992.

2. Grabb and Smith. In Smith JW, Astor SJ (eds): *Plastic Surgery,* 4th ed. Boston: Little, Brown, 1991.

3. McCraw and Arnold. McCraw JB, Arnold PG (eds): *Atlas of Muscle and Musculocutaneous Flaps*. Hampton Press Publishing, 1986.

4. Strauch B, Yu HL (eds): *Atlas of Microvascular Surgery*. New York: Thieme Medical Publishers, 1992.

See also Chapters 30, 31, 32, 35, 36, 39, 47 and 51.

SECTION 4B

Anorectal Pathology
Neoplastic

CHAPTER 43

Anal Canal Neoplasms

David E. Beck, M.D.

Refer to Algorithm 43–1.

A. The anal canal is the portion of the anus related to the internal sphincter. It runs from the anorectal junction (superior portion of the anal sphincter muscles) to the intersphincteric groove (approximately 2 cm distal to the dentate line). The lining transitions from squamous epithelium distally to columnar epithelium proximally. Lesions distal to the intersphincteric groove are located at the anal margin.

B. Most (65%) patients are female in the sixth to seventh decades of life. Presenting symptoms include bleeding (27–74% of patients) and pain or anal discomfort (21–39% of patients). Masses are located in the anal canal and are commonly firm and ulcerated.

C. One to two pieces of tumor are obtained from the edge of the lesion. A local anesthetic is seldom required.

D. It is essential to document the size, location, percent of anal circumference, and fixity of an anal canal lesion as the lesion may completely disappear after therapy.

E. This includes all the pathologic variations such as squamous cell, basoiloid, cloacogenic, basosquamous, epitheloid, transitional, and mucoepidermoid. These histologic subtypes respond in a similar manner to treatment and are thus managed in the same way.

F. Anal melanomas are rare locally invasive tumors with high metastatic potential. The lesions are usually elevated, and 34–75% are pigmented.

G. Anal adenocarcinomas are rare tumors arising from anal glands or chronic fistulas. They are slow-growing and locally invasive. An accurate diagnosis requires a deep biopsy.

H. Anal sarcomas produce symptoms similar to other anal tumors and may be intra- or extraluminal. They may show differentiation resembling any mesodermal tissue (leimyosarcoma, fibrosarcoma, liposarcoma, etc.) and are radioresistant.

Anal canal neoplasms

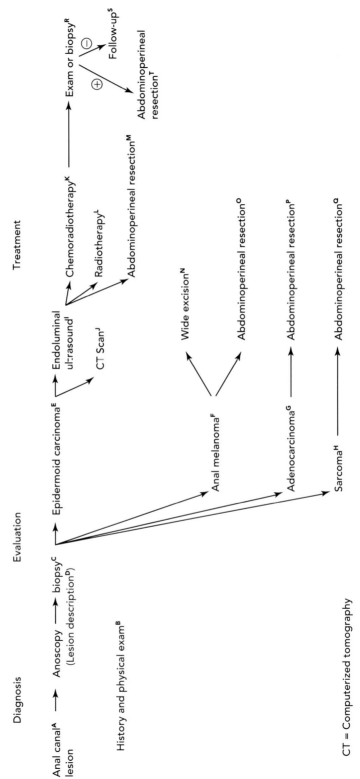

CT = Computerized tomography

ALGORITHM 43–1

I. Endoanal ultrasound identifies depth of tumor penetration and location and size of lymph nodes.

J. Computerized tomography (CT) scans are helpful to exclude hepatic or extra-pelvic disease.

K. Mitomycin-C (10 mg/m^2 body surface area intravenously) on day 1 of therapy. 5-Fluoro-uracil (5-FU) administered as a continuous intravenous infusion of 1,000 mg/m^2 body surface area on days 1–5 and days 31–36. External beam radiotherapy is administered in 2 Gy fractions concomitantly with chemotherapy to a dose of 30–45 Gy. This method of treatment is associated with a 12% local recurrence rate, a 5-year survival above 80%, and a continence rate of 80%.

L. High-voltage (2–4 mV) external beam radiotherapy to the pelvis. Total dose has varied from 45 to 60 Gy; this method is popular in Europe. Results include a 26% rate of local recurrence, a 5-year survival of 68%, a 9% major complications rate, and 73% of patients retain continence.

M. Persistent or recurrent cancer occurs in about 14% of patients after chemoradiation therapy. These patients are generally treated with an abdomino perineal resection (APR). However, some surgeons have tried modified "second try" chemoradiotherapy protocols. Such anecdotal reports do not represent the standard approach.

N. The majority of melanoma patients succumb from distal metastases. Wide excision can provide local control and most patients retain continence.

O. An abdominoperineal resection (APR) provides improved local control. Long-term survival has occurred only in patients with tumors < 3.0 mm in depth (5-year survival of 15%).

P. Survival even after an APR is worse than in patients who undergo an APR for care of rectal carcinoma.

Q. The 5-year survival in patients with sarcomas has varied from 20% to 39%.

R. Four to six weeks after treatment, the area of lesion is examined. This waiting period is necessary to allow resorption of nonviable tumor cells. Any residual lesion or scar tissue is biopsied to exclude persistent or residual tumor.

S. Recommended follow-up includes anal exam, endoanal ultrasonography, and biopsy of any suspicious lesions.

T. Recurrence or persistence of tumor is managed with an abdominoperineal resection.

BIBLIOGRAPHY

1. Beck DE, Wexner SW: Anal neoplasms. In Beck DE, Wexner SD (eds): *Fundamentals of Anorectal Surgery*. New York: McGraw-Hill, 1992.

2. Beck DE, Karulf RE: Combination therapy for epidermoid carcinoma of the anal canal. *Dis Colon Rectum* (in press).

3. Gordon PH: Current status—perianal and anal canal neoplasms. *Dis Colon Rectum* 33:799–808, 1990.

4. Nivatvongs S: Perianal and anal neoplasms. In Gordon PA, Nivatvongs S (eds): *Principles and Practice of Surgery for the Colon, Rectum, and Anus*. St. Louis: Quality Medical Publishers, 1992.

See also Chapter 35.

CHAPTER 44

Retrorectal Tumors

Charles O. Finne, M.D.

Refer to Algorithm 44–1.

A. The retrorectal space is a potential space bordered anteriorly by the rectum, posteriorly by the sacrum, superiorly by the peritoneal reflection and levators, and laterally by the iliac vessels, and ureters. It is embryologically derived from the area of the primitive pit and Hensen's node where cells differentiate into the three germ-cell layers. The anatomic proximity of these layers and the complicated tissue rearrangements that occur during development of the embryo give rise to an incredible variety of pathologic entities in this region. Lesions in this space are fortunately rare, but because they are unfamiliar, a structured approach to their management is required. Biopsy can be dangerous and is strictly contraindicated in most situations, hence a classification schema is useful to outline the most appropriate action. Evaluation of a lesion in the presacral space should include any of the procedures necessary to accurately classify a lesion as cystic, solid, or combination; soft tissue only (or associated indirectly with bony deformity); directly involving bone; or direct central nervous system (CNS) involvement. Bone or CNS involvement requires a multidisciplinary approach, and counseling of the patient about potential bladder and rectal sphincter dysfunction. Careful digital rectal examination, under anesthesia if appropriate, is very important to assessing the proper surgical approach. Lesions that are mostly transrectally palpable generally are located caudal to the S4 segment and rarely require either an abdominal approach or a laminectomy.

B. Plain radiographs of the sacrum are useful for showing congenital deformity that can be diagnostic (scimitar sacrum = sacral meningocele) or suggestive of a congenital lesion. Specific bony changes can be suggestive of primary bone tumors or metastatic disease. Ectopic bone or teeth may confirm a congenital lesion.

C. Abnormality of bone, or historic or physical findings suspicious of CNS involvement, require computerized tomography/magnetic resonance imaging (CT/MRI) scanning to delineate the extent of a lesion and the amount of sacrum or

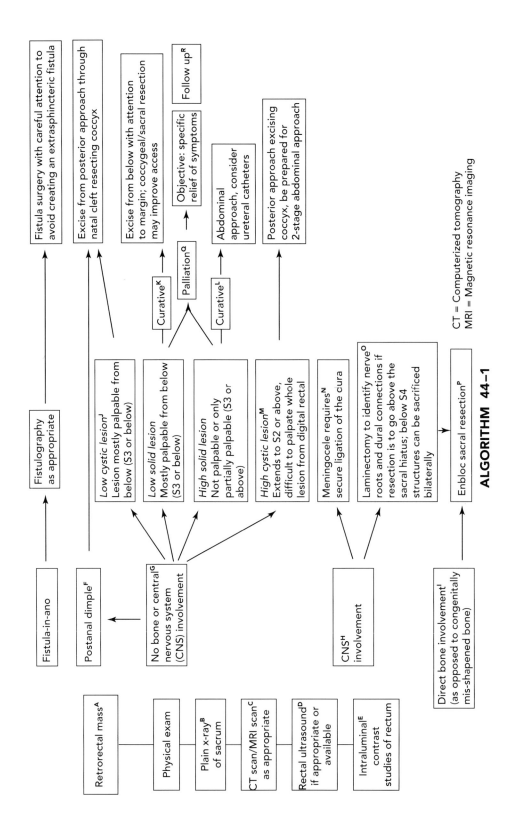

ALGORITHM 44–1

Retrorectal mass^A → Physical exam → Plain x-ray^B of sacrum → CT scan/MRI scan^C as appropriate → Rectal ultrasound^D if appropriate or available → Intraluminal^E contrast studies of rectum

Fistula-in-ano → Fistulography as appropriate → Fistula surgery with careful attention to avoid creating an extrasphincteric fistula

Postanal dimple^F → Excise from posterior approach through natal cleft resecting coccyx

No bone or central nervous system (CNS) involvement^G

Low cystic lesion^J Lesion mostly palpable from below (S3 or below)

Low solid lesion Mostly palpable from below (S3 or below) → Curative^K → Excise from below with attention to margin; coccygeal/sacral resection may improve access

High solid lesion Not palpable or only partially palpable (S3 or above) → Palliation^Q → Objective: specific relief of symptoms → Follow up^R

High cystic lesion^M Extends to S2 or above, difficult to palpate whole lesion from digital rectal → Curative^L → Abdominal approach, consider ureteral catheters

Posterior approach excising coccyx, be prepared for 2-stage abdominal approach

CNS^H involvement

Meningocele requires^N secure ligation of the cura

Laminectomy to identify nerve^O roots and dural connections if resection is to go above the sacral hiatus; below S4 structures can be sacrificed bilaterally

Direct bone involvement^I (as opposed to congenitally mis-shapened bone) → Enbloc sacral resection^P

CT = Computerized tomography
MRI = Magnetic resonance imaging

232

CNS involvement. Such investigation may help predict the likelihood of a complication such as a postoperative nerve deficit, adjacent organ involvement, the need for a combined abdominal–perineal approach, potential for dural injury, and the presence of an unanticipated second lesion (solid teratoma associated with a cystic lesion). Imaging of the retrorectal space may reveal an unsuspected cyst as the cause of a refractory fistula-in-ano. Ectopic bone may be more apparent on CT than on plain films.

D. Ultrasonic imaging of the rectum and anus can show intimate involvement of the rectal wall, may suggest direct derivation from the rectal wall, and can show an undetected internal opening of a fistula-in-ano. It may also suggest dual cystic–solid nature. Non palpable fistulas may be apparent with high-resolution scanning of the anal sphincter. Selected *solid* tumors may be accurately biopsied under ultrasonic guidance such as suspected metastatic disease or endometriosis. Transrectal biopsy of solid lesions under cover of antibiotics has proved safe, but biopsy should be avoided for any cystic lesion because of the risk of infection or fistula formation. In most cases, excision without either needle or incisional biopsy is the procedure of choice.

E. The importance of rectal contrast studies has been displaced by CT scanning, but there is still a role, particularly for a suspected fistula or perforation or to evaluate obstructive symptoms.

F. Postanal dimple is a rare finding, present in 6% of adult congenital cysts, but when present makes a benign diagnosis likely. These dimples can be confused with fistula-in-ano, and vice versa, and strongly imply the need to completely resect the coccyx to prevent recurrence.

G. Pure soft tissue lesions closely adjacent to the sacrum require careful evaluation, because chordoma is typically soft, feels cystic, and is easily confused with a benign cyst when evaluated by palpation alone. Lesions that are clearly separate from the sacrum and are cystic carry only a 10% chance of malignancy in the adult, but solid lesions carry a 60% risk of malignancy and should be approached with the intent of resection with a significant tumor-free surgical margin. Preoperative biopsy is *not* appropriate in the majority of instances, unless palliative treatment is the only option. The majority of these lesions should be approached with the idea of total excision for diagnosis. Meningitis frequently complicates any less than definitive procedure for sacral meningocele; chordomas implant along needle tracts, and have been shown to have poorer survival if biopsied preoperatively; unanticipated injury to pelvic or peripheral nerves can occur; infection of a cystic lesion is common, especially after transrectal biopsy and fistulas may result; biopsy of a vascular malformation or tumor may be complicated by hemorrhage; and finally, compromise of surgical margin may preclude the chance for curative excision. Solid lesions in the setting of an adult with previous cancer require metastatic workup. The presence of multiple lesions makes the diagnosis of metastatic disease very likely. Ultrasound directed needle biopsy is most appropriate in this circumstance.

H. CNS involvement of any kind requires special considerations to avoid complications and excessive neural injury. Occult dural injury may be difficult to recognize if proper attention is not rendered to likely places of injury. It may also result in spinal fluid leak, and frequently results in meningitis from Gram-negative organisms. Failure to recognize sacral meningoceles has resulted in reported mortality rates as high as 40%. Laminectomy is usually required to delineate nerve involvement and to identify the sacral nerves and preserve nerves that are not directly involved in a malignant process. Functional consequences of nerve sacrifice are described in paragraph O.

I. Direct bone involvement below the S4 (sacral hiatus) level may not require laminectomy, since sacrifice of these neural elements does not result in significant motor deficit. Involvement above this level should require laminectomy to assess what can be safely preserved, and sacral resections involving major portions of the second segment or above can result in pelvic instability.

J. The low cystic lesion is the most common of these tumors. A standard approach to these lesions is a transverse incision over the coccyx. The coccyx is divided from the anococcygeal ligament, disarticulated from the sacrum and left attached to the cyst for en-bloc resection. Scattered literature reports (mostly pediatric) suggest a 15% recurrence rate if the coccyx is left behind. There is no functional deficit after coccygeal resection, and for a larger lesion it does improve exposure.

Full bowel preparation is undertaken, and the rectum is irrigated with antibacterial or antiseptic irrigant. A digit in the rectum is very helpful to manipulate the tumor for better exposure and to avoid rectal injury. A rectal digit also facilitates recognition of a rectal injury should it occur. Often part of the muscular wall of the rectum is resected and subsequently closed separately. Topical antibiotics may be used in the irrigation. A suction drain is also a useful adjunct. The anococcygeal raphe is approximated to the sacrum using the parasacral fascia and periosteum. The skin is closed with a subcuticular synthetic absorbable suture, and an adhesive plastic film dressing is very useful. The drain is ideally removed before first bowel movement. Postoperative bowel confinement may be considered.

Sphincter dividing operations are generally unnecessary and, except for lesions directly involving the sphincter by local extension, should be shunned because of the added risk of incontinence if the repair fails.

K. Because of their risk of malignancy, solid lesions require more careful attention to surgical margins of normal tissue. Otherwise the same considerations as paragraph I apply. Sacral resections below the hiatus (S4 level) do not require laminectomy and may improve access.

L. The high presacral lesion often derives its blood supply from the middle sacral vessels that are inaccessible to early control. The surgical approach is facilitated by a modified lithotomy position using multiposition stirrups. The proximal sacrum is supported by a pad that allows the buttocks and coccyx to protrude over the edge of the operating table, allowing combined surgical access to the presacral space through the anococcygeal raphe. Such combined access is rarely necessary, but positioning the third operator between the legs allows better anterior retraction of the rectum, and allows access from below for air insufflation or other maneuvers to check rectal integrity. Bulky lesions may be difficult to expose and mobilize within the confines of the pelvis, ureteral catheters can be invaluable in speeding dissection and avoiding ureteral injury. The catheters can be removed at the conclusion of the procedure.

M. Because cystic lesions seldom have prominent blood supply, are rarely malignant, and require only limited margins, they are more likely to be removed from below despite their large size. Infrequent need for abdominal access and necessity for coccygeal resection make the initial approach from below much more efficient.

N. Sacral meningoceles are rare, usually associated with a characteristic "scimitar sacrum" deformity of the sacrum, and are associated with a high complication and morbidity rate, although most series in the literature antedate the present era of multiple effective antibiotics. Operations on unsuspected meningoceles have an alarming rate of Gram-negative meningitis associated with them, and every attempt should be made to anticipate this lesion and achieve secure ligation of the dura. Ten percent of sacral meningoceles have associated teratomas. The teratoma may be the only palpable part of the lesion and if solid, may be misleading for the unwary; hence it is important to consider meningocele in the differential diagnosis to avoid overlooking a meningocele. Sacral meningoceles rarely have significant neural elements within them and appear as a simple cyst when opened.

O. Anal sphincter and detrusor function depends on intact S2, S3, S4 nerve function. Unilateral loss of all of these roots results in hemianesthesia but is tolerated well and does not result in significant dysfunction. Bilateral S2 loss results in total absence of anal sphincter function. Unilateral loss of S2 results in ineffective sphincter closure and inability to discriminate rectal contents or distension. External sphincter response to cough and distension is lost, but internal sphincter sphincter tone remains intact, probably because it is mediated intramurally. Preservation of S3 bilaterally results in practically normal function. Unilateral preservation of S3 and all higher nerves results in acceptable function and sensation of rectal filling and discrimination. Preservation of at least one S3 is most desirable because it provides most of the anal sensory function and most of the external sphincter function.

P. Low sacral resection (S4 and below) using the sacral hiatus as the dividing point, is easily accomplished from the prone jackknife position with little risk of significant bleeding, unanticipated injury to the rectum, or loss of anal function. High sacral resection is a major undertaking with potential massive blood loss, and should be prepared for by assuring adequate resources for resuscitation, and adequate multidisciplinary support in the operating room. The techniques of resection are well described in the included references. In the event a combined abdominoperineal approach for sacral resection is necessary, exposure is better first performing the entire abdominal portion of the procedure, closing the abdomen, and then turning the patient to the prone jackknife position, repeating the prep, and proceeding with the perineal portion as a separate second stage. In a combined rectal and sacral resection, the posterior wound can be left open, protected, the patient repositioned on to a new operating table, reprepped, and redraped, with the sacral resection accomplished with good light and access by the surgeons. The prone position minimizes venous blood loss and provides much better access to neural structures for identification and preservation. The margin for sacral resection can be marked from the abdominal side by driving a K-wire through the lateral sacrum at the most cephalad margins and approaching this easily visible and palpable landmark with the patient prone. The main disadvantage of the prone position is the need to anticipate use of an omental sling to close the pelvic defect and lack of access to pelvic blood supply. Adequate dissection from the abdominal approach should secure good vascular control, however, except for bone and venous sinuses.

Q. The wide variety of tumor types encountered in the retrorectal group of tumors makes specific recommendation for palliative maneuvers impractical. Tumors in this space, if causing symptoms, tend to be large advanced lesions causing pain, incontinence, or obstruction. The role of radiation therapy, chemotherapy, incomplete resections, fecal diversion, ureteral stenting, or resection all have to be individualized based on tumor type, expected length of survival, and the specific symptom requiring palliation.

R. Completely treated benign disease probably requires no follow-up beyond ensuring operative recovery and resolution of complications. Follow-up for malignant disease is controversial, but I believe it should be directed toward potentially treatable recurrences in an individual with an otherwise uncompromised life expectancy. Usually this focuses attention on treatable local recurrence which can be diagnosed by digital rectal, vaginal examination, CT/MRI scanning, endorectal, or vaginal ultrasound examinations.

BIBLIOGRAPHY

1. Christiansen MA, Blatchford BJ: Presacral tumors in adults. In Beck DE, Wexner SD (eds): *Fundamentals of Anorectal Surgery.* New York: McGraw-Hill, Inc., 1992.

2. Finne CO: Presacral tumors and cysts. In Cameron J (ed): *Current Surgical Therapy–3.* Philadelphia: Decker, 1989.

3. Gordon PH: Retrorectal tumors. In Gordon PH, Nivatvongs S (eds): *Principles and Practice of Surgery for the Colon, Rectum, and Anus.* St. Louis: Quality Medical Publishing, 1992.

4. Gunterberg B, Kewenter J, Petersen I, et al: Anorectal function after major resections of the sacrum with bilateral or unilateral sacrifice of sacral nerves. *Br J Surg* 63:546–554, 1976.

5. Jao S, Beart R, Spenser RJ, et al: Retrorectal tumors. Mayo Clinic experience 1960–1979. *Dis Colon Rectum* 28:641–652, 1985.

6. Karakousis CP, Wabnitz RC: Tumor involving the sacrum. In Karakousis, CP (Ed). *Atlas of Operations for Soft Tissue Tumors.* New York: McGraw-Hill, 1985.

7. Uhlig BE, Johnson RL: Presacral tumors and cysts in adults. *Dis Colon Rectum* 18:581–596, 1978.

8. Wexner SD, Jagelman DG: Pilonidal sinus, pre-sacral cysts and tumors and pelvic pain. In: Zuidema GD, Condon RE (eds): *Surgery of the Alimentary Tract* (3rd ed) Philadelphia: WB Saunders Co. 1991; 390–405.

See also Chapters 6, 8, 43, 46 and 47.

CHAPTER 45

Rectal Polyps

Douglas R. E. Johnson, M.D.
and Robert D. Madoff, M.D.

Refer to Algorithm 45–1.

A. While several reports suggest an association between rectal hyperplastic polyps and proximal colon neoplasms, prospective, controlled studies have not confirmed this association. Thus, rectal hyperplastic polyps are not an indication for further evaluation of the colon.

B. Very distally located polyps, large polyps (> 2 cm) in the lower and middle thirds of the rectum and polyps involving less than half the circumference of the rectum are more suitable for transanal excision. Criteria for transanal excision include a soft freely movable nonulcerated lesion.

C. Endorectal ultrasound (ERUS) accurately detects submucosal invasion of rectal neoplasms, which bespeaks malignancy. The technique is not suitable for pedunculated polyps.

D. Adequately excised polyps recur in approximately 30% of patients and therefore regular follow-up examinations are essential (e.g., every 3 months for 2 years, then yearly)

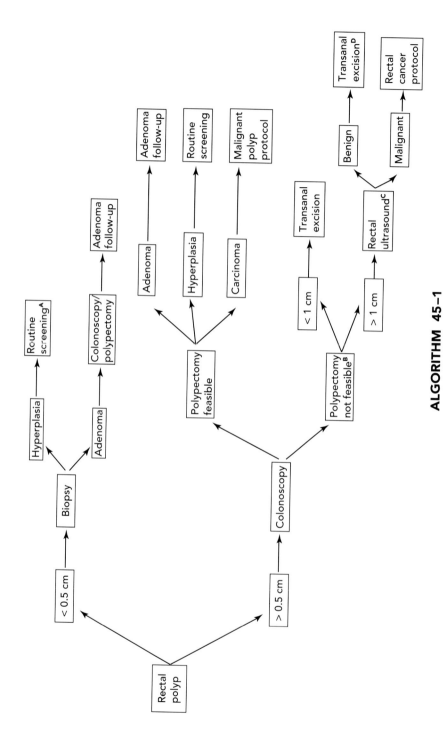

ALGORITHM 45–1

BIBLIOGRAPHY

1. Bond JH: Polyp guideline: diagnosis, treatment and surveillance for patients with non-familial colorectal polyps. *Ann Int Med* 119:836–843, 1993.

2. Nivatvongs S: Perianal and transanal techniques. In Gordon PH, Nivatvongs S (eds): *Principles and Practice of Surgery for the Colon, Rectum, and Anus.* St. Louis: Quality Medical Publishers, 1992.

3. Rex DK, Smith JJ, Ulbright TM, et al: Distal colonic hyperplastic polyps do not predict proximal adenomas in asymptomatic average-risk subjects. *Gastroenterology* 102:317–319, 1992.

4. Sakamoto GD, Mackeigan JM, Senagore AJ: Transanal excision of large, rectal villous adenomas. *Dis Colon Rectum* 34:880–885, 1991.

5. Wong WD, Orrom WJ, Jensen LL: Preoperative staging of rectal cancer with endorectal ultrasonography. *Perspectives Colon Rectal Surg* 3:314–334, 1990.

See also Chapters 46 and 47.

CHAPTER 46

Rectal Cancer—Local Surgical and Nonsurgical Therapy

Robin Phillips, M.S., F.R.C.S.

Refer to Algorithm 46–1.

A. There is no doubt that conventional surgery for rectal cancer in skilled hands can result in good cancer specific and functional results. Less radical operations must *always* be regarded as second best.

   When dealing with a fit patient, there are times when the perceived functional result of a low anastomosis for a small and favorable tumor may not have that good a prospect, particularly if the anus is already compromised (e.g., by a preexisting pudendal neuropathy). In these circumstances, a local excision may be a tempting alternative for both the patient and surgeon; but there is no doubt that taking such an approach in an otherwise fit patient *does* put the patient at an increased risk of death from cancer. Nevertheless, there are some patients, fully acquainted with the facts, who would choose this option.

B. For the remainder of patients who are not—or cannot be rendered—fit enough for conventional surgery, the choices are limited. Local excision for favorable tumors (not poorly differentiated), <3 cm in size, confined endosonographically or after histologic examination to the bowel wall becomes a good option; technical difficulties can be overcome either with the Buess instrument or by endoscopic transanal resection (ETAR). Photodynamic therapy after prior sensitization with a hematoporphyrin derivative is another consideration.

C. Less favorable tumors can be removed transsacrally under a light spinal anesthetic in the prone–jackknife position. Continuity is restored. However, the approach is unfamiliar to most surgeons, access is poor (but can be improved by removal of the coccyx and even the lower part of the sacrum), the amount of rectum that can be removed is limited, and disorientation may put the ureters at risk. Furthermore, older patients are at risk of a decubitus ulcer in the wound area. Should an anastomotic leak develop, the subsequent fecal fistula

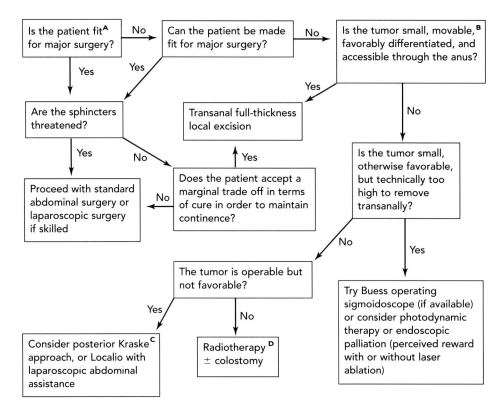

ALGORITHM 46–1

can be difficult to manage and almost always requires at least temporary fecal diversion. However, it is with a transsacral approach that a limited abdominal phase with the laparoscope holds great potential for facilitating mobilization and high ligation of the lymphovascular pedicle.

D. For the remainder, radiotherapy has the best hope of significant palliation. Other methods, such as laser and cryosurgical debulking, fail to treat the deeper parts of the tumor that can give rise to considerable pain. Many of these patients will require a colostomy, which can be achieved either by a trephine technique or a laparoscopic stoma.

It is tempting to consider the role of adjuvant chemotherapy, particularly with 5-fluorouracil and folinic acid, in these irresectable cases. However, these patients have been denied surgery *because* of their frailty, and many would not tolerate the rigors of chemotherapy either.

BIBLIOGRAPHY

1. Berry AR, Souter RG, Campbell WG, et al: Endoscopic transanal resection of rectal tumours—a preliminary report of its use. *Br J Surg* 77:134–137, 1990.

2. Bown SG, Barr H, Mathewson K et al: Endoscopic treatment of inoperable colorectal cancers with the Nd-YAG laser. *Br J Surg* 73:949–952, 1986.

3. Bright N, Hale P, Mason R: Poor palliation of colorectal malignancy with the neodymium yttrium-aluminium-garnet laser. *Br J Surg* 79:308–309, 1992.

4. Hughes EP, Veidenheimer MC, Corman ML, et al: Electrocoagulation of rectal cancer. *Dis Colon Rectum* 25:215–218, 1982.

5. Localio SA, Eng K, Coppa GF: Abdomino-sacral resection for mid rectal cancer. *Ann Surg* 198:320–324, 1983.

6. Lock MR, Ritchie JK, Hawley PR: Reappraisal of radical local excision for carcinoma of the rectum. *Br J Surg* 80:928–929, 1993.

7. Papillon J: The future of external beam irradiation as initial treatment for rectal cancer. *Br J Surg* 74:449–454, 1987.

8. Saclarides TJ, Smith L, Sung-Tao Ko, et al: Transanal endoscopic microsurgery. *Dis Colon Rectum* 35:1183–1191, 1992.

See also Chapters 45 and 47.

CHAPTER 47

Rectal Cancer—Radical Surgical Therapy

R. J. Heald, F.R.C.S.

Refer to Algorithm 47-1.

A. *Cancer of the rectum* is the most technique-dependent of all common malignancies. Most rectal cancers are adenocarcinomas. Irrespective of histologic grade, they all behave in a rather similar manner and can be treated similarly. No other cancer has so great a variation in outcome between surgeons. Understanding how to perform a curative operation requires comprehension of the regional anatomy. The rectum is generally defined as being that part distal to 15 cm from the anal verge. The true top of the rectum is really where the sigmoid colon with its teaniae becomes rectum with a continuous enveloping muscle coat.

B. The reference point for height is usually taken as the anal verge that is reliable and useful in the conscious patient. The dentate line, however, is more reliable and useful as a reference point in the anesthetized patient when the external sphincter retracts external to the internal sphincter.

The anatomy of the integral visceral mesentery of the rectum (mesorectum) is determined by its position deep in the back of the pelvis. *Anteriorly* are:

1. The intraperitoneal anterior wall of the upper rectum
2. The peritoneal reflection
3. Denonvillier's fascia behind the seminal vesicles, and which ends by fusing with the fascia on the back of the prostate

Posteriorly is the bulky bilobed "lipoma-like" structure that lies in the levator gutters and against the sacrum. *Distally* the mesorectum tapers onto the rectal muscle, which becomes the internal anal sphincter and is inserted into the pelvic floor, which comprises puborectal sling and external anal sphincter. Around the entire mesorectum lies the investing fascia of the hindgut. This plane may be used by the surgeon as the essential "guidance" for the operation

Rectal carcinoma [A] → Lesions below [B] 15 cm require specialized skilled surgery

Potentially curative surgery → Lesions below [B] 15 cm require specialized skilled surgery

12–15 cm [C] → Partial mesorectal [D] mobilization and division 5 cm below tumor Anterior resection + anastomosis (manual or stapled) at 9–10 cm

Lower edge above 4–5 cm (up to 11–12 cm) → Ultra-low AR + TME Long midline incision Ligation of IMA just clear of aorta or just distal to ALCA Ligation of IMV just clear of pancreas or just distal to ALCA crossing it.

Lower edge below 4–5 cm → Usually APR necessary

Total mesorectal [E] mobilization and excision (TME) including Denonvillier's fascia to level of prostate.

→ APR if [H] clamp beyond tumor is impossible

→ Clamp or staple[F] washout below clamp or manual purse string.

Colon → Splenic or flexure mobilization / Very long sigmoid

→ Circular staple to anorectal slump

Consider temporary loop [G] ileostomy for anastomosis below 5–6 cm

Consider [I] Adjuvant Therapy

IMA = Inferior mesenteric artery
IMV = inferior mesenteric vein
ALCA = ascending left colic artery
TME = total mesorectal excision
APR = abdominoperineal resection
AR = anterior resection

ALGORITHM 47–1

of total mesorectal excision. Waldeyer's fascia invests the front of the sacrum and fuses with the fascia on the pelvic floor. It lies outside the investing visceral fascia and provides some protection for the inferior hypogastric autonomic plexus on the side walls of the pelvis.

Lateral to the mesorectum the presacral nerves, bifurcating within the concavity of the aortic bifurcation, course across the pelvic side wall toward their distal anterolateral corner. As they do so, they are joined by the parasympathetic roots of the sacral nerves, particularly that of S3, the "exigent" nerve. S2 and S1 are much more slender autonomic contributions to a variable nerve plexus that ultimately joins with the presacral nerves. Ultimately, the "neurovascular bundles" that curve medially behind the vesicles, and then the prostate to which they are closely applied, become the erectile nerves of the corpora cavernosa.

C. The idea that all poorly differentiated tumors require an abdominoperineal resection (APR) has been generally abandoned. A small proportion of those lesions classified by the histopathologists as "high-grade" or "poorly differentiated" do behave in a highly malignant manner and appear to be uncontrollable by any available treatment. Nevertheless the idea that such cases should be managed differently from other rectal cancers is no longer widely supported.

In one large multisurgeon series only two histologic criteria emerged as highly significant indicators for local cure failure (locoregional recurrence): (1) lymph node status and (2) involvement of lateral resection margins. In the author's opinion prognostic indicator (2) is a measure in almost every case of the surgeon's failure to perform a *total* mesorectal excision. In the last 20 years APR has been replaced as the standard operation for most rectal cancers by sphincter-preserving anterior resection. Nevertheless sphincter preservation rates still vary from 30% to 90% according to the centre reporting the series.

D. The general principle in both colon and rectal cancer is that the tumor segment be removed with its relevant mesentery en bloc with 5 cm of mesentery distal to the lower edge of the cancer. In the lesions in the mid- and lower rectum the *whole* of the mesorectum should be excised. For lesions in the upper one-third of the rectum, the final decision about excision (TME) or transsection of the mesorectum can be made only after initial posterior and lateral mobilization before the so-called lateral ligaments are divided.

E. The question that determines this decision is whether 5 cm of mesentery can be removed, as anterior resection with mesorectal transection is a lesser procedure for the patient. The anastomosis can be effected either manually or with a stapling device. The decision between anterior resection (AR) + TME for most middle and low rectal cancers and APR for the lowest is more difficult and will vary somewhat from surgeon to surgeon. An APR is seldom indicated for lesions above 4–5 cm cephalad to the dentate line. Acceptable distal muscle tube margins for the pathologist have been progressively reduced in recent years. Most reports suggest that there is no increased local recurrence if the distal margin is 1–2 cm plus a clear "doughnut" from the stapler.

The "patient's muscle tube margin" can be so reduced that a staple line as low as the dentate line can be expected to give acceptable function in a motivated patient with a preoperative normal sphincter.

F. Progressive adaptation with reduction of fecal frequency and urgency can be expected for several years after ultralow anastomoses. Results during the first 1–2 years may be improved by creating a "J" colon pouch. This pouch must be much smaller (e.g. 2 × 8 cm) than the "J" pouches suitable for an ileoanal anastomosis. Larger colonic pouches have the risk of fecal retention and overflow incontinence.

G. The principal danger of low anastomosis to the anorectum (below 5–6 cm) is anastomotic leakage. In many series, including those of the author, this complication occurs in around 10% of cases where the anastomosis lies below 6 cm. Causes of anastomosic leakage include infected hematoma within the pelvis, relative ischemia of the colonic side of the anastomosis, and possibly diarrhea stressing such an anastomosis. The absence of a reservoir distal to the anastomosis and the temporary disappearance of the anorectal reflex may be contributory factors. For these reasons and because leakage can cause such insidious septicemia and peritonitis, the author considers temporary defunctioning to be desirable when the anastomosis is constructed very close to the anal canal (below 5 cm from the anal verge). Either a loop ileostomy or a loop transverse colostomy are viable options, although the former option is preferred.

H. Excision of the posterior vaginal wall as a part of an anterior or abdominoperineal resection is now generally limited to those cancers where there is invasion. Apart from this structure the general principle will be to excise en bloc with the primary cancer any other invaded organ. Fortunately, with midrectal cancer such invasion is rather uncommon as the tumor has usually spread elsewhere before it breaches its mesorectal outer envelope.

I. Radiotherapy is being increasingly used, particularly in the United States as a postoperative modality. Many others, however, prefer preoperative radiation.

The author's personal view is that high-dosage preoperative radiotherapy should be given only to rare cases. Fixation of the tumor with fear of involved margins at operation is the principal indication for preoperative radiotherapy. If appropriate surgery is performed, then the vast majority of patients do not require either pre- or postoperative radiotherapy.

Chemotherapy is also increasingly used in the United States. Measurable response rates to available agents still leave at least two-thirds or more of patients without benefit, and side effects are considerable. Actual proof of increased long-term survival has never been demonstrated. Nevertheless there is enormous medicolegal pressure on clinicians to give postoperative chemotherapy. In the author's unit such adjuvant therapy is restricted to Dukes "C" cases and certain Dukes "B" cases in the younger patient or the patient who requests it. However recurrence rates after TME are vastly superior to those noted after adjuvant therapy. In the hands of a skilled surgeon the benefits of the adjuvant therapy are far outweighed by the morbidity and the absence of any advantage relative to increased survival or decreased local recurrence.

BIBLIOGRAPHY

1. Cawthorn SJ, Parums DV, Gibbs NM, et al: Extent of mesorectal spread and involvement of lateral resection margins as a prognostic factor after surgery for rectal cancer. *Lancet* 335:1055–1059, 1990.

2. Hallbook O, Krog M, Pahlman L: Prospective randomized comparison between straight and colonic; J-pouch anastomosis after low anterior resection. *Dis Colon Rectum* April 1995 (Abstract).

3. Heald RJ: Towards fewer colostomies—the impact of circular stapling devices on the surgery of rectal cancer in the district hospital. *Br J Surg* 67:198–200, 1980.

4. MacFarlane JK, Ryall RDH, Heald RJ: Mesorectal excision for rectal cancer. Lancet 1993; 2:457–460.

5. Parc R, Tiret E, Frileux P, et al: Resection and coloanal anastomosis with colonic reservoir for rectal carcinoma. *Br J Surg* 73:139–141, 1986.

6. Quirke P, Dixon MF: Local recurrence of rectal adenocarcinoma due to inadequate surgical resection. *Lancet* 1:996–998, 1986.

7. Vernava AM III, Robbins PL, Brabbee GW: Restorative resection: coloanal anastomosis for benign and malignant disease. *Dis Colon Rectum* 32:690–693, 1990.

8. Wexner SD, Taranow D, Johansen OB, et al: Loop ileostomy: A safe alternative for fecal diversion. *Dis Colon Rectum* 36:349–354, 1993.

9. Williams NS, Dixon MF, Johnston D: Reappraisal of the 5 centimeter rule of distal excision for carcinoma of the rectum: a study of distal intranural spread and of patient's survival. *Br J Surg* 70:150–154, 1983.

See also Chapters 46 and 48.

CHAPTER 48

Adjuvant Therapy

James Weick, M.D.

Refer to Algorithm 48–1.

A. 95% of all rectal tumors are epithelial adenocarcinoma.
B. Complete blood count (CBC), Chemistries carcinoembryonic antigen (CEA).
C. Preoperation chest radiograph; computerized tomography (CT) of abdomen and pelvis suggested, especially if preoperative irradiation to be considered. Rectal ultrasound becoming more useful in assessing tumor node metastases (TNM) preoperatively.
D. Prognostic indicators:

Stage	Duration of symptoms
Age	Obstruction
Gender	Perforation
Perineural invasion	Location
Vascular invasion	Lymph nodes
Grade	Oncogene expression
Cell type	
Ploidy	

E. Recommended for Stage 2 and 3 (most patients with T_3 or T_4 and/or N_1) rectal cancers (NIH Consensus Conference 1990) using Hi Dose Pelvic Irradiation (45–55 Gy) and 5-fluorouracil. 5-Fluorouracil (5-FU) at 500 mg/m²/d × 5, D_1 and D_{28} by IV bolus, beginning 22–70 days after surgery. Irradiation to 5040 cGy in 180 fractions × 5 days weekly for 6 weeks, beginning day 56 after therapy initiated; 5-FU at 500 mg/m² days 1–3 of irradiation and last 3 days of irradiation; 5-FU at 400 mg/m²/d × 5 one month after irradiation completed and repeated in 4 weeks for 5 days at identical dose.
F. Endpoints of adjuvant treatment of rectal cancer can be evaluated by

1. Incidence of local recurrence
2. Time to relapse (DFS)
3. Overall survival

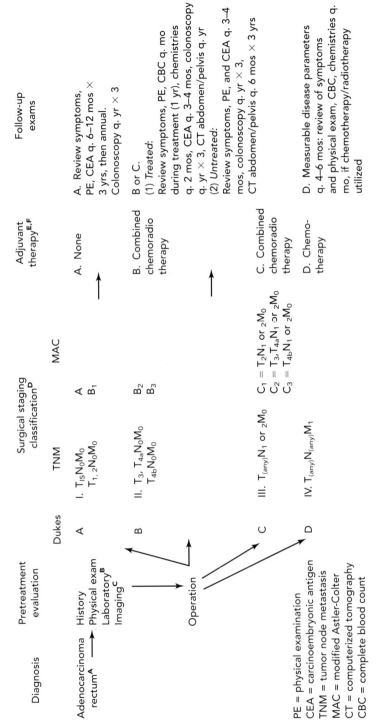

ALGORITHM 48-1

Diagnosis	Pretreatment evaluation	Surgical staging classification[D] Dukes	TNM	MAC	Adjuvant therapy[E,F]	Follow-up exams
Adenocarcinoma rectum[A]	History, Physical exam[B], Laboratory[C], Imaging[C] → Operation	A	I. $T_{IS}N_0M_0$, $T_{1,2}N_0M_0$	A, B_1	A. None	A. Review symptoms, PE, CEA q. 6–12 mos × 3 yrs, then annual. Colonoscopy q. yr × 3
		B	II. T_3, $T_{4a}N_0M_0$, $T_{4b}N_0M_0$	B_2, B_3	B. Combined chemoradio therapy	B or C. (1) *Treated:* Review symptoms, PE, CBC q. mo during treatment (1 yr), chemistries q. 2 mos, CEA q. 3–4 mos, colonoscopy q. yr × 3, CT abdomen/pelvis q. yr (2) *Untreated:* Review symptoms, PE, and CEA q. 3–4 mos, colonoscopy q. yr × 3, CT abdomen/pelvis q. 6 mos × 3 yrs
		C	III. $T_{(any)}N_1$ or $_2M_0$	$C_1 = T_2N_1$ or $_2M_0$, $C_2 = T_3,T_{4a}N_1$ or $_2M_0$, $C_3 = T_{4b}N_1$ or $_2M_0$	C. Combined chemoradio therapy	
		D	IV. $T_{(any)}N_{(any)}M_1$		D. Chemotherapy	D. Measurable disease parameters q. 4–6 mos: review of symptoms and physical exam, CBC, chemistries q. mo, if chemotherapy/radiotherapy utilized

PE = physical examination
CEA = carcinoembryonic antigen
TNM = tumor node metastasis
MAC = modified Astler-Colter
CT = computerized tomography
CBC = complete blood count

Single-modality adjuvants (irradiation *or* chemotherapy) don't achieve these endpoints

- Radiation diminishes local recurrences but does not change survival rate.
- Chemotherapy produces significant improvement in DFS and slight improvement overall survival.

Combined modality trials improve all three parameters.

BIBLIOGRAPHY

1. Buyse M, Zeleniuca-Jacquotte A, Chalmers T: Adjuvant therapy of colorectal cancer. *JAMA* 259:3571–3578, 1988.
2. Krook JE, Moertel CG, Gunderson LL, et al: Effective surgical adjuvent therapy for high risk rectal carcinoma. *N. Engl J Med* 324:709–715, 1991.
3. Moertel CG: Chemotherapy for colorectal cancer. *New Engl J Med* 330:1136–1142, 1994.
4. NIH Consensus Conference. Adjuvant therapy for patients with colon and rectal cancer. *JAMA* 264:1444–1450, 1990.
5. Schilsky R, Brachman D: Adjuvant chemotherapy and radiation therapy in colorectal cancer. *PPO Updates* 6(3): March 1992.
6. Sugarbaker PH, Gianola FJ, Dwyer A, et al: A simplified plan for followup of patients with colon and rectal cancer supported by prospective studies of laboratory and radiologic test results. *Surgery* 102:79–87, 1987.

CHAPTER 49

Postoperative Follow-up of Rectal Cancer

Anthony J. Senagore, M.D., M.S.

Refer to Algorithm 49-1.

A. Following operation for cure of rectal adenocarcinoma, a number of facts should be used to assess potential risks of local and locoregional recurrence. Factors adversely affecting survival include Duke's "C" stage, mucinous tumor, poorly differentiated neoplasms, diffusely infiltrating tumor, vascular, lymphatic or perineural invasion, and lower-third rectal lesions.

B. The pattern of recurrence of rectal cancer is affected primarily by the adequacy of the mesorectal dissection at the initial procedure. Very little influence is attributed by the anastomotic technique or the performance of a low anterior resection versus an abdominal perineal resection. Overall, the risk of local recurrence as the first sign of treatment failure occurs in 19-21% following abdominoperineal resection, 17-19% for sutured low anterior resections, and 12-24% for stapled low anterior resections. Overall, the risk is higher the more distal the primary lesion. Recurrence can be either distant (liver), local or both.

C. Patients should be interviewed for symptoms of weight loss, decreased appetite, decreased activity level, change in bowel habits, tenesmus, rectal bleeding, or pelvic pain. Abdominal examination for the presence of abdominal masses or organomegaly should be done at each follow-up visit. Digital rectal examination and perineal examination should be performed. In a female patient, vaginal exam is essential. Overall, history and physical examination identify 20-25% of recurrences. These visits should occur at 3-month intervals for 2 years, every 6 months for the next 2 years, and yearly thereafter prostatic specific antigen (PSA) screening for prostate cancer should be considered in males >50 years old following abdominoperineal resection (APR).

D. Rigid sigmoidoscopy should be performed at each office visit. Colonoscopy should be done at the first-year anniversary and if no adenomatous neoplasms are found, at 3-year intervals thereafter.

E. Carcinoembryonic antigen (CEA) determination should be made within 2-4 weeks postoperatively and then repeated at 3-month intervals at the time of each office visit. If an elevation is identified, the test should be repeated in 1 month to see if this is a true elevation. One elevation >10 mg/dL or 2 progres-

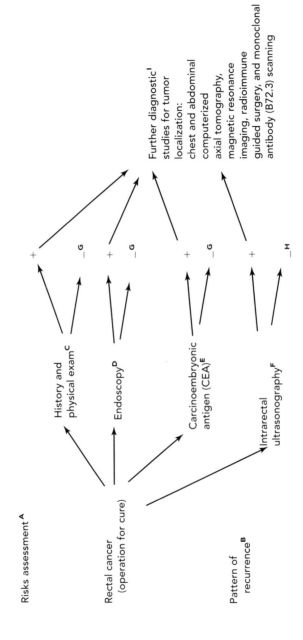

Postoperative follow-up of rectal cancer

Risks assessment ^A

History and physical exam^C

Endoscopy^D

Rectal cancer (operation for cure)

Carcinoembryonic antigen (CEA)^E

Pattern of recurrence^B

Intrarectal ultrasonography^F

Further diagnostic^I studies for tumor localization: chest and abdominal computerized axial tomography, magnetic resonance imaging, radioimmune guided surgery, and monoclonal antibody (B72.3) scanning

ALGORITHM 49–1

sive increases should lead to further investigations (see paragraph I). CEA elevation will be the initial indication of recurrent disease in 60–70% of patients.

F. Rectal ultrasound has been highly accurate in preoperative staging of rectal cancers. Postoperatively this tool has been used with success transanally or transvaginally (after APR in females) for the early identification of local recurrence. The study should be performed at 1–2 months following surgery to identify postoperative changes. Thereafter, 6-month intervals should be adequate. If a suspicious area is noted, intrarectal ultrasound guided biopsies can be performed.

G. Continue every 3 months for 2 years, then every 6 months for 2 years, then yearly thereafter.

H. Repeat every 6 months for 2 years, then annually for 2 years.

I. If recurrent disease is suspected based on clinical examination, CEA determination, endoscopy, or rectal ultrasound, localization of extensive disease is essential. The patient should undergo colonoscopy to exclude a metachronous neoplasm. In addition, chest, abdominal, and pelvic computerized tomography (CT) should be obtained. Magnetic resonance imaging (MRI) may be somewhat more accurate in assessing pelvic scar versus recurrent disease. The patient should also undergo a thorough medical evaluation if further surgery is considered. Recently, immunoscintigraphy with indium-labeled B72.3 monoclonal antibody has shown promise in localizing recurrent disease.

BIBLIOGRAPHY

1. Abdel-Nab HH, Doerr RJ: Multicenter clinical trials of monoclonal antibody B72.3-GYK-DTPA 111In (111In-CYT-103; OncoScint CR103) in patients with colorectal carcinoma. *Targeted Diagn Ther* 6:73–88, 1992.

2. Beynon J, Mortenson NJ McC, Foy DMA, et al: The detection and evaluation of locally recurrent rectal cancer with rectal endosonography. *Dis Colon Rectum* 32:509–517, 1989.

3. Chu DJ, Erickson CA, Russell MP, et al: Prognostic significance of carcinoembryonic antigen in colorectal carcinoma. *Arch Surg* 126:314–316, 1991.

4. Ferguson E Jr: Operations of choice for cancers of the colon and rectum: an overview. *Am Surg* 3:121–127, 1984.

5. Neville R, Fielding LP, Amendola C: Local tumor recurrence after curative resection for rectal cancer. *Dis Colon Rectum* 30:12–17, 1987.

6. Rocklin MS, Senagore AJ, Talbott TM: Role of carcinoembryonic antigen and liver function tests in the detection of recurrent colorectal carcinoma. *Dis Colon Rectum* 34:794–797, 1991.

7. Sugarbaker PH, Gianola FJ, Dwyer A, et al: A simplified plan for follow-up of patients with colon and rectal cancer supported by prospective studies of laboratory and radiologic test results. *Surgery* 102:79–87, 1987.

8. Thoeni R: Colorectal cancer: cross-sectional imaging for staging of primary tumor and detection of local recurrence. *Am J Radiol* 156:909–915, 1991.

9. Wolmark N, Gordon P, Fisher B, et al: A comparison of stapled and handsewn anastomoses in patients undergoing resection for Dukes' B and C colorectal cancer: an analysis of disease-free survival and survival from the NSABP prospective clinical trials. *Dis Colon Rectum* 29:344–350, 1986.

See also Chapters 46, 47, 48 and 50.

CHAPTER 50

Recurrent Rectal Cancer

Göran Ekelund, M.D. Mans Bohe, M.D. and Thomas Troeng, M.D.

Refer to Algorithm 50--1.

A. Recurrent rectal carcinoma may be suspected either because of symptoms or if found in asymptomatic patients during follow-up. The total recurrence rate after curative resection of rectal carcinoma is 20--50%. The longer the observation time and the higher the autopsy rate, the higher the observed rate of local as well as distant metastases. The recurrence is local pelvic in 25%, metastatic in 25%, and combined local and disseminated disease in 50%.

B. In patients with poor general health, or who are otherwise not suitable for either curative resection or radiotherapy, further evaluation of possibly resectable disease is unnecessary.

C. In patients operated on with sphincter-saving resection, local recurrences are often diagnosed endoscopically and confirmed with biopsy. In patients operated on with abdominoperineal resection biopsy from the perineum or vagina may be performed. Computed tomographic (CT) scanning as well as ultrasound may detect recurrent disease—if present—in the pelvis or in the liver and can be combined with fine-needle biopsy of any suspected mass. Pulmonary metastases are easiest detected with x-ray of the chest. Hepatic metastases less than 1 cm in diameter can rarely be detected.

D. In highly selected patients with no extrapelvic disease, a pelvic exenteration or abdominosacral resection has been reported.

E. For nonfixed local recurrences without signs of disseminated disease a curative abdominoperineal resection or a re-resection can be attempted with reported 5-year survival of 15--40%. Most of the local recurrences are detected during the first 2 years after resection. Most of the recurrences are due to tumor growth in the pelvis outside the bowel but may invade the wall and then be seen endoscopically. The anastomotic recurrence limited to the bowel wall is very rare.

F. Nonnarcotic analgesics can usually control mild cancer pain. In moderate to severe pain narcotic analgesics can be used. Good results are usually obtained

Recurrent rectal cancer

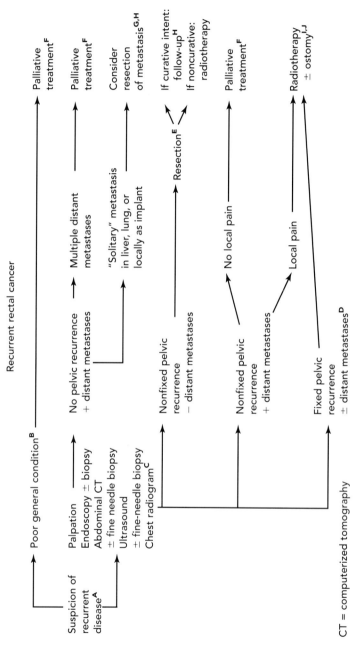

CT = computerized tomography

ALGORITHM 50–1

when analgesics are administered via an epidural catheter. Chemotherapy may be of value for palliative treatment of recurrent disease. Compared to untreated patients, a mean increase in survival of 2–5 months has been reported.

G. Patients with solitary hepatic or pulmonary metastases may be cured by resection with a 30–50% 5-year survival rate in selected series.

H. Although the results of the different types of operation for recurrent rectal carcinoma seem fairly good, this is so only in about 1% of all patients operated on for cure.

I. For inextirpable local recurrences, radiotherapy with a dose of 45 Gy will result in a good palliation in 80% of the patients, even if only temporary.

J. For patients with symptomatic stenosis or stricture of the rectum a sigmoidostomy may eventually be necessary for deviation of the fecal stream.

BIBLIOGRAPHY

1. Corman ML (ed): Carcinoma of the rectum, treatment of local recurrence. In *Colon and Rectal Surgery*. Philadelphia: Lippincott, 1993, Vol 3, pp 646–648.

2. Gordon PH, Nivatvongs S (eds): Malignant neoplasm of the rectum, recurrent disease, In *Principles and Practice of Surgery for the Colon, Rectum and Anus*. St. Louis: Quality Medical Publishing, 1992, pp 637–664.

3. Keighley M RB, Williams NS (eds): Recurrence of colorectal carcinoma. In *Surgery of the Anus, Rectum and Colon*. London: Saunders, 1993, Vol 1, pp 1073–1083.

4. Safi F, Link KH, Berger HG: Is follow-up of colorectal cancer patients worthwhile? *Dis Colon Rectum* 36:636–644, 1993.

5. Wanebo HJ, Gaker DL, Whitehill R: Pelvic recurrence of rectal cancer, option for curative resection. *Ann Surg* 12:482–495, 1987.

See also Chapter 49.

SECTION 5A

Colonic Pathology
Inflammatory Conditions

CHAPTER 51

Crohn's Colitis

David A. Rothenberger, M.D.

Refer to Algorithm 51–1.

A. *Crohn's Colitis.* While ileocolic Crohn's disease is the most common pattern, about 30% of cases involve only the large bowel. Two-thirds of such individuals will have total proctocolitis, while one-third will have segmental distribution of Crohn's colitis. About 3% of patients have Crohn's disease involving only the rectum and/or perianum. Surgeons must always be aware that patients may have other involved segments of bowel that can impact on surgical therapy.

B. *Clinical Evaluation.* Symptoms of Crohn's colitis are nonspecific, and other types of colitis must be considered and excluded. Pseudomembranous colitis is suspected by a history of prior antibiotic use. Infectious colitis can be suspected by an unusual travel history. Distinguishing Crohn's colitis from ulcerative colitis can be difficult and is sometimes impossible for the endoscopist and even for the pathologist. Physical examination provides critical information regarding the patient's overall status and is focused on abdominal findings. It is important not to neglect the perianal region, anal canal, and anal sphincter in assessing a patient with Crohn's colitis as the condition of these areas will have important implications for subsequent treatment. Extraintestinal manifestations of Crohn's disease should be noted.

C. *Ancillary tests.* Laboratory tests can confirm need for fluid resuscitation, transfusion, institution of nutritional support, and can help exclude other types of colitis. A flat and upright abdominal x-ray can exclude colonic distention, obstruction, or free air. A computerized tomography (CT) scan may identify an abscess amenable to percutaneous drainage and can warn the surgeon that a ureter or some other structure may be adjacent to or involved within a phlegmonous reaction from Crohn's disease. Contrast studies of the large and small intestine are of some value in assessing patients with concomitant small bowel disease or with suspected fistulas involving the colon and other viscera. Endoscopic examination is highly useful in making the initial diagnosis of Crohn's colitis and in determining its extent and severity. Biopsies may be

Crohn's Colitis[A]

ALGORITHM 51-5

Diagnosis	Triage[D]	Condition	Treatment

Diagnosis

Clinical evaluation[B]
- History
  - Symptoms
  - Past history
  - Current medications
- Physical examination
  - General
  - Abdomen
  - Anorectum

Ancillary tests[C]
- Laboratory
- Medical imaging
- Endoscopy

Triage[D] → Condition → Treatment

Emergency →
- Toxic colitis/megacolon → Resuscitation, antibiotics → Exploration → Segmental vs. total colectomy ± Drainage ± anastomosis vs. diversion
- Free perforation[E]
- Massive hemorrhage[F] → Resuscitation, identify source of bleeding, attempt nonoperative control →
  - Specific colonic hemorrhage → Segmental colectomy
  - Diffuse colonic hemorrhage → Total colectomy with ileostomy vs. ileorectal anastomosis
  - Minimal or no rectal hemorrhage, Normal sphincter
  - Diffuse colonic and rectal hemorrhage → Severe rectal disease and/or sphincter dysfunction → Total proctocolectomy with ileostomy
  - (Exploration if unstable, transfusions, rebleed)

Nonemergency, complicated[G] →
- Dysplasia, carcinoma[H] →
  - Exploration, curative intent
  - Exploration, palliative intent
- Fistula, abscess[I] → Control sepsis, define anatomy → Exploration
- Obstruction, stricture[J] → Exclude cancer, medical therapy ± balloon dilation → Exploration if fails
  - Minimal or no rectal disease, Normal sphincter → Segmental resection
  - Diffuse colitis and severe rectal disease and/or sphincter dysfunction → Total proctocolectomy + ileostomy vs. segmental resection

Nonemergency, Uncomplicated[K] →
- Severe colitis → Hospitalize for medical therapy
  - Improved → Outpatient medical therapy
  - Not improved → Exploration if fails
    - Sphincter dysfunction and/or severe rectal disease and normal proximal colon → Proctectomy + colostomy
- Moderate or mild colitis → Outpatient medical therapy

obtained but are often nonspecific, and the clinician's judgment as to the type of colitis is usually more useful. The surgeon must determine the extent and severity of Crohn's proctitis. Endoscopy in the setting of toxic megacolon is dangerous and, if performed, is limited to the rectum, which is examined without insufflating air.

D. *Triage.* Clinical evaluation and ancillary testing should provide the physician with sufficient information to properly triage the patient with Crohn's colitis. Emergency complications consist of toxic colitis: megacolon, free perforation, or massive hemorrhage. Nonemergency cases can be grouped as either complicated or uncomplicated.

E. *Free perforation.* Free perforation requires immediate resuscitation, institution of antibiotics, and exploration of the abdomen. Segmental colectomy is generally adequate, but if there is diffuse colonic disease, it is best to do a total colectomy. If there is an established abscess cavity, drainage is mandatory. No definitive guidelines are available to determine when a primary anastomosis following an emergency colectomy is safe. In the absence of significant peritoneal contamination, shock, severe malnutrition, or other systemic diseases that would impair healing, a primary anastomosis is likely safe. In critically ill patients, colectomy with ileostomy is preferred. In any event, a protectomy should not be performed in this setting.

F. *Massive hemorrhage.* Laparotomy for massive hemorrhage from Crohn's colitis is required if the patient remains unstable despite aggressive resuscitative efforts or if continued transfusions are necessary. Segmental resection is reasonable if a specific source of colonic hemorrhage is identified. Usually the bleeding is diffuse and total colectomy with ileostomy is advised. The rectum is rarely the source of uncontrolled major hemorrhage. Thus, a protectomy is almost never indicated and an ileoproctostomy can be performed after recovery.

G. *Complicated Crohn's colitis.* Infectious, obstructive, and neoplastic changes can complicate Crohn's colitis. Whenever possible, the surgeon should try to convert urgent surgery to elective laparotomy. Patients who are chronically ill may need correction of fluid and electrolyte imbalance, transfusion, and/or hyperalimentation. Preoperative education and marking for a temporary or permanent stoma will minimize patient anxiety and optimize stomal function. Ureteral stents should be considered in patients with an inflammatory or neoplastic mass. The rectum should be preserved when possible for subsequent ileoproctostomy.

H. *Dysplasia–Carcinoma.* Patients with long-standing Crohn's colitis have a significantly increased risk of developing carcinoma, especially if their disease onset was at an early age. Rectal cancer requires a radical resection. In the absence of metastases, a rectal cancer should be treated by radical proctectomy and total colectomy with ileostomy. There is controversy regarding the optimal treatment of a potentially curable carcinoma in the proximal colon. Some surgeons advocate a total colectomy and ileorectal anastomosis if the rectum is relatively normal and sphincter function is good. Others advise removal of all large bowel mucosa with a total proctocolectomy and ileostomy. Segmental resection is indicated for palliation.

I. *Fistula–abscess.* Sepsis from internal fistulas and walled-off abscess can often be controlled with systemic antibiotics and percutaneous CT-guided drainage. Most Crohn's colonic fistulas to the bladder, skin, stomach, small bowel, rectum, uterus, vagina, or ureter will ultimately require operative intervention. The goal of such surgery is to resect the diseased segment of colon and close the secondarily involved organ. Perianal and anal canal abscesses should be drained. Anorectal and anovaginal fistulas are often treated nonoperatively. For highly symptomatic patients, advancement endorectal flap repair is performed if the anorectum is relatively normal and sphincter function is normal. If severe anorectal Crohn's disease is present or if the patient is incontinent, proctectomy is indicated. A conservative, intersphincteric proctectomy is advised to minimize morbidity. On occasion a temporary loop ileostomy may allow healing of the perianal disease. Such a stoma is well suited to laparoscopic construction.

J. *Obstruction–stricture.* An element of obstruction often accompanies the infectious complications of Crohn's colitis and often requires a modification of the preoperative bowel preparation. Many strictures can be nonoperatively managed after excluding the presence of carcinoma. Endoscopic balloon dilations can be of value.

K. Noncomplicated Crohn's colitis. Patients with severe acute colitis should be hospitalized for intensive medical therapy, and after improvement, followed closely in the outpatient setting. If they fail to improve, operative intervention must be considered. The extent of the disease, and in particular the degree of involvement of the anorectum and anal sphincter function determine whether a proctectomy or a restorative procedure is indicated.

BIBLIOGRAPHY

1. Ekbom A, Helmick C, Zack M, et al: Increased risk of large bowel cancer in Crohn's disease with colonic involvement. *Lancet* 336:357–359, 1990.

2. Nogueras JJ, Rothenberger DA: Surgical management of anorectal Crohn's disease. *Prob Gen Surg* 10:169–179, 1993.

3. Strong SA, Fazio VW: Crohn's disease of the colon, rectum and anus. In Wolff BG (ed): *Inflammatory Disorders of the Colon.* Reprinted in *Surg Clin N Am* 73:933–963, 1993.

4. Williams JG, Wong WD, Rothenberger DA, et al: Recurrence of Crohn's disease after resection. *Br J Surg* 78:10–19, 1991.

See also Chapters 5, 20, 21, 40, 52, 54 and 55.

CHAPTER 52

Mucosal Ulcerative Colitis

R. J. Nicholls, M. Chir, F.R.C.S., and Friedrich Herbst M.D.

Refer to Algorithm 52-1.

Ulcerative colitis (UC) is a chronic inflammatory condition confined to the large bowel mucosa. The etiology and pathogenesis are under investigation. It probably occurs in a genetically susceptible subject as a result of the interaction between antigenic stimulus and cells of the immune system.

CLINICAL PRESENTATION

The disease is characterized by local symptoms of bloody diarrhea and mucus. Urgency is a common feature and is related to rectal inflammation. In patients with distal involvement only, constipation may occur and the stool may be normal. However, blood and mucus are typical. There is a relationship between the anatomic extent of the disease and the presence of systemic symptoms. In patients with extensive involvement of the large bowel, there may be evidence of malnutrition with anorexia, weight loss, and hypoproteinemia due to the protein-losing enteropathy. The disease may be chronic or acute. Patients with chronic disease may have acute exacerbations. There is a general tendency for periodicity with exacerbations and remissions. Extraintestinal manifestations, including skin, joint, eye or liver disease, may be present, usually in patients with extensive colitis. Anal lesions complicate severe diarrhea and are not primary manifestations of disease.

Severe acute colitis leading to fulminant colitis or toxic dilatation occurs in about 5-10% of cases, most commonly during the first attack. In this situation, malnutrition, water, and electrolyte depletion and toxicity may occur (see Chapter 54).

A. *Diagnosis.* The rectum is involved in all cases, and inflammation will be seen on rigid sigmoidoscopy. If rectal inflammation is absent, Crohn's disease or previous treatment with local steroids should be considered. Usually, there is

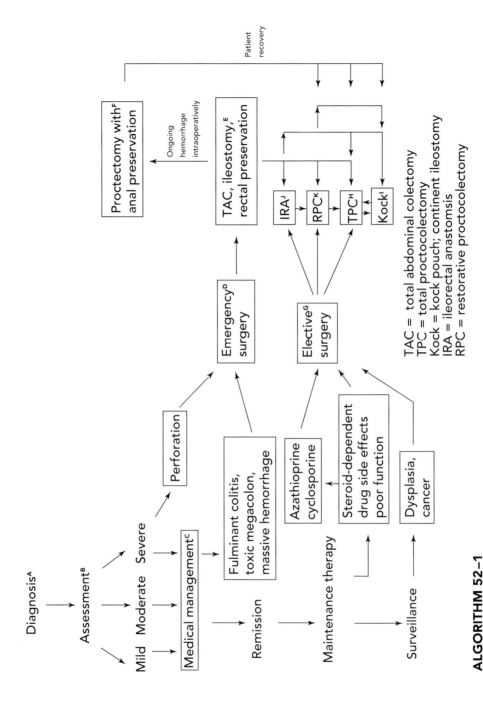

Patient recovery

Proctectomy with[F] anal preservation

Ongoing hemorrhage intraoperatively

TAC, ileostomy,[E] rectal preservation

IRA[J]   RPC[K]   TPC[H]   Kock[I]

Emergency[D] surgery

Elective[G] surgery

Perforation

Fulminant colitis, toxic megacolon, massive hemorrhage

Azathioprine cyclosporine

Steroid-dependent drug side effects poor function

Dysplasia, cancer

Diagnosis[A]

Assessment[B]

Mild   Moderate   Severe

Medical management[C]

Remission

Maintenance therapy

Surveillance

TAC = total abdominal colectomy
TPC = total proctocolectomy
Kock = kock pouch; continent ileostomy
IRA = ileorectal anastomsis
RPC = restorative proctocolectomy

ALGORITHM 52–1

diffuse hyperemia with contact bleeding and granularity due to mucosal edema; occasionally ulceration is evident. In patients with repeated acute exacerbations, pseudopolyps may be present. A stool sample and a biopsy should be taken to exclude infection (e.g., clostridium–difficile) particularly amebiasis. A barium enema is an extremely useful investigation tool as it will demonstrate the anatomic extent of the disease. Blood tests for hemoglobin, albumen, and platelets, will indicate the severity of systemic involvement. A biopsy may not distinguish between ulcerative colitis and Crohn's disease. Under this circumstance, further biopsy is necessary and small bowel radiology should be undertaken. Clinical features, including the presence of anal disease, should be taken into account in distinguishing between Crohn's disease and ulcerative colitis. Histologic indeterminate colitis is reported most commonly in colectomy specimens obtained after emergency surgery (see below).

B. *Assessment.* Assessment is the key to management. Anatomic extent is related to the severity of disease. Radiologic or endoscopic examination of the colon is essential. At presentation 50% of patients have disease confined to the rectum, 30% confined to the left colon, and in 20% inflammation extends beyond the splenic flexure (extensive disease). Severity of symptoms, including frequency of defecation, urgency with urge incontinence, or blood on each defecation all indicate severe local symptoms. Weight loss, anorexia, anemia, and hypoproteinemia are important markers of systemic involvement. Ulcerative colitis predisposes to cancer. This development is confined to patients with extensive disease or rarely those with left-sided colitis. The incidence within 10 years from onset of symptoms is negligible. Because the risk increases at 1% per year, annual colonoscopic surveillance is obligatory. Multiple biopsies should be reviewed by the pathologist for the presence of dysplasia.

MANAGEMENT AND SURGICAL TREATMENT

C. *Medical.* Medical management is the mainstay of treatment. When local symptoms exist alone, topical steroids or 5-aminosalicylic acid (5-ASA) medication (enemas or suppositories) combined with oral 5-ASA should be given. Patients with more severe disease, including systemic involvement, should be treated by oral or intravenous steroids according to severity. In these cases a starting dose of prednisolone 40 mg is appropriate. However if oral 5-ASA and tapered steroids are added, remission may be possible even while the steroids are tapered. In patients with chronic disease requiring long-term steroids, azathioprine may be useful in reducing steroid dependence. Patients with acute severe colitis require admission to hospital. They will have severe local symptoms and systemic features. Close monitoring of vital functions including pulse, blood pressure, and temperature is undertaken. Such patients may develop toxic dilatation leading to perforation. Monitoring of the abdomen is therefore essential. This care requires regular clinical examination of the abdomen and daily plain radiographs to assess colonic diameter. A diameter of ≥ 7 cm is taken to indicate dilatation. If intravenous steroids in high doses (e.g., prednisolone $\geqq$ 60 mg) are given, 70% of patients will respond within a week. In these patients the dose of prednisolone can be gradually reduced over a period of several weeks. Such patients should be managed jointly by gastroenterologist and surgeon. Response to treatment is monitored by improvement in vital signs and symptoms. If response does not occur within a few days, surgery is indicated. Recently cyclosporine has been used in the acute case with encouraging results. Patients with chronic colitis managed by steroids should also receive nutritional supplements, including iron. Individuals with extensive colitis should enter into a colonoscopic surveillance program. Most patients can be medically managed throughout their lives, but the proportion referred for surgery has increased in the last 15 years with the introduction of restorative proctocolectomy. The indications can be divided into emergency and elective.

D. *Emergency.* The indications for emergency surgery include acute severe colitis unresponsive to medical treatment, toxic megacolon, perforation, and massive hemorrhage. If appropriate medical treatment of acute severe colitis does not lead to improvement within 24–48 hours or the patient worsens (develops toxic colitis), surgery is indicated. Frequent careful monitoring, preferably by the same surgeon, is required to reduce delay and to avoid toxic dilatation or perforation. About 70% of patients requiring emergency surgery are in this category; 20% have toxic dilatation that itself is an indication for surgery; and perforation occurs in about 10% of patients undergoing emergency surgery. Massive bleeding is a rare indication for surgery. When it occurs, it usually arises from ulceration in the rectum.

E. The choice of operation is now generally agreed to be colectomy with ileostomy and preservation of the rectal stump. In patients with toxic megacolon, great care should be taken to avoid damage to the friable bowel wall. In patients with perforation, despite peritoneal irrigation, a mortality of 30–40% is common. The distal sigmoid may be exteriorized to the mucous fistula or closed, according to the condition of the bowel wall. If there is any doubt of the capability of the bowel to take sutures owing to edema or friability, a mucous fistula must be carried out. This operation leads to recovery of the general health of the patient in almost all cases and leaves all subsequent therapeutic operations as options.

F. Where bleeding is the indication, it will be necessary to resect the area of ulcerated bowel. This exceedingly rare situation may well require a rectal excision as well as a colectomy. In this circumstance the anal canal and pelvic floor should always be preserved.

G. *Elective.* There are three chief indications for elective surgery: failed medical treatment, retardation of growth in a child, and the development of dysplasia or invasive cancer. Other less frequent indications include intolerance to medical management (such as side effects) or extraintestinal manifestations of inflammatory bowel disease (IBD) unresponsive to medical management. Failure of medical treatment may be difficult to judge. The patient may not be objectively aware of the severity of local or systemic symptoms. As a general guide, however, chronic symptoms including anemia leading to invalidity at work or home, recurrent severe acute attacks, severe symptoms, usually urgency or frequency even without systemic illness, and the presence of certain extraalimentary manifestations, are all indications for surgery. Excision of the disease will help the activity related polyarthropathy and about 50% of patients with pyoderma gangrenosum, but will not influence parenchymal liver disease, sclerosing cholangitis, or sacroileitis ankylosing spondylitis types of arthropathy. Retardation of growth in a child is a most important indication. Percentile chart analysis is essential. Steroids themselves can lead to early fusion of the epiphyses with dwarfism. It is now recognised that dysplasia of any type, high or low, may give a similar risk of invasion having already occurred.

CHOICE OF OPERATION

There are four elective operations available including conventional proctocolectomy with permanent ileostomy (TPC); colectomy with ileorectal anastomosis (IRA); restorative proctocolectomy (RPC), and continent ileostomy (KOCK). Each procedure involves a complete colectomy. The issues at stake are whether the rectum, including anal canal, should be preserved, whether the anal canal should be retained or whether both should be removed.

H. *Total proctocolectomy.* Total proctocolectomy (TPC) with permanent ileostomy became the standard operation in the early 1950s with the development of the everted spout (Brooke) ileostomy. It is a safe and curative operation; a close rectal dissection combined with an intersphincteric removal of the anus will avoid pelvic nerve damage. However, this technique should not be undertaken in patients with dysplasia since malignant invasion is possible. Complications include intestinal obstruction due to adhesions, delayed healing of the perineal wound, and ileostomy complications requiring revision. The cumulative revision rate over a 5-year period is between 20% and 30%. Despite the availability of sphincter saving operations, TPC still has a place for patients who do not wish to undergo the potential morbidity of restorative proctocolectomy or those candidates with poor sphincters. Clearly a patient with carcinoma in the lower rectum should have a total proctocolectomy.

I. *Kock ileostomy.* This operation is a modification applied to patients having had a total proctocolectomy. The operation was developed before restorative proctocolectomy became generally available and it has subsequently been relegated to an almost historical role. It has a complication and reoperation rate almost identical to those associated with restorative proctocolectomy. Therefore it should be advised to patients who are motivated to accept these possibilities for the potential improvement in the quality of life that the operation offers. It was the first reservoir operation developed and its success led to the introduction of restorative proctocolectomy (RPC). The 45 cm of terminal ileum are used. A two-loop reservoir is fashioned and a distal limb (15 cm) is invaginated into the reservoir to form an inverted nipple valve. This valve is held in place by four applications of linear staplers. The terminal ileum is brought out via an abdominal stoma just above the inguinal ligament. Cosmetically as well as functionally it is therefore preferable to a conventional ileostomy. Patients evacuate the reservoir 2–4 times per day with a catheter and do not require a stoma appliance. Currently, candidates are mainly patients who have already had a TPC or who are unsuitable for an RPC owing to poor sphincter function. It may also be used as a salvage following failed RPC. Motivation and competence to catheterize the pouch are required. The main disadvantage of the procedure is a high reoperation rate owing to subluxation of the nipple valve. When this happens, continence is lost. Reoperation rates to restore the valve are in the range 10–50%. Other complications include pouchitis, stricture of the stoma, and fistula formation. The operation is almost never appropriate as the first surgical alternative in the young patient with mucosal ulcerative colitis (MUC) and should never be knowingly offered to patients with Crohn's disease.

J. *Ileorectal anastomosis.* Ileorectal anastomosis (IRA) either after abdominal colectomy or following an initial total abdominal colectomy (TAC), is indicated where the rectum is thought to be satisfactory. Failure of the operation over a 5–10-year period is 20–50%. Reasons for failure include persistent disease or neoplastic transformation. The criteria thus include a rectum with minimal inflammation that has adequate reservoir capacity, absence of dysplasia, and adequate anal sphincters. Rectal capacitance and sphincter function can be tested by preoperative physiological examination. After IRA patients must be regularly assessed by sigmoidoscopy with rectal biopsy for the development of dysplasia. If the patient is unlikely to comply with this demand, the operation is contraindicated. The anastomosis is performed at the level of the sacral promontory without pelvic dissection. In patients who have previously had an emergency colectomy with partial removal of the rectum, it is preferable to advise a restorative proctocolectomy. In general, IRA offers low operative and perioperative morbidity.

K. *Restorative proctocolectomy.* Today the most frequently performed elective operation for ulcerative colitis is restorative proctocolectomy (RPC). The reason for its popularity is that it eradicates virtually all diseased mucosa and avoids a permanent stoma. The operation involves excision of the colon and rectum with transection of the gut tube at the level of the anorectal junction. Classically a mucosectomy of the anorectal stump is performed leaving a short muscular cuff. A reservoir of terminal ileum using two, three, or four loops is made and is joined to the anus just above the dentate line using an endoanal technique. Modifications have included construction of the reservoir using staples and stapled ileoanal anastomosis without mucosectomy. In the latter circumstance, care must be taken not to employ a pouch-rectal anastomosis. For many years the operation was covered by a defunctioning ileostomy. More recently this step has been omitted in selected cases. However, there is a learning curve, and complications are common, with rates of 25–40%. There is a reoperation rate of 15–25% and an overall failure rate within the first year of 5–15%. At a median of 8 years, failure with the need to establish a permanent ileostomy is approximately 5–15%. It is very important to adopt strict indications for this procedure. Crohn's disease must be excluded; an acutely ill patient should have an initial TAC. The anal sphincters should be adequately assessed, when possible, by preoperative manometry. Patients with carcinoma in the lower rectum should be excluded unless the lesion is early. Patients must be fully aware of the possible complications and time scale of the operation. They should not be pressured in their decision and should have every opportunity of being informed and seeing patients who have already had the procedure. In most series about 50% of patients have had a previous TAC. There is no contraindication on the basis of physique, but obese or tall patients or those previously operated on may have a relatively short mesentery; age is no contraindication. Patients with indeterminate colitis in whom there are no clinical or radiological stigmata of Crohn's disease are still candidates for RPC. In cases with dysplasia, a mucosectomy should be employed.

RESULTS

Complications are common. The most important early examples include pelvic sepsis (5–10%), almost always due to some degree of breakdown of the ileoanal anastomosis. In females this complication may lead to pouch vaginal fistula. During long-term follow-up, small bowel obstruction occurs in approximately 20% of patients, half of whom need a laparotomy. Pouchitis is a long-term complication occurring cumulatively over a 5-year period in up to 30% of patients. Pouchitis causes increased frequency of defecation with the passage of stool more fluid than usual, sometimes associated with malaise, fever, abdominal colics, and intestinal manifestations, particularly arthropathy. The condition is intermittent and may indeed occur only once. Patients likely to be at risk for developing pouchitis can be recognized by histologic examination of a biopsy taken within 3–6 months of closure of the ileostomy. Treatment of pouchitis includes antibacterial agents such as metronidazole or ciprofloxacin and conventional antiinflammatory treatment with 5-ASA and steroids. Overall most patients obtain a good functional result, frequency of evacuation decreases with time. Urgency occurs in less than 5% of patients, and continence is normal in 70–90% of patients. Fecal leakage is rare, but flatus incontinence or mucous leakage occur in 10–30% of patients. Some patients experience night leakage. In these individuals, ambulatory studies have demonstrated a poor sphincter response to increases in pouch pressure. After adaptation of up to a year, most patients will have a mean evacuation frequency of 3–7 times per 24 hours. The most important predictors of frequency are pouch capacity and compliance, the absence of pelvic sepsis and pouchitis. Autonomic nerve damage is very rare. Recently laparoscopic assisted RPC has been tried but in a controlled study it has not resulted in benefit for patients apart from a smaller incision.

CONCLUSIONS

Ulcerative colitis is managed in most cases by medical treatment. The indications for surgery require experience to define patients in whom medical treatment has not been successful. The choice of surgery does offer most patients the opportunity of avoiding a permanent ileostomy. Patients should be advised as to the various merits and problems of each option. They should also be encouraged to speak with other patients who have undergone the various options. No single procedure is uniformly applicable. Care must be taken in correct case selection, and the surgeon must be prepared and able to manage complications after restorative proctocolectomy should they occur.

BIBLIOGRAPHY

1. Jorge JMN, Wexner SD, James K, Nogueras JJ, et al: Recovery of anal sphincter function after the ileoanal reservoir procedure in patients over the age of 50. *Dis Colon Rectum* 37:1002–1005, 1994.

2. Jorge JMN, Wexner SD, Morgado PJ Jr.: Optimization of sphincter function after the ileoanal reservoir—a prospective randomized trial. *Dis Colon Rectum* 37:419–423, 1994.

3. Keighley MRB, Williams NS, (eds): *Surgery of the Anus, Rectum and Colon*. London: Saunders 1993.

4. Morgado PJ Jr., Wexner SD, James K, et al: Ileal pouch and anastomosis (IPAA): is preoperative anal manometry predictive of postoperative functional outcome? *Dis Colon Rectum* 37:224–228, 1994.

5. Nicholls RJ, Bartolo DCC, Mortensen NJMcC, (eds): *Restorative Proctocolectomy*. Oxford; Blackwell Scientific Publications, 1993.

6. Schmitt SL, Cohen SM, Wexner SD, et al: Does laparoscopic assisted ileal pouch anal anastomosis reduce the length of hospitalization? *Int J Colorect Dis* 9:134–137, 1994.

7. Schmitt SL, Wexner SD, James K, et al: The retained mucosa after double-stapled ileal reservoir and ileoanal anastomosis. *Dis Colon Rectum* 35:1051–1056, 1992.

8. Targan SR, Shanahan F, (eds): *Inflammatory Bowel Disease—from Bench to Bedside*. Baltimore: Williams & Wilkins, 1994.

9. Wexner SD, Rothenberger DA, Jensen L, et al: Ileal pouch vaginal fistulae: incidence etiology and management. *Dis Colon Rectum* 32:460–465, 1989.

See also Chapters 5, 20, 21, 40, 51, 54 and 55.

CHAPTER 53

Extraintestinal Manifestations of Inflammatory Bowel Disease

Bruce A. Kerner, M.D.

Refer to Algorithms 53--1 through 53--4.

Increasing evidence supports the statement that inflammatory bowel disease (IBD) of the intestine is a systemic problem rather than one localized to the gastrointestinal tract. Extraintestinal manifestations in patients with IBD occur frequently, often complicate their management, and are a significant source of morbidity and mortality. There are approximately 100 systemic complications of inflammatory bowel disease involving most organ systems of the body. At least one extraintestinal manifestation occurs in 25--35% of patients with IBD. The organ systems most frequently affected (in decreasing order) are musculoskeletal, dermatologic, hepatobiliary, and ophthalmologic.

Extraintestinal manifestations can be divided into three categories: (1) those intimately related to the activity or extent of disease and responding to therapy directed at the bowel disease, (2) those whose course is independent of the underlying bowel disease, and (3) those that are direct sequelae of the underlying bowel disease.

A. Musculoskeletal manifestations
B. Four categories of arthritis have been described.
C. A characteristic peripheral arthritis, often called "colitic or enteropathic," is observed in 15--20% of patients with inflammatory bowel disease. This form of peripheral arthritis is rheumatoid-factor-negative, polyarticular, migratory, and asymmetric, affecting mostly the large joints of the lower extremities. The knees are most commonly affected, with hips, ankles, wrists, and elbows following in decreasing frequency. The onset of inflammation seen with "colitic" arthritis tends to be abrupt, often peaking within 24 h. It is accompanied by overlying warmth, erythema, and pain.
D. Enteropathic peripheral arthritis typically flares coincident with exacerbations of IBD and is more common in patients with chronic IBD. Enteropathic arthritis

Musculoskeletal manifestations[A]

Complications of IBD[J]

Symptoms	Location	Labs	Diagnosis	Therapy

History of IBD with joint pain[B]

Active or quiescent

Active disease →

Migratory polyarticular asymmetrical[C] → Knees > ankles > elbows → RF − , ANA − X-ray − soft tissue swelling, no joint destruction → Enteropathic peripheral arthritis[D]

1. Underlying bowel disease
2. Corticosteroids
3. Physical therapy
4. Colectomy for refractory cases[E]

Low-back pain "stooped posture" (dorsal kyphosis) "morning stiffness"[F]

SI joint vertebrae (cervical spared) → HLA-B27 + X-ray − symmetric SI joint distortion, marginal bridging of spine → Ankylosing spondylitis

Hips, shoulders, knees[G] → HLA-B27 − X-ray − symmetric SI joint distortion, no vertebral involvement[H] → Sacroiliitis

1. Physical therapy
2. NSAID[I]

IBD = Inflammatory bowel disease
RF = Rhematoid factor
ANA = Antinuclear antibody
NSAID = Nonsteroidal antiinflammatory drugs
SI = Sacroiliac

ALGORITHM 53–1

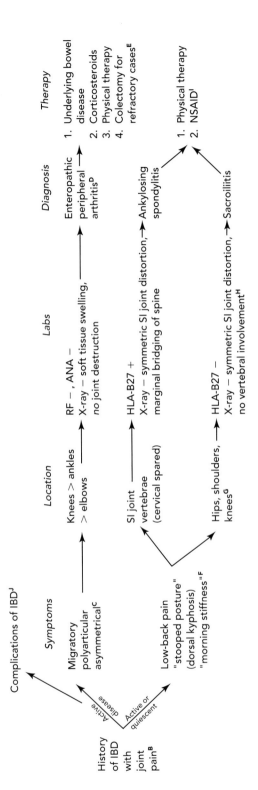

Dermatologic manifestations[K]

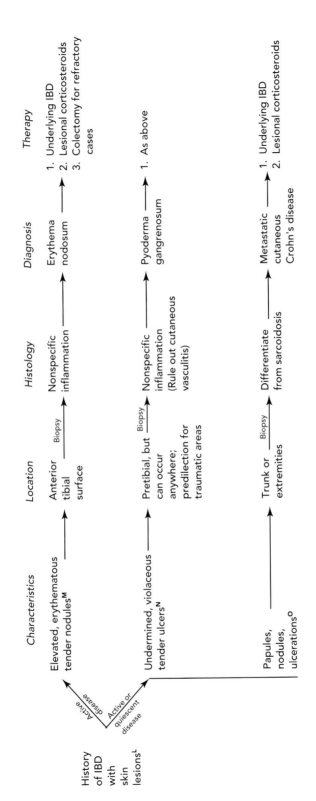

Characteristics		Location		Histology	Diagnosis	Therapy
Elevated, erythematous tender nodules[M]	→	Anterior tibial surface	Biopsy →	Nonspecific inflammation	Erythema nodosum →	1. Underlying IBD 2. Lesional corticosteroids 3. Colectomy for refractory cases
Undermined, violaceous tender ulcers[N]	→	Pretibial, but can occur anywhere; predilection for traumatic areas	Biopsy →	Nonspecific inflammation (Rule out cutaneous vasculitis)	Pyoderma gangrenosum →	1. As above
Papules, nodules, ulcerations[O]	→	Trunk or extremities	Biopsy →	Differentiate from sarcoidosis	Metastatic cutaneous Crohn's disease →	1. Underlying IBD 2. Lesional corticosteroids

History of IBD with skin lesions[L]

Active disease

Active or quiescent disease

IBD = inflammatory bowel disease

ALGORITHM 53–2

279

Hepatobiliary manifestations[P]

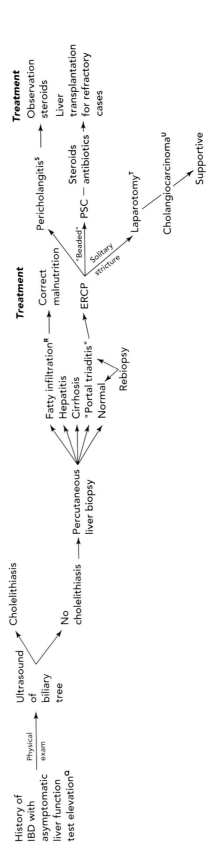

History of IBD with asymptomatic liver function test elevation[Q] —Physical exam→ Ultrasound of biliary tree

Ultrasound of biliary tree → Cholelithiasis

Ultrasound of biliary tree → No cholelithiasis → Percutaneous liver biopsy

Percutaneous liver biopsy →
- Fatty infiltration[R]
- Hepatitis
- Cirrhosis
- "Portal triaditis"
- Normal

Normal ⇄ Rebiopsy

Treatment

Fatty infiltration[R] → Correct malnutrition

"Portal triaditis" → ERCP

ERCP → "Beaded" PSC
ERCP → Solitary stricture → Laparotomy[T]

"Beaded" PSC — antibiotics → Pericholangitis[S]

Treatment

Pericholangitis[S] →
Observation
steroids
Liver transplantation for refractory cases

Steroids

Laparotomy[T] → Cholangiocarcinoma[U] → Supportive

IBD = inflammatory bowel disease
ERPC = endoscopic retrograde cholangiopancreatography
PSC = primary sclerosing cholangitis

ALGORITHM 53–3

Ophthalmologic manifestations[V]

Symptoms	Split-Lamp Exam	Diagnosis	Therapy
Photophobia, blurred vision, headache	Perilimbic edema "Flare" Conjunctival + scleral injection	Uveitis[X]	1. Pupillary dilatation 2. Eye patching 3. Steroid ophthalmic solution 4. Underlying IBD
Burning, itching	Conjunctival + scleral injection	Episcleritis[Y]	1. Steroid ophthalmic solution 2. Underlying IBD

History of IBD with reddened eye[W]

Active or quiescent

Active disease

IBD = inflammatory bowel disease

ALGORITHM 53–4

is more likely to occur in conjunction with other extraintestinal complications of IBD, such as erythema nodosum, pyoderma gangrenosum, aphthous ulcers, and uveitis. This type of arthritis typically does not deform or distort joints.

E. Because flares of enteropathic arthritis correlate so closely with the activity of underlying bowel disease, therapy is typically directed against the latter. Corticosteroids are frequently used, and it appears that the peripheral arthritis is steroid-responsive. Improvement may result from a direct steroid effect on the synovial tissue or a decreased immunologic stimulus for continued arthritis as the bowel disease becomes quiescent. Colectomy universally cures the peripheral arthritis in patients with ulcerative colitis. Surgical resection is less successful in Crohn's disease because it usually is incapable of removing all of the diseased tissue.

Patients with enteropathic arthritis whose bowel disease is difficult to control, who do not respond optimally to conservative measures, present therapeutic dilemmas. The bowel problems, not the joint disease, usually dictate the corticosteroid dose. Although increased corticosteroid dosages may occasionally be necessary to treat refractory enteropathic arthritis, steroids should rarely be instituted or increased to treat spondylitis. Nonsteroidal antiinflammatory drugs (NSAIDs) are potentially beneficial but must be used with great caution.

F. A clinical picture identical to idiopathic ankylosing spondylitis occurs in 3–6% of patients with IBD. Ankylosing spondylitis is defined as an inflammatory process involving one or more vertebrae and a sacroiliac joint. In addition, the upper vertebrae are spared with the axial arthropathy associated with IBD. The symptoms and features of spondylitis are similar to those seen with idiopathic ankylosing spondylitis: namely, low-back pain that is insidious in onset associated with significant morning stiffness. The back pain is usually relieved with exercise, worsened with rest and involves the entire lower back.

G. Arthritis of the hip, shoulder, and knees may be seen in association with spondylitis and IBD. Asymptomatic sacroileitis occurs with an incidence of 4–18% of patients with IBD.

H. Whereas 90% of patients with ankylosing spondylitis are associated with the human antigen leukocyte HLA-B27, isolated, asymptomatic sacroileitis is not. Unlike patients with "colitic" arthritis, those with spondylitis or sacroileitis often present with rheumatologic symptoms prior to the onset of bowel symptoms. Axial arthritis may be destructive, progresses independently of underlying IBD, and have a genetic pathogenesis.

I. The treatment of ankylosing spondylitis in IBD is notoriously poor. Salicylates and other associated anti-inflammatory medications help relieve pain and stiffness but do not arrest the disease process. Physical rehabilitation is usually the best approach. Surgical treatment has no effect on axial arthropathy associated with IBD.

J. The fourth category consists of complications of IBD and its therapy, which include granulomas of the joints, amyloidosis, septic arthritis, and hypertrophic osteoarthropathy. Finger clubbing is a form of hypertrophic osteoarthropathy. This condition correlates with disease activity and is accompanied by periosteal new bone formation that may or may not be symptomatic.

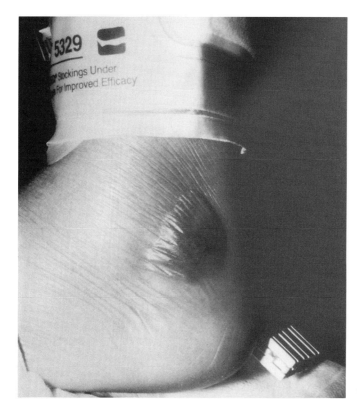

FIGURE 53-1 Pyoderma gangrenosum of the left lower extremity.

K. Dermatologic Manifestations

L. A host of dermatologic manifestations may be seen with either ulcerative colitis or Crohn's disease. The most common lesion is erythema nodosum; the most severe is pyoderma gangrenosum (Fig. 53-1). Although both of these conditions occur primarily in patients with colitis, they seldom present in the same patient, and their clinical courses differ.

M. The lesions of erythema nodosum are characterized as elevated, red, tender nodules ranging in size from 1 cm to several centimeters. They are characteristically located on the anterior tibial surfaces. In patients with active IBD, erythema nodosum is frequently associated with other extraintestinal manifestations such as arthritis and uveitis. Its clinical course parallels that of active bowel inflammation, and erythema nodosum lesions generally resolve without scarring in a few days.

N. Pyoderma gangrenosum is an ulcerative cutaneous lesion usually found on the extremities; the most common location is the anterior tibial area. However, the ulcers can also occur on the trunk and buttocks. There is a predilection for areas of previous trauma. Usually there are only one or two lesions, but they may be of considerable size. The lesion usually begins as an erythematous papule or nodule and then ulcerates, creating a characteristic undermined and violaceous margin. The lesions are extremely tender to palpation. Pyoderma gangrenosum lasts longer and is more difficult to manage than erythema nodosum. In contrast to erythema nodosum, pyoderma gangrenosum may be related to diseased bowel activity or may occur with quiescent bowel disease. Treatment for both of these dermatologic conditions includes therapy for underlying bowel disease in combination with systemic, topical, or intralesional corticosteroids. Topical disodium cromoglycate, azathioprine, and cyclosporine have also been used in treating pyoderma gangrenosum. Colectomy is reserved only for the rare, severe, refractory cases.

O. Cutaneous granuloma formation, or granulomatous dermatitis, occurring remote from or noncontiguous with the bowel lesions in Crohn's disease, has been termed *metastatic cutaneous Crohn's disease*. These lesions are quite varied and have included ulcerations, papules, and nodules found on the trunk or extremities. Biopsy is required to establish the diagnosis with differentiation from sarcoidosis. Treatment includes not only that of the underlying IBD but also interstitial corticosteroid therapy that can provide transient improvement.

P. Hepatobiliary Manifestations

Q. Hepatic diseases are frequently found in patients with IBD. Up to 50% of patients with ulcerative colitis have minor hepatic abnormalities. The spectrum of hepatobiliary disease ranges from relatively benign disorders such as fatty infiltration of the liver and cholelithiasis to more aggressive ones such as primary sclerosing cholangitis and cholangiocarcinoma. With the exception of fatty infiltration of the liver, hepatobiliary complications do not appear to correlate with disease activity, duration, or severity of IBD.

R. Fatty degeneration of the liver is probably the most frequently encountered microscopic abnormality. This condition is a nonspecific, reversible, lesion that by itself does not lead to fibrosis. The pathogenesis is not known but probably is a result of a combination of chronic illness, malnutrition, and corticosteroid therapy, rather than representing a true extraintestinal manifestation of IBD. The overwhelming majority of patients are asymptomatic, with only incidental hepatomegaly. Liver enzymes and serum bilirubin are usually within the normal range, although elevation of serum alkaline phosphatase has been reported. Treatment is directed toward the correction of malnutrition.

S. Another common hepatobiliary disorder in patients with IBD is "pericholangitis." Considerable debate continues as to whether "pericholangitis" is a distinct entity or is part of the syndrome of sclerosing cholangitis. Histologically, "pericholangitis" is a portal triaditis with acute inflammation surrounding the portal venules, bile ductules and lymphatics. Despite the high incidence of "pericholangitis" in IBD, it is recommended that if the presence is suspected a liver biopsy and endoscopic retrograde cholangiopancreatography (ERCP) should be performed to rule out concomitant sclerosing cholangitis. Because no specific therapy exists for asymptomatic "pericholangitis," the prognosis is not known. Therapy for "pericholangitis" is rarely indicated, but steroids have been used.

T. Primary sclerosing cholangitis (PSC) is a chronic cholestatic disorder of unknown etiology. This condition is characterized by fibrosing inflammation of the biliary tract with resulting bile duct obliteration, sclerosis, and subsequent hepatic failure. PSC occurs in 1–4% of patients with IBD, and 70% of cases are associated with ulcerative colitis. There is no correlation between PSC and the onset, duration, activity, or extent of ulcerative colitis. The clinical presentation of PSC is variable. Patients may be asymptomatic, or present with constitutional symptomatology or symptoms of severe liver disease. The procedure of choice for diagnosis of PSC is ERCP. This demonstrates diffuse, multifocal, short strictures of the intrahepatic and extrahepatic ducts resulting in a "beaded" appearance. The natural history of this lesion is poorly defined. In general, PSC is a progressive disease, but the rate of progression is unpredictable. Treatment with corticosteroids, antibiotics, or colectomy are palliative in nature. Patients progressing to severe sclerosis and liver failure may be candidates for liver transplantation.

U. Cholangiocarcinoma is a well-recognized but rare complication of IBD. Biliary tract carcinoma usually complicates extensive colitis of long-standing duration. Curiously, it may develop many years after proctocolectomy without preceding evidence of hepatic dysfunction. The usual clinical presentation is that of general malaise, pyrexia, and right upper quadrant pain followed by the development of progressive obstructive jaundice. Tumors are usually adenocarcinomas, multicentric in origin, and commonly involve the extrahepatic biliary tree. Patients in whom a solitary biliary stricture is detected on ERCP should be considered for a laparotomy to rule out cholangiocarcinoma. The prognosis with this tumor is poor.

V. Ophthalmologic Manifestations

W. There is a wide range of ocular manifestations reported in patients with IBD, ranging from 4% to 10%. The most common ocular manifestations include episcleritis and uveitis. Infrequent ocular complications include conjunctivitis, cataracts, and keratopathy. In contrast to other extraintestinal manifestations, ophthalmic manifestations appear to be more common in the first several years of symptomatic IBD. There is also an association between eye complications and other extraintestinal manifestations, especially peripheral arthritis and erythema nodosum. Eye complications are known to parallel the activity of large bowel inflammation.

X. Uveitis, or iritis, involves inflammation of the anterior chamber and perilimbic erythema. This condition presents with a reddened eye in conjunction with the acute onset of blurred vision, eye pain, photophobia, and headache. Diagnosis is achieved by slit-lamp examination. Perilimbic edema and "flare" in the anterior chamber, in addition to conjunctival injection, are the usual findings. Urgent therapy to prevent scarring and visual impairment consists of pupillary dilatation, eye patching, and administration of topical steroids in conjunction with treatment of the underlying GI disease. Uveitis may occur whether the underlying IBD is symptomatic or in remission and is not an accepted indication for colectomy.

Y. Episcleritis is a benign disorder occurring predominantly with Crohn's colitis. Patients present with hyperemia of the conjunctiva and sclera in combination with ocular burning and itching. Corticosteroid ophthalmic solution administered concomitantly with treatment of underlying IBD is effective in managing the patient.

BIBLIOGRAPHY

1. Corman, ML: *Colon and Rectal Surgery,* third ed. Philadelphia: Lippincott, 1993, pp 1035–1047.

2. Flamm S, Chopra S: Inflammatory bowel disease management issues, hepatobiliary manifestations. *Seminars Colon Rectal Surg* 4:62–71, 1993.

3. Jacoby R, Kraft S: Extraintestinal manifestations. In Gitnick G: *Inflammatory Bowel Disease; Diagnosis and Treatment.* New York: Ingaku-Shoin, 1991, pp 523–531.

4. Kantrowitz F: Inflammatory bowel disease management issues, arthritic manifestations. *Seminars Colon Rectal Surg* 4:55–61, 1993.

5. Mayer L, Janowitz H: Extraintestinal manifestations of inflammatory bowel disease. In Kirsner, RG: *Inflammatory Bowel Disease,* third ed. Philadelphia: Lee and Febiger, 1988, pp 299–317.

6. Rankin G: Extraintestinal and systemic manifestations of inflammatory bowel disease. *Med Clin N Am* 74:39–49, 1990.

7. van Erpecum KJ, van Berge Henegouwen GP: Hepatobiliary abnormalities in inflammatory bowel disease. *Neth J Med* 35:S40–S49, 1989.

See also Chapters 51 and 52.

CHAPTER 54

Toxic Colitis

Alejandro González Padrón, M.D. and
David A. Cherry, M.D.

Refer to Algorithm 54‑1.

A. *Toxic colitis:* Toxic colitis is an acute presentation of colitis with systemic manifestations of toxicity. Generally, it is an exacerbation of a previous inflammatory process in the colon, but can also be seen in patients without a history of colonic disorders. Causative agents or related pathologies can be numerous (Table 54‑1), and because this condition may be life-threatening, correct diagnosis and treatment must be immediately established.

B. *History:*

1. *Familial or personal history of IBD.* The incidence is 0‑10% in the majority of patients with ulcerative colitis, although there has been an increase in patients with Crohn's disease.

2. *Exposure to infectious agents.* Focus on patients in endemic areas of amebiasis, poor hygienic habits, possible ingestion of contaminated food, hospitalized patients under antibiotic regimen (*Clostridium difficile*), immunodepressed patients, or patients who practice anal receptive intercourse.

3. *Ischemic colitis.* Colitis can manifest after aortic surgery or aortography in patients with fibrillation or with recent myocardial infarction, history of diabetes, vasculitis, and collagen disease (especially systemic lupus erythematosus), colonic venous thrombosis in young female patients taking oral contraceptives, and chronic renal disease.

4. *Patients undergoing chemotherapy.*

C. *Signs and symptoms include*

- Multiple bowel movements or bloody diarrhea
- Temperature > 100.5°F
- Tachycardia > 100 min

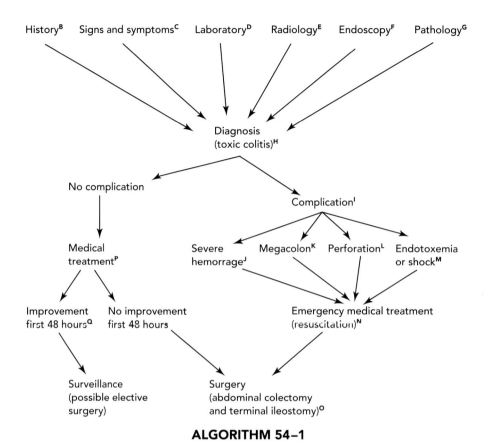

ALGORITHM 54–1

- Weight loss
- Anorexia
- Abdominal colic
- Tenesmus
- Pallor, dehydration, or shock
- Abdominal distension
- Localized or generalized tenderness

D. *Abnormal laboratory findings can be*

- Anemia
- Leukocytosis
- Hypoalbuminemia
- Hypogammaglobulinemia
- Hyponatremia

TABLE 54–1 ETIOLOGY OF TOXIC COLITIS

Inflammatory bowel disease
  Ulcerative colitis
  Crohn's disease
Infectious colitis
  Bacterial:
    Shigella (bacillary dysentery)
    Salmonella (typhoid fever)
    Clostridium-difficile (pseudomembranous colitis)
    Campylobacter jejuni
    Invasive *E. coli*
    Yersinia
  Parasitic:
    Entamoeba histolytica (amebiasis)
  Sexually transmitted:
    Herpes simplex
    Gonococcus
    Cytomegalovirus
    Lymphogranuloma venereum
    Chlamydia
Ischemic colitis
Antineoplastic agents

- Hypokalemia
- Hypochloremia
- Hypoprothrombinemia

E. *Radiologic studies are generally very valuable.* Barium enema is contraindicated; investigation should be limited to plain abdominal x-rays. Thicker haustral margins can be seen with a tendency of disappearing with progressive dilatation. Dilatation normally starts in the splenic flexure and extends proximally to the transverse colon, although the cecum and ascending colon may occasionally be involved. If perforation occurs, free air may be present; however, air delineating the borders of the colon may indicate that the perforation was sealed.

F. *Endoscopy:* One must limit endoscopy to proctoscopy only, without air insufflation; Colonoscopy is contraindicated. Vascular congestion, supuration, and ulcerations are usually present. Aspirate testing for bacterial cultures, *C. difficile,* and parasites help to diagnose infectious agents.

G. *Pathology.* Patterns of IBD are recognizable; however, differentiating between ulcerative colitis and Crohn's can sometimes be very difficult. The mucosal surface is intensely hyperemic and the entire colon may be involved imitating ulcerative colitis disease. However, when the transverse and sigmoid colon are more severely affected, this gives the appearance of distal sparing, imitating Crohn's disease. Multiple deep fissures surrounded by necrotic tissue are seen in Crohn's disease with single or few seen in ulcerative colitis.

H. *Diagnosis.* A diagnosis can be made once all of the previously mentioned investigations are undertaken. Fulminant disease is present with one or more of the following findings:

- > 6–8 evacuations/day
- Hematocrit < 30
- Temperature > 100.5°F
- Weight loss > 10% of premorbid weight
- Tachycardia > 100/min
- Sedimentation rate > 30
- Albumin < 3
- Barium enema investigation must be avoided in this scenario.

I. *Complications.* Depending on the severity and progression of the disease, complications may be present and include

- Severe hemorrhage
- Megacolon
- Perforation
- Endotoxemia or shock

J. *Severe hemorrhage.* Intense vascular congestion, erosion, and ulceration through mucosa and submucosa, compromising abundant vessels, results in severe hemorrhage.

K. *Megacolon.* Megacolon can be diagnosed when the transverse colon is > 7 cm in diameter and may be caused by the inflammation and destruction of the colonic muscle and/or the inflammation of the myenteric and submucosal nerve plexuses. With megacolon, physical examination will normally reveal distention in the upper abdomen; however, when pain is present, perforation may be a possibility.

L. *Perforation.* As mentioned previously, perforation can be frequently seen in the presence of toxic megacolon; however, it is not exclusive of this condition. Because of the severity of the inflammatory process, transmural ulceration can produce perforation of the colonic wall without any dilatation. This perforation can be sealed by the omentum or other contiguous organs without many abdominal symptoms, or can remain open, causing peritonitis.

M. *Endotoxemia/shock.* This is the result of toxins released into the systemic circulation, resulting in hypoperfusion, tissue ischemia, single or multiple organ failure, hyperdynamic state, and severe hypotension.

N. *Emergency medical treatment.* Primarily, medical treatment focuses on stabilizing the patient's clinical condition and normalizing the laboratory values. If, however, any of the previously mentioned complications are present, resuscitation must be performed immediately and surgery is recommended.

O. *Surgery.* The operation of choice is total abdominal colectomy with construction of a terminal ileostomy. Proctocolectomy or terminal ileostomy is not recommended because of the increased mortality and morbidity in an emergency setting. Further reconstruction can be performed at a later date after the patient's condition has improved with a sphincter-saving operation. If dilatation is present, intraoperative decompression of the colon is performed with a colonoscope. For this reason, it is recommended that all patients be preoperatively placed in the modified lithotomy position. On very rare occasions, the Turnbull blowhole procedure may be useful. In this operation, antimesenteric blowhole transverse and sigmoidostomies and a loop ileostomy are fashioned.

P. *Medical treatment.* If no complications are present, depending on the patient's response, the first 3–5 days of medical treatment are crucial in determining the next step. Medical treatment may consist of

- Hydration and electrolyte balance
- Broad-spectrum antibiotics
- Steroids or azulfidine as necessary
- Avoiding anticolinergic agents and opiates
- Blood transfusion
- Total parenteral nutrition
- Nasogastric tube
- Immunosuppressive agents (cyclosporine, methotrexate)

If no improvement is achieved with medical treatment in the first 48 hours, surgery is indicated.

Q. *Improvement.* If improvement is achieved in the first 48 hours of medical treatment, continued medical management, surveillance, and possible elective surgery is recommended.

BIBLIOGRAPHY

1. Binderow SR, Wexner SD: Current surgical therapy for mucosal ulcerative colitis. *Dis Colon Rectum* 37:610–624, 1994.
2. Jagelman DG (ed): *Mucosal Ulcerative Colitis.* New York: Futura Press, 1986.
3. Keighley MRB, Williams NS (eds): *Surgery of the Anus, Rectum and Colon.* London: Saunders, 1993, Vol 2.

See also Chapters 5, 20, 21, 40, 51, 52 and 55.

CHAPTER 55

Infectious Colitis

José R. Cintron, M.D. and Russell K. Pearl, M.D.

Refer to Algorithm 55–1.

A. Recent travel of migration should suggest traveler's diarrhea; different organisms predominate in different regions. Bacterial enteropathogens cause at least 80% of traveler's diarrhea. The principal agents in most of the high-risk areas are as follows: enterotoxigenic *E. coli*, Shigella species, *Campylobacter jejuni*, aeromonas species, *Plesiomonas shigelloides*, salmonella species, and noncholera vibrios. Parasitic etiologies should be considered in tropical or Asiatic travel or migration.

B. Very important aspect of the history since even a single dose of antibiotics within 6 weeks of presentation may cause pseudomembranous colitis due to *C. difficile.*

C. Immunoincompetent individuals are more likely to develop life-threatening sepsis from their infectious colitis due to deficient humoral or cellular immunity. Therefore, a more aggressive approach is warranted under most circumstances, especially in the use of antimicrobial therapy. Patients with immunodeficiencies caused by the HIV virus present with a wide variety of opportunistic infections, many of which affect the gastrointestinal tract.

D. High relapse rates in patients with a history of sexually transmitted diseases (STDs) warrant retesting for cure of STD such as syphilis. Furthermore, all sexual contacts must be treated to prevent recurrence.

E. Homosexuals, bisexuals, women who practice anal receptive intercourse, and high-risk heterosexuals (prostitutes, drug addicts, or sexually promiscuous individuals) should be counseled regarding human immunodeficiency virus (HIV) testing. All patients should be investigated for STDs.

F. Severity and duration of diarrhea, assessment of skin turgor, and presence of orthostasis may alert the physician as to the severity of dehydration. Acute bacterial diarrhea can be classified into toxigenic types, in which an enterotoxin is the major if not exclusive pathogenic mechanism, and inva-

Infectious colitis

Workup

History and physical exam
Recent travel or migration[A]
Recent antibiotic use[B]
Immunocompromised status[C]
History of sexually transmitted disease[D]
Sexual preferences practices and contacts[E]
Presence of diarrhea[F]
Fever, emesis, abdominal cramps[G]
Occult or grossly bloody stools[H]
Weight loss[I]

Diagnosis

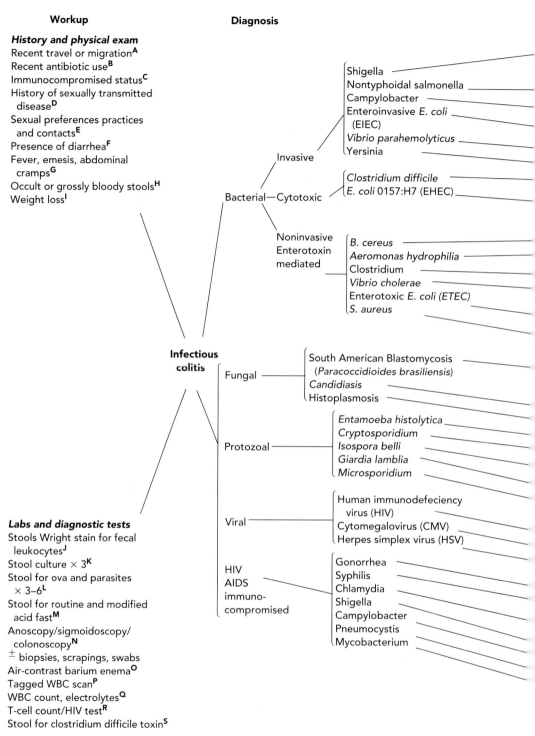

Infectious colitis

Bacterial
- Invasive
  - Shigella
  - Nontyphoidal salmonella
  - Campylobacter
  - Enteroinvasive *E. coli* (EIEC)
  - *Vibrio parahemolyticus*
  - Yersinia
- Cytotoxic
  - *Clostridium difficile*
  - *E. coli* 0157:H7 (EHEC)
- Noninvasive Enterotoxin mediated
  - *B. cereus*
  - *Aeromonas hydrophilia*
  - Clostridium
  - *Vibrio cholerae*
  - Enterotoxic *E. coli* (ETEC)
  - *S. aureus*

Fungal
- South American Blastomycosis (*Paracoccidioides brasiliensis*)
- *Candidiasis*
- Histoplasmosis

Protozoal
- *Entamoeba histolytica*
- *Cryptosporidium*
- *Isospora belli*
- *Giardia lamblia*
- *Microsporidium*

Viral
- Human immunodeficiency virus (HIV)
- Cytomegalovirus (CMV)
- Herpes simplex virus (HSV)

HIV AIDS immunocompromised
- Gonorrhea
- Syphilis
- Chlamydia
- Shigella
- Campylobacter
- Pneumocystis
- Mycobacterium

Labs and diagnostic tests
Stools Wright stain for fecal leukocytes[J]
Stool culture × 3[K]
Stool for ova and parasites × 3–6[L]
Stool for routine and modified acid fast[M]
Anoscopy/sigmoidoscopy/ colonoscopy[N]
± biopsies, scrapings, swabs
Air-contrast barium enema[O]
Tagged WBC scan[P]
WBC count, electrolytes[Q]
T-cell count/HIV test[R]
Stool for clostridium difficile toxin[S]

TB = Tuberculosis
WBC = White blood cell

ALGORITHM 55–1

Treatment

Nonspecific therapy/symptomatic shigellosis-fluoroquinolones, i.e. (ciprofloxacin 500 mg[T] PO b.i.d. 7 days)—expensive therapy for third-world countries; cartilage toxicity in children; alt.: trimethoprim-sulfamethoxazole (TMP/SMX) 1 double-strength tablet PO b.i.d. 5–15 days or ampicillin 500 mg PO q.i.d. 5 days—resistance commonplace in developing countries.

Nonspecific therapy; antimicrobial therapy not recommended except in unusual cases (see Table 55–2).

Nonspecific therapy; antimicrobials only if started within 3 days of symptoms but generally not recommended; treat in cases of traveler's diarrhea[U]

Nonspecific therapy; antimicrobial use inconclusive; TMP/SMX[V]

Nonspecific therapy; antimicrobial therapy inconclusive[W]

Nonspecific therapy; antimicrobial use inconclusive[X]

Discontinue implicated antimicrobial agent; supportive measures; avoid antimotility agents; enteric isolation precautions for hospitalized patients; see text[Y]

Nonspecific therapy; antimicrobial therapy not generally recommended[Z]

Self-limited; no antimicrobials indicated; can be a cause of foodborne outbreaks[AA]

Nonspecific therapy; specific treatment when indicated-fluoroquinolones; alt. TMP/SMX; resistant to B-lactams; implicated in traveler's diarrhea[BB]

Self-limited; usually implicated in foodborne outbreaks; toxin affects primarily terminal ileum[CC]

No colitis; enterotoxin affects small intestine; supportive care, doxycycline or fluoroquinolone[DD]

Nonspecific therapy; primarily affects small intestine; common cause of traveler's diarrhea in which antimicrobial therapy is occasionally recommended[EE]

Supportive care; no specific therapy indicated[FF]

Ketoconazole 400 mg/d for 6–18 mos or Amphotericin B total dose 1.5–2.5 gm; may also be treated with sulfa drugs alone or combined with trimethoprim.; sulfadiazine 4–6 g/day for several weeks, then 500 mg/d for 3–5 yrs[GG]

Amphotericin B[HH]

Amphotericin B[II]

Metronidazole 750 mg PO t.i.d. 10 days followed by iodoquinol 650 mg PO t.i.d. 20 days[JJ]

No antimicrobial agents indicated; usually self-limited; AIDS and immunocompromised patients may benefit from octreotide[KK]

TMP 160/SMX 800 mg PO q.i.d. 10 days, then b.i.d. 3 weeks; AIDS patients require maintenance[LL]

Metronidazole 250 mg PO t.i.d. 5 days[MM]

No effective antimicrobials in controlled trials; TMP/SMX anecdotal improvement[NN]

Antiretroviral therapy as indicated, otherwise supportive treatment[OO]

Ganciclovir (5 mg/kg) q.12h 14–21 days[PP]

Symptomatic therapy; acyclovir 200 mg PO 5x qday 10 days and topical acyclovir[QQ]

Ceftriaxone 250 mg IM × 1 plus doxycycline 100 mg PO b.i.d. 7 days[RR]

Benzathine penicillin G 2.4 million units IM × 1 if disease < 1 year; if disease > 1 year, then benzathine penicillin G 2.4 million units IM × 1 every week × 3 weeks[SS]

Doxycycline 100 mg PO b.i.d. 7 days or azithromycin 1 g PO × 1; LGV strains require longer therapy[TT]

See "A" above[UU]

Fluoroquinolones see "C" above[VV]

Antipneumocystis therapy; TMP/SMX; pentamidine[WW]

Increased incidence in HIV+ and AIDS; increased incidence of multidrug resistance; M. avium-intracellulare resistant to all standard TB drugs except cycloserine—optimal regimens not defined[XX]

sive types, in which the organism penetrates the mucosal surface as the primary event. By definition, traveler's diarrhea occurs in a person who normally resides in an industrialized region and who travels to a developing tropical or semitropical country and passes at least three unformed stools in a 24-hour period together with nausea, emesis, abdominal pain or cramps, fecal urgency, tenesmus, or the passage of bloody or mucoid stools.

G,H,I. The presence of high fever, systemic illness, and bloody diarrhea may suggest dysentery secondary to shigella. Avoid antimotility agents and narcotics since they can prolong diarrhea and provoke toxic megacolon. Weight loss may be seen in significant dehydration, chronic colitis, or immunodeficient individuals.

J. A useful rapid and inexpensive technique to establish a presumptive diagnosis in infectious diarrhea. Use 2 drops of Loeffler's methylene blue mixed with a small amount of stool on a slide and search for leukocytes and erythrocytes.

K. Most patients with infectious diarrhea, even with a recognized pathogen, have a mild self-limited course. However, all patients who are HIV-positive, have AIDS, are immunocompromised, are homosexual, or who have fever, systemic illness, tenesmus, bloody diarrhea, dehydration, and a prolonged course need standard stool cultures and fecal exams for ova and parasites.

L. Especially important in patients with overseas travel and in immigrants. Also important in HIV/AIDS and other immunocompromised patients. The parasitologic examination in the HIV/AIDS patient should include saline, iodine, trichrome, and acid-fast preparations of direct or concentrated samples or both from each stool specimen. Mineral oil, tetracyclines, and residual barium may give a false-negative result. Microscopic exam of repeated (3–6) fresh stool specimens will establish a diagnosis in the majority of symptomatic cases.

M. Primarily important in the HIV/AIDS patients in order to detect isospora, cryptosporidium, and mycobacteria as the etiologies of infectious diarrhea.

N. Lubrication of the anoscope or sigmoidoscope with anything other than water is not advisable since many lubricants and creams contain antibacterial agents that can interfere with cultures. Swabbing of pus in the anorectum under direct visualization will significantly increase yields on Gram stain and cultures. In most of the infectious diseases biopsy has a secondary role. It is unusual to detect parasitic diseases in endoscopic biopsies when stool examinations are negative with the exception of microsporidiosis and adenovirus in AIDS. This diagnosis needs to be made in glutaraldehyde fixed biopsy specimens processed for electron microscopy. Colonic biopsy specimens in the AIDS patient should be cultured for cytomegalovirus, adenovirus, mycobacteria, and herpes simplex virus. Colonic tissue biopsy specimens should also be examined for histologic changes and the presence of viral inclusion cells, mycobacteria, and invasive and noninvasive protozoa through the use of hematoxylin eosin, Grocott, methenamine silver or Giemsa, and Fite stains. Endoscopic and histologic features of infectious colitis may be indistinguishable from ulcerative colitis, Crohn's colitis, or other specific colitis.

O. Obtain all stool collections prior to air-contrast barium enema (BE) studies to avoid false-negative results. Avoid BE studies in patients with severe acute colitis since it may precipitate toxic megacolon or perforation.

P. A noninvasive method that may ascertain presence and or extent of inflammation.

Q. Leukocytosis may be present in infectious colitis, although it is nonspecific. Eosinophilia may be present in some parasitic infections. Leukopenia, thrombocytopenia, and anemia are often recognized in asymptomatic HIV+ (HIV-positive) individuals or in patients with more advanced HIV-related disorders. Electrolyte determination may be useful in patients with severe fluid losses in order to direct appropriate replacement.

R. CD4 counts (helper cell T-lymphocyte) may provide information on the degree of immunoincompetency, morbidity, and mortality. Certain pathogens are less likely to be implicated with higher CD4 counts; for instance, *Mycobacterium avium*-intracellulare is seldom seen in patients with CD4>100 mm^{-3}. Additionally, CD4 counts may provide some prognostic information in HIV+ patients requiring surgery due to complications of their infectious colitis. All patients with sexually transmitted diseases, and those in high-risk categories, should be counseled to undergo HIV testing.

S. Stool should be obtained for cytotoxic products, especially if *C. difficile* is suspected because of recent antibiotic use history within the past 4--6 weeks. The preferred method to establish the diagnosis of pseudomembranous colitis is with endoscopy. Up to $^{1}/_{3}$ of patients may have lesions restricted to the right side of the colon, necessitating colonoscopy.

T. Antimicrobial therapy recommended in symptomatic patients. Hemolytic uremic syndrome (HUS) may occur with *S. dysenteriae* type 1 infection and may require dialysis. Antibiotic unresponsive toxic megacolon with or without perforation is often managed with colectomy. Nonspecific therapeutic agents for infectious diarrhea are listed in Table 55--1. Antimotility drugs *should not* be used when this condition is suspected or in patients with bloody diarrhea, fecal leukocytes, or substantial abdominal pain. Although

TABLE 55–1 NONSPECIFIC THERAPY OF INFECTIOUS DIARRHEA

Fluid
  Intravenous
  Oral rehydration therapy (recommendations by World Health Organization)
Food
  Continue nutrition intake
  Avoid lactose, caffeine, and methylxanthines
Antimotility drugs
  Codeine, paregoric, tincture of opium
  Loperamide
  Diphenoxylate
Bismuth subsalicylate

TABLE 55–2 ANTIMICROBIAL THERAPY RECOMMENDATIONS

Lymphoproliferative disorders	Prosthetic devices
Malignancies	Hemolytic anemia
Immunosuppression	Extreme ages of life
Abnormal cardiovascular system	Severe sepsis or toxicity
Heart valves	
Grafts	
Aneurysms	

the use of antimotility agents is controversial in certain bacterial diarrheas, most patients will derive considerable symptomatic benefit. Recommendations for antimicrobial therapy are listed in Table 55–2.

U. Campylobacter jejuni is second only to *Giardia lamblia* among recognized causes of waterborne diarrheal disease outbreaks in the United States. Common cause of traveler's diarrhea especially in the drier winter season, at least in semitropical Morocco and Mexico. Prophylactic treatment of traveler's diarrhea is controversial (see list of self-therapy agents in Table 55–3). Acute therapy for this pathogen in AIDS patients is erythromycin (250–500 mg orally q.i.d. for 7 days) or ciprofloxacin (500 mg orally twice daily for 7 days)

V. Produces a shigella-like toxin with cytotoxic, neurotoxic and enterotoxic properties.

W. Associated with seafood ingestion such as raw fish or shellfish. Recognized as an important pathogen in the Far East. In the United States, usually reported in the coastal states.

X. Reported more frequently in Scandianavian and European countries than in the United States. Enterocolitis occurs more frequently in children and can be confused with the diagnosis of appendicitis leading to laparotomy. Radiographically can simulate Crohn's disease of terminal ileum.

Y. Treatment recommendations for *C. difficile*-induced diarrhea and colitis are listed in Table 55–4.

Z. This specific serotype causes acute hemorrhagic colitis. Associated with hemolytic uremic syndrome.

AA. Associated with two clinical types of food poisoning: a diarrhea syndrome and a vomiting syndrome.

BB. A principal agent in traveler's diarrhea in high-risk areas, especially Thailand. Infections most likely associated with drinking untreated well water or spring water.

CC. Major foodborne pathogen that causes vomiting and diarrhea. Usually associated with roasted, boiled, stewed, or steamed meats and poultry as the vehicle of infection. No specific therapy since symptoms rarely last longer than 24–36 hours.

DD. The entire disease consists of intestinal fluid loss secondary to adherence of the organism to the upper small bowel and elaboration of an enterotoxin. Mainstay of therapy is hydration.

TABLE 55–3 CURRENT PHARMACOLOGIC SELF-THERAPY OF TRAVELER'S DIARRHEA BASED ON CLINICAL FEATURES

Clinical Syndrome	Probable Cause	Agent Recommended
Watery diarrhea (no blood in stool or fever)	Bacteria	Antibacterial drug[a] plus (for adults) loperamide
Dysentery (passage of bloody stools) or fever $T > 37.8°C$	Invasive bacteria	Antibacterial drug[a]
Vomiting, minimal diarrhea	Viruses; preformed toxin (food poisoning)	Bismuth subsalicylate (for adults): 30 mL or 2 tablets every 30 min for 5 doses; may repeat on day 2
Diarrhea in infants (<2 years old)	Bacteria	Fluids and electrolytes
Diarrhea in pregnant women	Bacteria	Fluids and electrolytes; consider attapulgite
Diarrhea despite TMP/SMX prophylaxis	Unknown, drug-resistant bacteria?	Fluoroquinolone, with loperamide if no fever/blood
Diarrhea despite FQ prophylaxis	Unknown	Bismuth subsalicylate

[a] The recommended antibacterial drugs are as follows: TMP/SMX DS for inland Mexico during the summer; and norfloxacin (400 mg), ciprofloxacin (500 mg), ofloxacin (300 mg), or fleroxacin (400 mg) for other areas in other seasons. The drugs should be taken in these doses twice daily for 3 days for more sever illness. For milder illness, single-dose therapy is effective.

TABLE 55–4 TREATMENT ALTERNATIVES IN CLOSTRIDIUM-DIFFICILE DIARRHEA[a]

Antimicrobial agents
    Vancomycin 125 mg PO q.i.d., 7–14 days.
    Metronidazole 250 mg PO t.i.d., 7–14 days.
    Bacitracin 25,000 units PO q.i.d., 7–14 days.
Anion-exchange resins
    Cholestyramine 4 g PO t.i.d., 5–10 days.
    Cholestipol 5 g PO t.i.d., 5–10 days.
Alter fecal flora
    Lactinex (or lactobacillus preparation) 1 g PO q.i.d., 7–14 days.
    Fecal enema (fresh stool via enema 1 or 2 × separated by 3 days

[a] Toxic colitis or megacolon unresponsive to antimicrobial therapy warrants colectomy.

EE. One of the most common enteropathogens implicated in traveler's diarrhea. Refer to paragraph CC in text and CC in Algorithm 55-1 for causes of traveler's diarrhea.

FF. Second most common cause of food poisoning in the United States since 1973.

GG. Primarily geographically limited to Latin America from Mexico to Argentina. Reportedly not contagious from person to person. Males are more commonly affected with a ratio of 15:1. When gastrointestinal (GI) involvement occurs, most commonly it involves the appendix, cecum, and anorectal areas.

HH. Only occasionally involves the colon and rectum and may involve other portions of the GI tract as part of a disseminated infection, particularly in immunocompromised individuals. May present as ulceration, bleeding, obstruction, or a protein-losing enteropathy.

II. Disseminated *H. capsulatum* infection is emerging as an important opportunistic infection in patients with AIDS who reside in endemic areas. GI involvement is detected by evaluation of biopsy specimens in approximately 70% of patients, but GI symptoms are present in only about 10% of patients. Most patients with GI manifestations have colonic involvement.

JJ. Important to distinguish amebiasis from inflammatory bowel disease such as ulcerative colitis or Crohn's colitis, because steroids are often prescribed in the latter and these drugs may be lethal in patients with acute invasive amebiasis. Microscopic exam of 3-6 fresh stool specimens will establish the diagnosis in 90% of patients. The cecum is involved in 90% of cases of chronic amebiasis and can become concentrically narrowed (i.e., the "coned cecum"). Rarely, a patient may progress to fulminant colitis before anti-amebic therapy takes effect and can be indistinguishable from fulminant ulcerative colitis. If examination and abdominal x-rays (transverse colon diameter >9 cm) show no improvement over several days, then subtotal colectomy should be considered. Other intestinal complications that may require surgery include perforation or ameboma, although the latter can be managed by medical means the majority of the time.

- *Asymptomatic intestinal infection.* Iodoquinol 650 mg PO t.i.d., 20 days, alt.: furamide or paromomycin.

- *Mild to severe dysenteric infection.* Metronidazole 750 mg PO t.i.d. 10 days followed by iodoquinol 650 mg PO t.i.d. 20 days.

KK. Cryptosporidium infection is among the most common causes of enteric disease in patients with AIDS, occurring in 10-20% of patients with AIDS and diarrhea in the United States and in up to 50% of patients with AIDS in developing countries. Also implicated as a cause of traveler's diarrhea especially in Russia, particularly St. Petersburg.

LL. Causes GI infection in patients with AIDS in approximately 1-3% in the United States but in 15-19% of patients in developing countries. Clinically resembles cryptosporidiosis. Although heavily concentrated in the small intestine, the organism can be identified throughout the GI tract.

MM. The most frequently reported gut parasite in the United Kingdom. Important cause of traveler's diarrhea in mountainous areas of North America and Russia, especially Leningrad. High incidence in campers and backpackers in the mountainous West such as Rocky Mountains and northern Cascades. Frequently spread by sexual or other close person to person contacts.

NN. Identified in as many as 33% of patients with AIDS who have chronic unexplained diarrhea. Difficult to identify because of small size and poor staining qualities, and diagnosis usually is based on electron-microscopic identification.

OO. AIDS-associated enteropathy may be caused by the HIV virus itself but is still controversial.

PP. One of the most common and potentially serious opportunistic pathogens of the GI tract in AIDS patients causing severe or life-threatening enteric disease in 2.2% of patients. The most common manifestation is colitis characterized by diarrhea, fever, hematochezia, and abdominal pain. The colon is particularly susceptible to ischemic necrosis and perforation, and under these circumstances subtotal colectomy and end ileostomy should be performed.

QQ. The three major manifestations of herpes simplex virus (HSV) infection in patients with AIDS are perianal lesions, proctitis, and esophagitis. Patients occasionally present with a lumbosacral radiculopathy caused by HSV infection characterized by urinary dysfunction, sacral paresthesias, impotence, or pain in the lower abdomen, thigh, and buttocks. Sigmoidoscopy is required to diagnose herpetic proctosigmoiditis and reveals friable mucosa, diffuse ulcerations, and occasional vesicles and pustules. Scrapings or biopsy from the ulcer reveal intranuclear inclusion bodies and multinucleated giant cells. Viral culture and direct immunofluorescence staining of vesicular fluid are also diagnostic. A chronic relapsing course occurs in 40%. In severe HSV proctitis: acyclovir IV 5 mg/kg q. 8h 5–7 days, otherwise oral acyclovir 200–400 mg PO 5× q.day for 10 days may be given. Perianal HSV infection is treated symptomatically in addition to the above with sitz baths, lidocaine ointment, oralanalgesics, and topical acyclovir. Suppressive oral acyclovir therapy may be given to suppress recurrences.

RR. Probably most common STD in homosexual men. Transmission via anal receptive intercourse. Diagnosis via Gram stain and culture of rectal swab under direct vision. Patients should be tested for cure in 3 months since failure rate with initial therapy can be as high as 35%.

SS. Syphilitic involvement of the colon usually occurs by direct inoculation of the anus or rectum during passive anal intercourse, so that the inflammatory reaction is confined to the distal 10–15 cm of the colon; a diffuse colitis does not occur.

TT. Most common STD in the United States' Chlamydial proctitis may coexist with gonorrhea and other STDs and is seen in up to 15% asymptomatic homosexuals. Patients may have suppurative inguinal adenopathy. Sigmoidoscopy may reveal severe nonspecific granular proctitis, intraluminal stricture, or mass. Biopsies are consistent with infectious proctitis. Microimmunofluorescent antibody titers are the most sensitive serotyping test. Can also perform biopsy for culture via direct tissue culture inoculation, but this is not readily available. Serotypes D through K are responsible for proctitis, while serotypes L_1, L_2, and L_3 are responsible for lymphogranuloma venereum (LGV). Treat for 7–14 days for non-LGV and 21 days for LGV+ serotypes. Rectal strictures are treated depending on symptomatology:

- *Asymptomatic*—no therapy required. Rule out IBD, ischemia, malignancy.
- *Symptomatic*—3-week course of doxycycline; if no improvement, then perform sphincter-sparing procedure.

UU. See paragraph A in text and A in Algorithm 55-1.

VV. See paragraph C in text and A in Algorithm 55-1.

WW. Pneumocytis colitis is extremely unusual in AIDS patients but has been reported. Diagnosis was made by colonoscopic biopsy that revealed *Pneumocystis carinii* organisms in the lamina propria of the cecum, descending colon, and sigmoid colon. The diarrhea and other manifestations should resolve with antipneumocystis therapy.

XX. The most common cause of systemic bacterial infection in HIV-infected persons identified primarily in patients with AIDS. Infection of the GI tract is associated with diarrhea, abdominal pain, malabsorption, weight loss, and fever. The small intestine is involved more commonly than the colon. Endoscopy may reveal erythema, edema, friability, and in some cases, small erosions and fine white nodules. Diagnosis is based on acid-fast organisms in stool and tissue (touch preparation and fixed) specimens. Surgical complications in descending order include obstruction, fistulas, bleeding, and perforation.

BIBLIOGRAPHY

1. Dryden MS, Shanson DC: The microbial causes of diarrhea in patients infected with the human immunodeficiency virus. *J Infect* 17:107–114, 1988.

2. DuPont HL, Ericsson CD: Prevention and treatment of traveler's diarrhea. *N Engl J Med* 328:1821–1827, 1993.

3. Janoff EN, Smith PD: Perspectives on gastrointestinal infections in AIDS. *Gastroenterol Clin N Am* 17:451–463, 1988.

4. Masur H: Therapy for AIDS. In Mandell GL, Douglas RG, Bennett JE (eds): *Principles and Practice of Infectious Diseases,* 3rd ed. New York: Churchill Livingston; 1990, pp 1102–1111.

5. Owen RL, Gorbach SL, Masur H, et al: In Sleisenger MH, Fordtran JS (eds): *Gastrointestinal Disease,* 4th ed. Philadelphia: Saunders, 1989, pp 1153–1274.

6. Pickering LK, Dupont HL, Olarte J, et al: Fecal leukocytes in enteric infections. *Am J Clin Pathol* 68:562, 1977.

7. Quinn TC, Stamm WE, Goodell SE, et al: The polymicrobial origin of intestinal infections in homosexual men. *N Engl J Med* 309:576–582, 1983.

8. Smith PD, Janoff EN: Infectious diarrhea in human immunodeficiency virus infection. *Gastroenterol Clin N Am* 17:587–598, 1988.

9. Smith PD, Quinn TC, Strober W, et al: Gastrointestinal infections in AIDS: NIH conference. *Ann Int Med* 116:63–77, 1992.

10. Wexner SD: Sexually transmitted diseases of the colon, rectum, and anus: The challenge of the nineties. *Dis Colon Rectum* 33:1048–1062, 1990.

11. Wexner SD, Smithy WB, Trillo C, et al: Emergency colectomy for cytomegalovirus ileocolitis in patients with the acquired immune deficiency syndrome. *Dis Colon Rectum* 31:755–761, 1988.

See also Chapters 20, 37, 51, 52 and 54.

CHAPTER 56

Diverticulitis

Angelita Habr-Gama, M.D. and Magaly Gemio Teixeira, M.D.

Refer to Algorithm 56-1.

A. Although diverticulae may be present throughout the colon, the muscle abnormality is limited in the great majority of patients to the sigmoid colon. Moreover, the condition is usually asymptomatic. When symptoms are present, they may or may not be associated with complications that include acute peridiverticulitis, perforation, fistula, obstruction, and bleeding.

B. History and physical examination is the essential key for correct diagnosis of diverticulitis and also for selection of appropriate treatment.

C. Uncomplicated symptomatic diverticular disease of the colon (DDC) may be suspected by the presence of left iliac fossa or lower abdominal pain and alteration of bowel habits (alternation between constipation and episodes of loose stools). Less frequently, abdominal distension or mucous discharge may be present. Physical examination is usually normal.

D. Flexible sigmoidoscopy with air-contrast barium enema or total colonoscopy is mandatory when there is suspicion of DDC, not only to confirm this possibility but also to exclude the presence of colonic carcinoma.

E. Treatment of complicated DDC is conservative and includes recommendation of high-fiber diet to improve bowel habit, stool consistency, and transit time, and to prevent development of complications. Antispasmodics and antidiarrheal agents may be useful in certain patients.

F. Inflammation may occur by retention of feces within the diverticular sac and subsequent obstruction of the neck. The process may be limited to the diverticulum, or it can spread to surrounding tissues, producing peridiverticulitis, which represents the first stage of acute diverticulitis. Acute left iliac fossa pain and tenderness, fever, and tachycardia are the most common symptoms and signs of this complication.

G. Clinical diagnosis of acute diverticulitis is often inaccurate since other acute abdominal conditions such as ischemic colitis, carcinoma, or inflammatory bowel disease may have similar presentation. Ultrasound (US) and computerized tomography (CT) scan are important not only for the diagnosis but

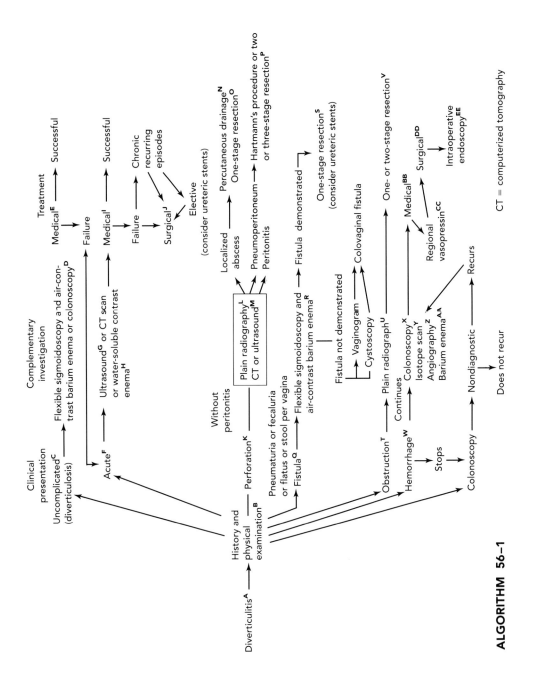

ALGORITHM 56-1

304

also to differentiate disease confined to the colonic wall from pericolic extension or an abscess that requires drainage. US, as a noninvasive method, is practical for detection of inflammation of the diverticulum, hypertrophy of the intestinal wall, and pericolic disease.

H. Air-contrast barium enema provides information on the extent of the disease, presence of stenosis, abscesses, or fistulas; however, in acute disease, it is preferable to use water-soluble enemas to limit morbidity in case perforation is present. Furthermore, a water-soluble contrast enema will allow other diagnoses to be pursued if diverticulitis is not demonstrated.

I. Patients must be admitted into the hospital for intravenous fluids and antibiotics. After recovery, either colonoscopy or air contrast barium enema are necessary to confirm the diagnosis and to exclude other diseases.

J. Conservative treatment may be considered as failed after a few hours or days, depending on the patient's condition. Elective surgery should be considered in patients under 55 years of age after the first attack of acute diverticulitis and after the second attack for those over 55 years. Many patients recover from a single acute attack but continue to have outpatient treatment of multiple "minor attacks" or relapses. Surgery may also be justifiable in these patients. The use of intraoperative ureteric stents is quite valuable as a fibrotic pelvic and left iliac fossa phlegmon is often present. Even in cases of elective resection, all patients should be consented and marked for possible fecal diversion. If unanticipated sepsis is encountered, either a sigmoidectomy with an end descending colostomy or a coloproctostomy with protective loop ileostomy may be undertaken.

K. Perforation may occur as a localized inflammatory mass or as free perforation into the peritoneal cavity that originates as either purulent or fecal peritonitis. Higher rates of free perforation, greater need for surgery, and increased morbidity and mortality are seen in immunocompromised patients with acute diverticulitis. Perforation may occur suddenly or may be preceded for some days by a less severe attack of acute diverticulitis. Localized peritonitis is commonly associated with abdominal pain, tenderness, and eventually, urinary symptoms. Purulent peritonitis is associated with fever, dehydration, diffuse abdominal pain, tenderness, and absence of bowel sounds. In addition, patients with fecal peritonitis may present with sepsis and circulatory collapse. The latter constellation of symptoms are absolute surgical indications.

L. Plain abdominal radiography may demonstrate abscess, fistula, or pneumoperitoneum. The latter finding warrants immediate laparotomy.

M. CT or US may demonstrate a localized abscess or extracolonic septic extension.

N. Percutaneous drainage guided by US or CT scan is the method of choice. Surgery can be postponed, and the patient can be operated on as an elective procedure after bowel preparation, thus avoiding multistage procedures.

O. Patients with pericolic abscess may be managed safely, after abscess drainage and subsequent bowel preparation, by a one-stage resection and anastomosis. Intraoperative colonic irrigation may be necessary.

P. In fecal peritonitis, Hartmann's operation is the safest procedure. In purulent or localized peritonitis, it is also well indicated; however, resection and anastomosis protected by an ostomy or even (rarely) a colostomy and drainage without resection may be indicated according to the degree of contamination and general condition of the patient.

Q. A diverticular or pericolic abscess may discharge directly into the viscus or out of the skin surface of the abdomen or perineum. Complaints including passage of air and/or stool per vagina or per urethra should lead one to suspect the presence of a fistula. The fistula most commonly seen is colovesical followed by colovaginal, colocutaneous, and coloileal. They may occur spontaneously or after operative procedures. Vaginography may reveal a colovaginal fistula. Alternatively, a methylene blue enema can be administered after insertion of a vaginal tampon. A colovesical fistula can sometimes be seen on cystography. Usually, however, cystoscopy reveals only an area of bullous edema at the dome of the bladder. If neither cystography nor cystoscopy reveals a suspected fistula, then activated charcoal or methylene blue can be ingested. The urine is subsequently analyzed for the respective compound. Lastly, after barium enema, a urine sample can be centrifuged and then radiographed to reveal a barium pellet. However, in some patients, the diagnosis of colovesical fistula remains a clinical one until laparotomy. Ureteric stents are a valuable adjunct during elective resection for colovesical or colovaginal fistulae.

R. Air-contrast barium enema can demonstrate a sinus or fistulous tract.

S. One-stage resection is the procedure of choice for patients who can be submitted to previous bowel preparation.

T. Complete large bowel obstruction is rare, and when it occurs, it is usually insidious and develops after repeated episodes of inflammation that gradually encase the colon. Obstruction of the small bowel by adherence to an inflammatory mass is more common. Increased constipation, mucous discharge, gaseous distension, and progressive abdominal pain, bloating, vomiting, and ileus are noted.

U. Radiography demonstrates a distended colon and absence of gas in the rectum. Attention to closed loop obstruction is important.

V. Primary resection and anastomosis may be safe in selected patients if intraoperative colonic irrigation is performed. A protective proximal stoma is indicated in high-risk patients or when adequate bowel preparation cannot be achieved.

W. Massive bleeding can occur from vessels that supply the mucosa. Usually the patient's condition is relatively stable and complete evaluation is possible. Often bleeding ceases spontaneously, but recurrent episodes are common. Such recurrences are a surgical indication.

X. If a rapid cleansing of the colon with an osmotically balanced purgative is possible, an emergent colonoscopy should be the first diagnostic procedure.

Y. Technetium-99m (^{99m}Tc)-labeled red cell scan is a noninvasive method which may help in localizing the site of bleeding even with rates of bleeding as low as 0.05–0.10 mL/min. However, interpretations may be difficult, and therefore it is more indicated as a screening procedure in acute bleeding before angiography.

Z. Selective angiography may demonstrate the site of bleeding if blood loss is > 0.5 mL. Radiographic findings are more helpful for differentiation of vascular ectasia. However, selective angiography is both invasive and expensive, and, therefore, should be indicated only in cases of persistent, massive bleeding.

AA. Air-contrast barium enema should not be indicated in the acute episodes of bleeding since it makes subsequent attempts at angiography and colonoscopy impossible. It can be justified only for the elective investigation of chronic disease.

BB. Blood replacement, volume stabilization, and correction of clotting abnormalities are fundamental adjunct measures.

CC. Injection of vasopressin if an experienced radiologist is available may stop bleeding, temporarily saving time for preparation for surgery.

DD. Intraoperative panendoscopy is indicated in patients with unexplained severe bleeding.

EE. In about 80% of the patients, the bleeding stops spontaneously or after only a few units of blood; if more than 8 units are required over a period of 48 hours, patients may require surgical treatment. If the bleeding point has been demonstrated prior to surgery, segmental resection is indicated.

BIBLIOGRAPHY

1. Alanis A, Papanicolau GK, Tadros RR, et al: Primary resection and anastomosis for treatment of acute diverticulitis. *Dis Colon Rectum* 32:933–939, 1989.

2. Ambrosetti P, Robert J, Witzig JA, et al: Prognostic factors from computed tomography in acute left colonic diverticulitis. *Br J Surg* 79:117–119, 1992.

3. Eaton AC: Emergency surgery for acute colonic hemorrhage—a retrospective study. *Br J Surg* 68:109–111, 1981.

4. Eisenstat TE, Rubin RJ, Salvati EP: Surgical management of diverticulitis. The role of the Hartmann procedure. *Dis Colon Rectum* 26:429–431, 1983.

5. Forde KA: Intraoperative colonoscopy. In Hunt RH, Waye JD (eds): *Colonoscopy: Techniques, Clinical Practice, and Colour Atlas.* London: Chapman & Hall, 1981, pp 189–198.

6. Killingback M: Management of perforative diverticulitis. *Surg Clin N Am* 63:97–115, 1983.

7. Practice Parameters for Sigmoid Diverticulitis-Supporting Documentation. Prepared by The Standards Task Force of the American Society of Colon and Rectal Surgeons. *Dis Colon Rectum* 38(2):126–132, 1995.

8. Rodkey GV, Welch CE: Changing patterns in the surgical treatment of diverticular disease. *Ann Surg* 200:466–478, 1984.

9. Schwerk WB, Schwartz S, Rothmund M: Sonography in acute colonic diverticulitis. A prospective study. *Dis Colon Rectum* 35:1077–1084, 1992.

10. Tyau ES, Prytowsky JB, Joehl RJ, et al: Acute diverticulitis. A complicated problem in the immunocompromised patient. *Arch Surg* 126:855–859, 1991.

11. Waye JD: A diagnostic approach to colon bleeding. *Mt Sinai J Med,* 51:491–499, 1984.

12. Wexner SD, Dailey TH: The initial management of left lower quadrant peritonitis. *Dis Colon Rectum* 29:635–638, 1986.

See also Chapters 10, 11, 12A, 12B, 13, 14, 15, 16, 20 and 21.

CHAPTER 57

Pouchitis

Paul Belliveau, M.D.

Refer to Algorithm 57–1.

As our experience with ileoanal reservoirs increases, so does the number of long-term sequelae. One of these complications, pouchitis, presents with a sudden or gradual change in the general state of well-being, increased stool frequency, lower abdominal cramping, reduction in continence, and occasionally fever. In the majority of cases, the patients will have a prior history of ulcerative colitis as only rare instances in familial polyposis have been reported. Interestingly, reappearance of arthritic symptoms similar to those occurring prior to colectomy are not infrequent. Approximately 20–30% of patients will experience such episodes of pouch enteritis; two-thirds of these attacks occur only once. It is important to recognize this condition as effective therapy is available for the majority of cases and will promptly restore satisfactory bowel control.

Pouchitis may be classified as acute, acute relapsing, subacute, or chronic. The etiology is unclear; studies of bacteriology, inflammatory cellular infiltrates, platelet-activating factor, emptying of the reservoir, ischemic changes, short-chain fatty acids, bile acids, and others have been researched. It is quite possible that pouchitis represents yet another manifestation of idiopathic inflammatory bowel disease.

A. History and physical exam of the abdomen, rectal area, and joints is the first step, and history of recent travel or use of antibiotics prior to the onset of diarrhea may lead to a specific cause. Other historical factors include any changes in diet or specific causes leading to malaise, loss of usual bowel control, or cramping abdominal pains. It is mandatory to exclude anal stricture and anal, pouch–anal, or cuff abscess–fistula. In general, digital examination and anoscopy allow exclusion of these etiologies.

B. Either rigid sigmoidoscopy (15-mm diameter) or flexible endoscopy may be used to make the diagnosis. Quantitative stool culture may reveal bacterial overgrowth (10^8 colony forming units/g). Aerobic counts may be elevated proportionally more than anaerobic counts in those with pouch inflammation.

C. Endoscopy will confirm redness, scattered whitish small plaques, edema, friability, ulcerations of various degrees (usually minute), and a watery exu-

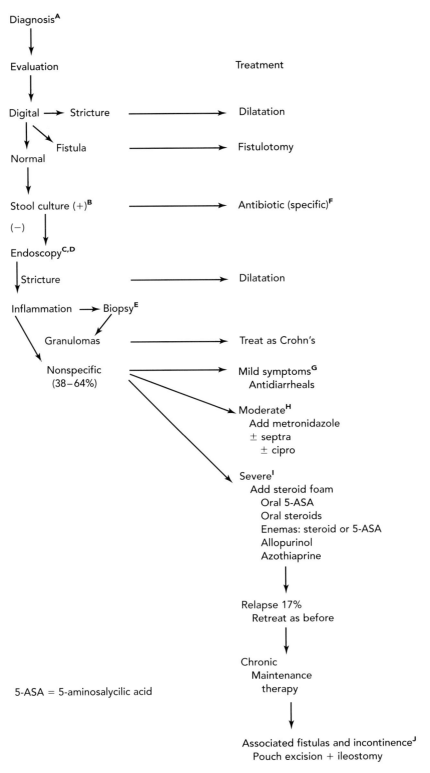

Diagnosis[A]

Evaluation   Treatment

Digital ⟶ Stricture ⟶ Dilatation

Fistula ⟶ Fistulotomy

Normal

Stool culture (+)[B] ⟶ Antibiotic (specific)[F]

(−)

Endoscopy[C,D]

Stricture ⟶ Dilatation

Inflammation ⟶ Biopsy[E]

Granulomas ⟶ Treat as Crohn's

Nonspecific ⟶ Mild symptoms[G]
(38–64%)   Antidiarrheals

Moderate[H]
Add metronidazole
± septra
± cipro

Severe[I]
Add steroid foam
Oral 5-ASA
Oral steroids
Enemas: steroid or 5-ASA
Allopurinol
Azothiaprine

Relapse 17%
Retreat as before

Chronic
Maintenance
therapy

5-ASA = 5-aminosalycilic acid

Associated fistulas and incontinence[J]
Pouch excision + ileostomy

ALGORITHM 57–1

date. The inflammation may be diffuse and patchy or may involve only the lower third or outlet of the pouch.

D. Diarrhea, weight loss, or anemia may herald Crohn's disease in the small bowel despite a pathologic diagnosis of ulcerative colitis in the colectomy specimen. Thus a small bowel series is indicated. Other causes of diarrhea include diet changes or intolerances to food such as lactose, fructose, or sorbitol; these problems should be excluded with appropriate tests.

E. Biopsy of patients with refractory pouchitis or unusual ulcerations may be helpful to confirm a diagnosis of Crohn's disease.

F. Specific infectious diseases respond to appropriate antibacterials, as discussed in Chapter 55.

G. In very mild cases, no treatment may be necessary as some episodes are self-limiting. Indeed, the finding of inflammation in an otherwise asymptomatic individual is not an indication for treatment. However, symptoms may be improved with nonspecific antidiarrheals. Dosages vary, but loperamide 2–4 mg, diphenoxylate 5 mg, or bismuth subsalicylate 3 mL once or twice a day can be employed.

H. For more severe symptoms, a course of metronidazole 250 mg by mouth t.i.d. for 14 days should be initiated. Alternatives include trimethoprime 160 mg + sulfamethoxazole 800 mg b.i.d. for 14 days or ciprofloxacin 500 mg b.i.d. for 10 days.

I. In severe cases the dose of antidiarrheals can be increased, or one can pre-scribe codeine 30 mg 4–6 times a day, administer metronidazole 250 mg t.i.d. for 14 days, or add topical steroid foam preparations b.i.d. Other alternatives are oral 5-aminosalicilic acid (5-ASA) 500 mg t.i.d., prednisone 10–20 mg daily, allopurinol 300 mg b.i.d. Azathioprine immunosuppression is advised only for advanced severe cases and requires close monitoring of blood parame-ters.

J. Pouchitis alone rarely requires pouch excision; indeed, chronic diarrhea states may persist despite the permanent ileostomy.

BIBLIOGRAPHY

1. Fozard BJ, Pemberton JH: Results of pouch surgery after ileoana anastomosis: the implications of pouchitis. *World J Surg,* 16:880–884, 1992.

2. Heppell J, Belliveau P, Taillefer R, et al: Quantitative assessment of pelvic ileal reservoir emptying with a semisolid radionuclide enema: a correlation with clinical outcome. *Dis Colon Rectum* 30:81–85, 1987.

3. Luukkonen P, Valtonen V, Sivonen A, et al: Fecal bacteriology and reservoir ileitis in patients operated on for ulcerative colitis. *Dis Colon Rectum* 31:864–867, 1988.

4. Mortensen NJ McC, Madden MV: Pouchitis—acute inflammation in ileal pouches. In Nicholls J, Bartolo D, Mortensen N (eds): *Restorative Proctocolectomy.* London: Blackwell Scientific Publications, 1993, pp 119–131.

5. Nicholls RJ, Belliveau P, Neill M, et al: Restorative proctocolectomy with ileal reservoir: a pathophysiological assessment. *Gut* 22:462–468, 1981.

6. Parks AG, Nicholls RJ, Belliveau P: Proctocolectomy with ileal reservoir and anal anastomosis. *Br J Surg* 67:533–538, 1980.

7. Wexner SD, Wong WD, Rothenberger DA, Goldberg SM: The ileoanal reservoir. *Am J. Surg* 159:178–185, 1990.

See also Chapters 52, 55 and 93.

Colonic Pathology
Miscellaneous Nonneoplastic Conditions

CHAPTER 58

Management of Volvulus

Susan A. Sgambati, M.D. and
Garth H. Ballantyne, M.D.

Refer to Algorithm 58-1.

A. Volvulus is the abnormal rotation of a segment of bowel around its mesentry, resulting in occlusion of the proximal and distal ends with a closed-loop obstruction. Vascular compromise and increased intraluminal pressure lead to gangrene and perforation if the volvulus is not reduced. The incidence of colonic volvulus varies worldwide. In the United States, colonic volvulus accounts for 1–3% of all large bowel obstructions; 80% of these occur in the sigmoid colon, 15% in the cecum, 3% in the transverse colon, and 2% in the splenic flexure. Among certain populations in Africa, Iran, and western Europe, volvulus is the most common cause of intestinal obstruction. All patients with a volvulus should undergo surgery during their initial hospitalization. The timing of the operation is based on two considerations: (1) the viability of the involved colon and (2) the outcome of endoscopic decompression of the volvulus. In the presence of signs and symptoms of gangrenous bowel (fever, peritonitis, leukocytosis, acidosis), urgent exploration is *always* indicated.

B. In the United States, volvulus occurs in patients over age 60 and affects men and women equally. Racial differences have been noted in the United States, with over two-thirds of cases occurring in blacks. Sigmoid volvulus is associated with numerous neuropsychiatric disorders including Parkinson's disease, multiple sclerosis, traumatic paralysis, dementia, and chronic schizophrenia. A chronic bedridden state, psychotropic drugs, and sedatives are thought to contribute to colonic dysmotility. Excessive use of laxatives, enemas, and cathartics is also associated with volvulus, but may represent a manifestation of chronic constipation and prolonged recumbency. In developing countries, a high-fiber diet is implicated in the acquired redundancy of the sigmoid mesentery. Additionally, volvulus is the most common cause of intestinal obstruction in the pregnant female. The most common symptoms of colonic volvulus include abdominal pain, distension, and obstipation. Because of the frequent

315

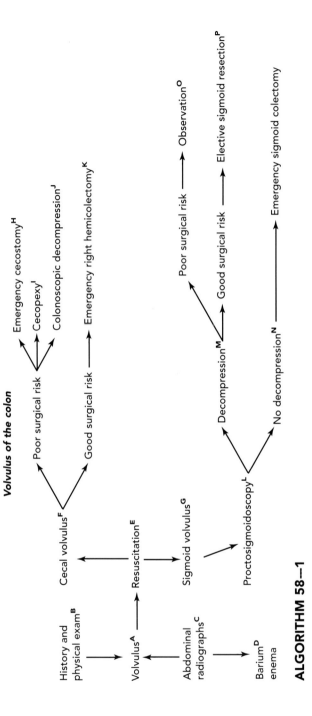

Volvulus of the colon

History and physical exam[B] → Volvulus[A] → Resuscitation[E]

Abdominal radiographs[C] → Volvulus[A]

Barium[D] enema

Cecal volvulus[F]
- Poor surgical risk
  - Emergency cecostomy[H]
  - Cecopexy[I]
- Good surgical risk
  - Colonoscopic decompression[J]
  - Emergency right hemicolectomy[K]

Sigmoid volvulus[G] → Proctosigmoidoscopy[L]
- Decompression[M]
  - Poor surgical risk → Observation[O]
  - Good surgical risk → Elective sigmoid resection[P]
- No decompression[N] → Emergency sigmoid colectomy

ALGORITHM 58—1

association with neuropsychiatric diseases, a reliable history may not be obtainable; when it is available, most patients have a history of previous self-limited episodes consistent with colonic obstruction. Physical examination reveals a massively distended abdomen with tympanitic bowel sounds over the dilated, gas-filled loop of bowel; the rectal vault is usually empty. Abdominal tenderness is worrisome, as it may represent peritoneal irritation from underlying ischemic or perforated bowel. Systemic toxicity varies according to the extent and duration of obstruction and ischemia.

C. Diagnosis of colonic volvulus is usually confirmed by a plain abdominal radiograph, which reveals the characteristic "omega" or "inverted loop" sign represented the volvulized colon with markedly dilated proximal bowel and an empty rectum (Fig. 58–1).

D. Barium enema demonstrates the characteristic "bird's beak" at the apex of a sigmoid volvulus (Fig. 58–2). Barium enema effectively reduces sigmoid volvulus in approximately 5% of cases. In cecal volvulus, utilization of radiologic contrast studies is controversial. The high pressures required to fill the right colon may cause perforation, and the presence of barium may jeopardize a primary anastamosis should the patient require resection. Additionally, any contrast study will severely impair endoscopic assessment of the colon, and should be reserved for cases in which the diagnosis remains elusive despite endoscopic evaluation. If it is absolutely essential to obtain contrast radiography, then a water soluble agent should be used.

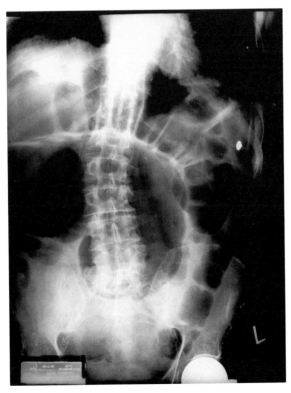

FIGURE 58–1 A radiograph depicting an omega sign.

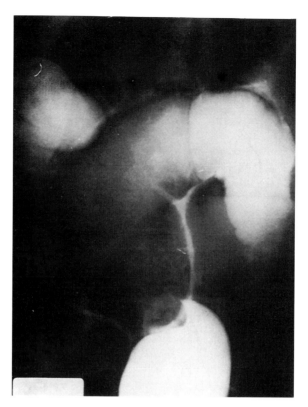

FIGURE 58–2 Barium enema depicting a bird-beak sign.

E. The initial priority is resuscitation of the patient. Vomiting and third space fluid losses result in hypovolemic shock, and intravenous fluid resuscitation must be initiated before any attempts at decompression. Broad-spectrum antibiotics are administered, as with any intestinal obstruction. The patient should be placed in the left lateral decubitus position to improve venous return, which may be compromised secondary to massive abdominal distention. Oxygen is administered, as diaphragmatic excursion is limited by the expanded intraabdominal contents. A Foley catheter is inserted in order to accurately monitor fluid balance, and a nasogastric tube inserted to decompress the stomach and prevent aspiration of enteric contents.

F. Cecal volvulus is a congenital condition, resulting from the failure of the parietal peritoneum to fuse to the cecum and ascending colon. The mobile right colon is free to torse axially about its mesentery. Cecal volvulus is less common and occurs in younger patients than does sigmoid volvulus.

G. Sigmoid volvulus is an acquired condition, occurring in the setting of an elongated, redundant sigmoid loop with a narrowed mesenteric base.

H,I. Options for surgical treatment of cecal volvulus in the poor-risk patient include cecostomy and cecostomy with cecopexy. The former procedure adequately decompresses the colon and fixes the cecum in the right lower quadrant. Recurrences following cecostomy are rare. Cecostomy contaminates the peritoneal cavity, the laparotomy incision, and the cecostomy site with stool; however, difficulties in decompressing the right colon through the cecostomy tube make the procedure significantly less attractive. Cecostomy tube placement is thus reserved for patients in whom right hemicolectomy with primary anastamosis is inadvisable.

J. Colonoscopic decompression of cecal volvulus is extremely difficult and is reserved for the highly skilled endoscopist. Attempts at colonoscopic decompression should not delay surgical exploration. If colonoscopic decompression is successful, the patient should undergo elective operative therapy during the same hospitalization after receiving a standard bowel preparation.

K. Right hemicolectomy decompresses the colon and precludes recurrence. Resection is required in the presence of colonic gangrene. Mortality rates for cecal volvulus vary with respect to operative findings. The average mortality in patients with a viable cecum at laparotomy is 12%; the mortality for those with cecal gangrene is 32%.

L. Rigid proctosigmoidoscopy is indicated for all cases of suspected sigmoid volvulus.

M. Once the site of torsion is encountered, decompression with either the sigmoidoscope or rectal tube is attempted. Endoscopic reduction is successful in 59% of patients. If unsuccessful, decompression with a flexible endoscope can be attempted. The combination of the rigid and flexible endoscopy should successfully reduce approximately 90% of nonstrangulated volvulus of the sigmoid colon.

N. In cases in which endoscopic decompression is unsuccessful, emergent surgery is indicated. The sigmoid colon must be resected and primary anastamosis in these emergent circumstances is generally contraindicated. A sigmoid colectomy with an end-descending colostomy is performed. The mortality rate for emergent sigmoid resection following volvulus is high, ranging from 25% to 50%.

O. Over 90% cases of sigmoid volvulus are successfully decompressed endoscopically. Following resuscitation and 3–4 days of observation, patients receive the standard mechanical and chemical bowel preparation and undergo an elective sigmoid resection with primary anastamosis. Given the anatomy of the disease and the population in which sigmoid volvulus occurs, these patients are ideal candidates for laparoscopic sigmoid resection. Under these circumstances, mortality is similar to that for other elective colonic resections.

P. Although not recommended, observation following successful endoscopic decompression of sigmoid volvulus is an option in the very poor-risk surgical patient. Recurrence following endoscopic reduction without resection ranges from 55% to 90%, and mortality with recurrent sigmoid volvulus is 20–30%.

BIBLIOGRAPHY

1. Ballantyne GH: Volvulus of the splenic flexure: case report and review of the literature. *Dis Colon Rectum* 24:630–632, 1984.

2. Ballantyne GH: Review of sigmoid volvulus: history and results of treatment. *Dis Colon Rectum* 25:82–88, 1982.

3. Ballantyne GH: Review of sigmoid volvulus: clinical patterns and pathogenesis. *Dis Colon Rectum* 25:823–830, 1982.

4. Ballantyne GH, Brander MD, Beart RW Jr, et al: Colonic volvulus: incidence and mortality. *Ann Surg* 202:83–92, 1985.

5. Burke JB, Ballantyne GH: Cecal volvulus: low mortality in a city hospital. *Dis Colon Rectum* 27:737–740, 1984.

6. Wexner SD, Dailey TH: The initial management of left lower quadrant peritonitis. *Dis Colon Rectum* 29:635–638, 1986.

See also Chapters 62, 64 and 76.

CHAPTER 59

Colorectal Trauma

Richard L. Whelan, M.D. and Karen D. Horvath, M.D.

Refer to Algorithm 59–1.

A. Antibiotics with adequate Gram-negative and anaerobic coverage should be given preoperatively and continued for 24–48 hours. If intraoperative blood loss is excessive, doses should be repeated at earlier intervals to compensate for the dilutional effects of large-volume crystalloid and colloid administration. Contingent on the degree of contamination, antibiotics may need to be continued postoperatively for several additional days.

B. Fecal soiling predisposes patients to the development of postoperative septic complications. After major bleeding has been addressed, control of contamination is the next priority and should be accomplished with atraumatic clamps and expeditious suture closure of perforations.

C. Civilian penetrating colon injuries are currently associated with a mortality rate of 10% and a septic complication rate of 18–26%.

D. Includes any limited colon injury not requiring resection where the blood supply to the injured segment remains intact.

E. Significant advances have occurred in the management of civilian penetrating colon trauma over the past 20 years, with a present emphasis on primary repair of most injuries. During World War II, exteriorization of the injured segment or colostomy formation became the standard management for all traumatic colon wounds. The logic underlying this conservative management scheme was to avoid intraabdominal suture line dehiscence and peritoneal sepsis. It was felt that the suture line in a primarily repaired injury was at high risk for leakage, or might dissolve secondary to intraabdominal infection. This theory has not been substantiated in studies performed over the past 20 years. The risk factors most closely associated with postoperative intraabdominal septic complications are hypotension and transfusion requirement. However, multiple reports have demonstrated the efficacy of primary repair over colostomy, even in the presence of these and other "risk factors," such as associated injuries and fecal contamination. The reported suture line failure rate in this

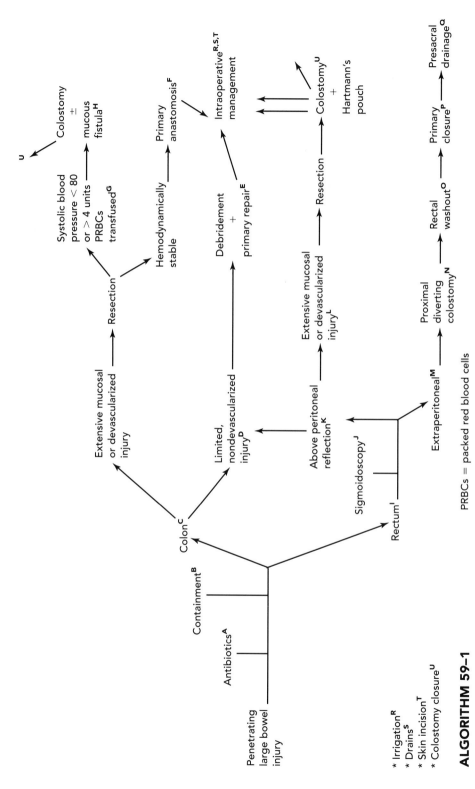

ALGORITHM 59–1

PRBCs = packed red blood cells

* Irrigation[R]
* Drains[S]
* Skin incision[T]
* Colostomy closure[U]

setting is only 0–1%. Thus, it appears that the method of colon wound management does not influence the infectious complication rate. The determinants of successful colon wound healing remain adequate blood supply, tension-free closure, and meticulous surgical technique. Right- and left-sided colon wounds are treated similarly. Care should be taken to delineate the entire injury. Missed injuries can occur at the mesenteric border and along the appendices epiploicae. Devitalized tissue at the wound edges must be debrided to bleeding tissue. A two-layer closure of the defect is recommended.

F. Resection with primary anastomosis in *unselected* patients (i.e., including hemodynamically unstable patients) is associated with an 8–10% leakage rate.

G. To date, no studies have assessed sizable numbers of the most severely injured patients with high transfusion requirements and hypotension. It is not clear whether resection and primary anastomosis is safe in this group of patients. These patients are most likely to become hypotensive postoperatively, creating a low-flow state that might place the anastomosis at risk. Additionally, limiting the length of the operation is important in this severely injured group of patients. Resection with anastomosis would lengthen the procedure. For these reasons it is recommended that patients requiring colon resection who are hypotensive pre- or intraoperatively to a systolic blood pressure < 80 or who require transfusion of > 4 units blood be managed with a colostomy.

H. End colostomy with a mucous fistula or a Hartmann's pouch.

I. Rectal injuries are suspected with penetrating injury to the suprapubic area, pelvis, flank, lower back, and buttocks. The presence of blood on rectal examination, or hematuria are signs that the rectum may have been injured. In the operating room, the patient should be placed in the modified lithotomy position to allow access to the rectum.

J. Sigmoidoscopy is absolutely essential to document the injury, even when there is already an indication for laparotomy. Patients are best examined under general anesthesia in the operating room. Adequate visualization may be difficult with a reported false-negative rate of 30%. At-risk patients in whom an injury cannot be definitively excluded should be treated as if an injury were present.

K. Limited intraperitoneal rectal injuries are treated like colon injuries.

L. For intraperitoneal rectal injuries requiring resection, formation of a colostomy, and Hartmann's pouch is advised. There are no data to support the performance of a rectal anastomosis in the trauma setting.

M. There is no role for expectant management in the treatment of patients with full-thickness extraperitoneal rectal injuries. The classic treatment includes (1) proximal colostomy, (2) rectal washout, (3) primary repair of the injury, if possible, and (4) presacral drainage.

N. A loop or stapled, sigmoid loop colostomy should be performed to assure complete fecal diversion. One advantage of a loop colostomy in the trauma setting is that it provides proximal access to the distal segment, which facilitates rectal washout.

O. As mentioned above, prograde rectal washout can be undertaken through a loop colostomy. Alternatively, after anal dilatation, a retrograde cleanout can be performed by irrigating residual fecal material from the distal rectal stump.

P. Primary closure of rectal injuries should be attempted but is usually quite difficult and probably not necessary.

Q. For posterior injuries involving the distal two-thirds of the rectum, presacral drainage is indicated. Closed-suction drains are placed into the presacral space through an incision made between the coccyx and the anus. Wounds involving the posterior proximal third of the rectum are best drained transabdominally. The need to place presacral drains in patients with a limited anterior wall injury is unclear. An anterior abscess would not be well drained through a posterior drain.

R. The abdominal cavity should be copiously irrigated with 4–6 liters of warm saline to remove gross contamination, dilute the bacterial inoculum, and increase core temperature.

S. Transabdominal drains are associated with a fourfold increased risk of infection in colostomy patients and a twofold increased risk in patients after primary closure. They should not be used except if necessary for an associated intraabdominal injury. In this case, it should be closed-suction and placed as far from the colostomy as possible.

T. Primary closure of skin incisions should be reserved for uncomplicated cases with minimal fecal contamination. All other wounds should be allowed to heal by secondary intention or delayed primary closure.

U. Colostomy closure, in the posttraumatic setting, is associated with a 10% morbidity, most complications are minor. Takedown should be performed no sooner than 6–8 weeks after injury in uncomplicated cases, and about 3–6 months postoperatively in patients who have had intraabdominal septic complications. This period will give the densely vascular and edematous adhesions that follow peritonitis time to resolve into the filmy adhesions that are easy to lyse. Prior to closure both the proximal colon and the Hartmann's pouch should be evaluated by either endoscopy, radiography, or both investigations. In older patients, pre-closure manometry may be warranted to document adequate sphincter function and rectal capacity and compliance.

BIBLIOGRAPHY

1. Chappuis CW, Frey DJ, Dietzen CD, et al: Management of penetrating colon injuries, a prospective randomized trial. *Ann Surg* 213:492–498, 1991.

2. Fabian TC, Croce MA: Management of penetrating colon injury. *Perspect Colon Rectal Surg* 5:24–49, 1992.

3. George SM, Fabian TC, Voeller GR, et al: Primary repair of colon wounds, a prospective trial in nonselected patients. *Ann Surg* 209:728–734, 1989.

4. Stone HH, Fabian TC: Management of perforating colon trauma, randomization between primary closure and exteriorization. *Ann Surg* 190:430–436, 1979.

5. Whelan RL, Scalea TM: Colorectal trauma. *Prob Gen Surg.* 9:623–633, 1992.

See also Chapter 36.

CHAPTER 60

Management
of Endometriosis
of the Intestine

H. Randolph Bailey, M.D.

Refer to Algorithm 60–1.

A. Evaluation consists of bidigital exam of the cul-de-sac and rectovaginal septum, rigid sigmoidoscopy and possibly barium enema (solid column) and intravenous pyelogram (IVP). Mucosal evaluation is necessary to rule out primary colorectal carcinoma.

B. The major symptom requiring colorectal resection for endometriosis is pain, either pelvic or rectal. Dyspareunia is highly predictive of cul-de-sac involvement. Obstructive symptoms and changes in the bowel habit occur with menses. Bleeding, if it occurs, is either from the anal canal and unrelated, or, rarely, sign of mucosal involvement by the endometriosis.

C. Hormonal suppression may result in resolution of small peritoneal implants and/or decrease vascularity of larger lesions. Rarely do significant ovarian or bowel endometriomas resolve. Commonly used agents include Danazol and gonadotropin-releasing hormone agonists such as Synarel and Lupron. Hormones are administered for periods ranging from 1 to 6 months preoperatively. Side effects and cost limit the use of these agents.

D. All patients suspected of severe pelvic endometriosis undergo mechanical bowel prep preoperatively. Those with significant findings of intestinal involvement receive oral antibiotics. Intravenous antibiotics are administered perioperatively.

E. Conservative gynecologic procedure is defined as leaving the uterus and at least one tube and ovary. In our series, 49% of women attempting pregnancy following bowel resection and conservative gynecologic procedures were able to conceive.

Management of endometriosis of the intestine

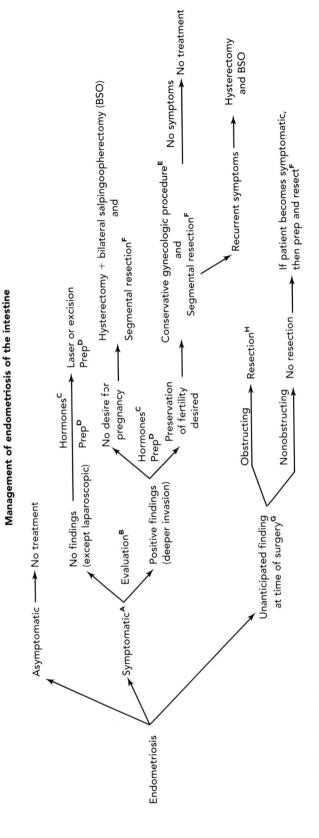

ALGORITHM 60–1

F. Occasionally a small, deeply infiltrating lesion may be managed by full-thickness disk excision. This procedure carries approximately the same risk as resection and anastomosis. Dissection of larger endometriomas from the bowel wall may result in recurrence due to indistinct margins and a bloody imprecise dissection. We prefer segmental resection in most cases for the above reasons. There have been a limited number of reports of colorectal endometriomas resected laparoscopically or with laparoscopic assist. While laparoscopic resection of endometriosis has been performed successfully, it has been done by extremely skilled laparoscopists, whose enthusiasm and technical proficiency far exceed mine and most others interested in this disease. Since the major site of involvement is the cul-de-sac, and obliteration of the normal planes of dissection is common, we feel that these techniques are of limited value.

G. Unanticipated finding of significant bowel involvement at time of laparotomy in a patient without mechanical bowel prep may result in confusion with carcinoma. Intraoperative sigmoidoscopy or colonoscopic examination of the mucosa may rule out colorectal carcinoma.

H. If the patient has obstruction and unprepped bowel, the options are similar to those for obstructing carcinoma or diverticulitis. These include resection with colostomy (Hartmann), on-table lavage with resection, primary resection with proximal stoma, or decompressing stoma followed by prep and resection a few days later.

BIBLIOGRAPHY

1. Bailey HR: Colorectal endometriosis. *Perspect Colon Rectal Surg* 5:251–259, 1992.

2. Coronado C, Franklin RR, Lotze EC, et al: Surgical treatment of symptomatic colorectal endometriosis. *Fertil Steril* 53:411–416, 1990.

3. Farinon AM, Vadora E: Endometriosis of the colon and rectum: an indication for peroperative coloscopy. *Endoscopy* 12:136–139, 1980.

4. Nezhat F, Nezhat C, Pennington E, et al: Laparoscopic segmental resection for infiltrating endometriosis of the rectosigmoid colon: a preliminary report. *Surg Laparosc Endosc* 2:212–216, 1992.

5. Prystowsky JB, Stryker SJ, Ujiki GT, et al: Gastrointestinal endometriosis. Incidence and indications for resection. *Arch Surg* 123:855–858, 1988.

6. Sharpe DR, Redwine DB: Laparoscopic segmental resection of the sigmoid and rectosigmoid colon for endometriosis. *Surg Laparosc Endosc* 2:120–124, 1992.

7. Weed JC, Ray JE: Endometriosis of the bowel. *Obstet Gynecol* 69:727–730, 1987.
See also Chapters 6, 14 and 62.

CHAPTER 61

Adult Hirschsprung's Disease

Sergio W. Larach, M.D. and Thomas B. Blake, III, M.D.

Refer to Algorithm 61-1.

A. Adult Hirschsprung's disease is congenital megacolon in which there is absence of ganglion cells in Meissner's submucosal plexus and Auerbach's intermyenteric plexus affecting the rectum and colon.
B. The history generally includes lifelong refractory constipation without fecal soilage with reliance on enemas and cathartics for bowel function. Abdominal pain (38%) and distension (66%) with history of prior hospitalizations for symptoms of partial bowel obstruction are also common features.
C. Examination typically reveals a distended abdomen with large firm fecal masses palpable through the abdominal wall with flaring of the ribs and an empty rectal vault on digital exam.
D. Plain abdominal x-rays reveal a massively dilated colon proximal to the aganglionic segment.
E. Barium enema is performed in unprepped bowel so that the transition zone is not altered by mechanical prep.
F. Absence of rectoanal inhibitory reflex has a reported accuracy rate of >90% in the diagnosis of Hirschsprung's disease.
G. The transition zone is typically a cone shaped narrowed rectum with markedly dilated proximal colon.
H. There is a 20% false-negative rate in which the transition zone is not visualized. If the diagnosis is in question, anorectal manometry and rectal biopsy should be undertaken.
I. The definitive diagnosis is a full-thickness 1 cm x 5 cm strip rectal biopsy performed beginning 2-3 cm from the anal verge.
J. If the diagnosis is in doubt, the rectal biopsy should be reviewed as to adequacy sampling. Other causes of megacolon may include disorders of the central nervous systems, Chagas' disease, volvulus, anorectal obstruction, or idiopathic megacolon.

Adult Hirschsprung's disease[A]
(age > 10 years)

History[B]

+

Physical[C]
exam

Abdominal[D]
x-ray (megacolon)

Barium
enema[E]

Anal manometric
studies[F]

(+) Transition
zone[G]

(−) Transition
zone[H]

Absent
rectoanal
reflex

Rectal[I]
biopsy

Ganglia
present
(consider other
diagnosis)[J]

Ganglia
absent[K]

Diverting
colostomy[L]

Definitive treatment[M]
Duhamel retrorectal
pull-through[N]
Swenson and Bill
abdominal pull-through[O]
Soave endorectal
pull-through[P]
Posterior anorectal myectomy[Q]
Posterior anorectal myectomy
with low anterior resection[R]
Low anterior
resection[S]
Colectomy[T]

ALGORITHM 61–1

K. The biopsy is diagnostic if there is absence of ganglia cells, hyperplasia, or hypertrophy of nerve fibers and increase of acetylcholinesterase-positive fibers in the muscularis mucosa and lamina propia.

L. A diverting colostomy may be the most important contribution to a successful outcome. It allows for adequate mechanical bowel prep and return of hypertrophied bowel to normal size as well as improvement in nutritional status.

M. Definitive treatment requires adequately mechanically prepped bowel. The goal of surgical therapy is to remove the aganglionic segment including the nonfunctioning part of the internal sphincter and megacolon. All surgical procedures have reported good results and appear to be dependent on the surgeon's experience.

N. The Duhamel pull-through is considered the operation of choice. Results are good in 91% of patients with 2% minor and 10% major complication rates. It avoids extensive pelvic dissection and injury to sensory fibers of the rectum.

O. The Swenson and Bill procedure has resulted in good results in 80% of patients with a 33% major and 7% minor complication rate. A draw back of this approach is a 7% incidence of impotence.

P. After the Soave pull-through, good results were noted in 85% of cases. A 25% major and a 13% minor complication rate and a 13% incidence of postoperative stricture and 16% includes an anastomotic leak rate.

Q. Posterior anorectal myectomy is advocated as initial treatment in short segment aganglionosis. 55% of patients have reported good results and 40% with poor results have required another procedure.

R. Anorectal myectomy performed followed with low anterior resection was associated with good results in 100% of patients without complications.

S. Low anterior resection alone has achieved good results in 72% of patients with a 6% mortality.

T. A subtotal or left hemicolectomy has achieved 67% good results and a 7% death rate.

BIBLIOGRAPHY

1. Jorge JMN, Wexner SD: A practical guide to anal manometry. *S Med J* 86:924–931, 1993.

2. Lavery IC: Hirschsprung's disease—current therapy. In Fazio VW (ed): *Colon and Rectal Surgery*. Philadelphia: Decker, 1990, pp74–82.

3. Luukkonen P, Heikkiner M, Huikuli K, et al: Adult Hirschsprung's disease. Clinical features and functional outcome after surgery. *Dis Colon Rectum* 33:65–69, 1990.

4. Oakley JR, Lavery IC: Etiology of congenital colorectal disease. In: Wexner SD, Bartolo DCC: *Constipation: Etiology, Evaluation, and Management*. London: Butterworth-Heinemann 1995, p9–16.

5. Schouter WR, Gordon PH: In Gordon PH, Nivatvongs S (eds): *Principles and Practice of Surgery for the Colon, Rectum and Anus*. St. Louis: Quality Medical Publishing, 1992, p907–953.

6. Wheatley MJ, Wesley JR, Coran AG, et al: Hirschsprung's disease in adolescents and adults. *Dis Colon Rectum* 33:622–629, 1990.

See also Chapters 3, 17 and 18.

SECTION 5C

Colonic Pathology
Ischemia, Obstruction and Stricture

CHAPTER 62

Colonic Obstruction

Joji Utsunomiya, M.D., Ph.D. and T. Yamamura, M.D., Ph.D.

Refer to Algorithm 62–1.

A. Mechanical large bowel obstruction differs significantly from small bowel obstruction in many aspects, including the etiology, pathophysiology, and principal management. As shown in Table 62–1, 50% of cases are attributed to colorectal cancer and most of the remaining to volvulus, diverticulosis, and fecal impaction. While the patient with colonic obstruction usually gives a history of progressive constipation, abdominal pain, and distension, vomiting starts quite late and eventually becomes feculent. Fever, tachycardia, abdominal tenderness, muscle guarding, and a palpable mass are suggestive of impending perforation in cases of strangulation, volvulus, intussusception, or a closed-loop obstruction due to a competent ileocecal valve. All of these scenarios demand immediate resuscitation and emergency laparotomy prior to the patient's progression into septic shock (see paragraph C).

B. Digital examination of the rectum may demonstrate an impacted fecal bolus, a rectal tumor, disseminated carcinoma in the Douglas pouch (Blumer's shelf), or a gynecologic neoplasm. A ballooning of the rectum indicates chronic proximal obstruction (Hochenneg's sign).

C. The patient with severe obstruction (Table 62–2) who shows septic and toxic systemic symptoms requires immediate intravenous hydration and broad spectrum antianaerobic and anti-aerobic antibiotics; vomiting indicates the need for a nasogastric tube. Preexisting cardiac disease suggests that central venous pressure monitoring is necessary.

D. Plain abdominal films will generally show large-bowel distension as isolated in 26%, or as combined with the small bowel in 58% of cases. In 16% of patients, however, the distension is seen exclusively in the small bowel, which presents diagnostic difficulty. Alternatively, the "coffee-bean" or "bent inner tube" sign suggests a volvulus.

E. In closed-loop obstruction in the patient with a competent ileocecal valve, a cecal diameter of 9–12 cm suggests that the risk of perforation is significant.

335

Colonic obstruction

Diagnosis

History → Plain → Colon → Contrast → Endoscopy^G → Tumor^H → Right-sided
and   film^D enema^F
physical
examination^A

Digital   Water-soluble
exam^B

Closed-loop obstruction^E → see Chapter 76

Small intestine → preparation for emergency laparotomy^C

Severe obstruction

Evaluation

Left-sided^K

Other mechanicals obstruction^I
Impacted feces → enema
Inflammation → biopsy
Extramural → CT

Endoscopic repositioning

Volvus → see Chapter 58
Diverticulosis → see Chapter 56
Intussusception
Pseudoobstruction → see Chapter 63

Slight
or   →
moderate

Severe

Treatment

One-stage^J
1. Right hemicolectomy
2. Colectomy with on-table lavage^L
3. Subtotal colectomy and anastomosis^M

Two-stage^N
1. Colectomy, colostomy, and mucous fistula; or
2. Hartmann procedure followed by delayed anastomosis

Three-stage^O
Diverting transverse colostomy, colectomy and delayed anastomosis, closure of colostomy

CT = Computerized tomography

ALGORITHM 62–1

TABLE 62–1 CLASSIFICATION OF LARGE BOWEL OBSTRUCTION BASED
ON LOCAL AND SYSTEMIC EFFECT (MODIFIED FROM
P. FIELDING)

Manifestation and Pathophysiology	Severity of Obstruction		
	Mild	**Moderate**	**Severe**
Abdominal film			
Solid	+	+	+
Fluid and gas	–	+	+
Systemic toxicity	–	–	+
Pathophysiology			
Bacteriology overgrowth	–	+	++
Peritoneal translocation	–	–	+
Colon wall change			
Edema	–	+	++
Congestion	–	+	++
Ischemic colitis	–	(+)[a]	(+)[a]
Fluid and electrolyte balance			
Intralulminal sequestation	–	+	++
Cardiorespiratory imbalance	–	–	+

[a] Parentheses indicate potential positivity.

Such radiographic demonstration of gaseous distension demands immediate laparotomy for decompression.

F. When the plain films suggest colonic obstruction, or cannot define the causative site, a gentle water-soluble contrast enema is always performed to locate the site and to identify the lesions such as tumor, diverticulosis, or volvulus (bird's beak sign) (see Fig. 62–1). The contrast enema will also help exclude pseudo-obstruction and may be therapeutic in that setting.

G. A flexible sigmoidoscopy is gently performed without insufflation to observe mucosal changes such as inflammation or ischemia and to exclude rectal neoplasia. Furthermore, sigmoidoscopy can decompress a sigmoid volvulus.

H. Between 5% and 40% of patients with colorectal cancer initially present with the symptoms of obstruction. Acceptable intraoperative therapy includes preliminary diversion with subsequent resection, subtotal colectomy with ileoproctostomy, segmented colectomy with a stoma, or segmental colectomy with intraoperative colonic lavage and primary anastomosis. Selection of treatment alternatives is based on each patient's circumstances.

I. Other causes of mechanical obstruction in adults (classified in Table 62–1) are managed as mentioned in the corresponding chapter algorithms.

J. For right colon cancer, one-stage right hemicolectomy with primary ileocolic anastomosis is generally justified, because the dilated colon is removed and the small intestine is usually suitable for anastomosis.

TABLE 62-2 CLASSIFICATION OF CAUSES OF MECHANICAL LARGE BOWEL OBSTRUCTION IN ADULT

Cause	See Chapter
Intraluminal—obstruction	
Fecal impaction[a]	
Inspissated barium	
Gallstone	
Foreign body	
Mural	
Neoplasia[a]	70
Endometroisis	60
Inflammation	
Diverticular disease[a]	56
Crohn's disease	51
Ulcerative colitis	52
Toxic megacolon	54
Tuberculosis	55
Schistosomiasis	55
Lymphogranuloma venereum, etc.	55
Congenenital: adult Hirschsprung's	61
Ischemic colitis	64
Intussusception	33
Radiation colitis	77
Anastomotic stricture	92
Other stricture	65
Extramural	
Adhesion	58
Volvulus[a]	76
Tumor and its spread	71
Inflammation: abscess	94
External and internal hernias	58

[a] The four most common obstructing conditions are fecal impaction, diverticular disease, neoplasia, and volvulus.

K. For the remaining 70% in the left colon and rectum, the general trend is changing from delayed resection by multistage surgery to one-stage primary resection. Selection of the surgical option differs depending on the degree of the obstruction (categorized in Table 62–2).

L. If the obstruction is slight or moderate, one-stage colectomy and primary anastomosis is now favored by an increasing number of surgeons provided the proximal colon is cleansed by "on-table" lavage. A large-bore (No. 20 French) Foley catheter or chest tube is inserted into the cecum usually via appendicostomy. Alternatively an ileostomy can be made. A disposable plastic corrugated anesthetic tube is inserted and secured into the distal end of the divided proximal loop. About 4 liters of warm balanced saline solution are infused

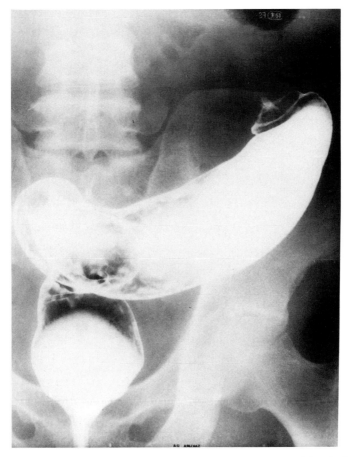

FIGURE 62–1 The contrast enema shows the typical bird-beak finding.

from the cecum to wash out the content into a closed-circuit bag (see Fig. 62–2). The proximal colon can be inspected by a fiberscope inserted through the tube to identify associated tumor or obstructive colitis and to verify adequate preparation.

M. If these adjunctive measures are not available or a proximal associated lesion is suspected, subtotal colectomy and primary ileosigmoidostomy is the choice. An exception to this choice is the patient with decreased anal continence.

N. Severe obstruction is an indication for delayed anastomosis in two-stage surgery. The first stage involves segmented colectomy with construction of an end-colostomy and a sigmoid mucous fistula or Hartmann-type pouch.

O. In selected critically ill patients being treated by an inexperienced surgical team, the classical three-staged procedure may be appropriate. The first stage constitutes of an initial diverting transverse colostomy, followed by colectomy and then by closure of the colostomy. This alternative is rarely indicated and has the disadvantage that the neoplasm or septic process causing the obstruction is left in situ.

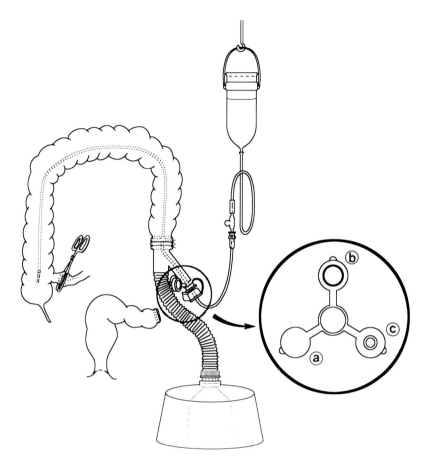

Intraoperative bowel preparation set.
(Create Medic CO., Ltd. Tokyo)

Insert : Triple Caps ⓐ for occlusion
                      ⓑ for endoscopy
                      ⓒ for irrigation

FIGURE 62–2 The equipment for on-table lavage.

BIBLIOGRAPHY

1. Fielding LP: Large bowel obstruction. In Fazio VW (ed): *Current Therapy in Colon and Rectal Surgery*. Philadelphia: Decker, 1990, pp246–253.
2. Welch JP: Mechanical obstruction of the small and large intestine. *Dis Intestinal Tract.* 766–785.
3. Williams NS: Large bowel obstruction. In Keighley MRB (ed): *Surgery of the Anus, Rectum and Colon*. London: Saunders, 1993, Vol 2, pp1823–1866.

See also Chapters 56, 58, 63 and 76.

CHAPTER 63

Acute Colonic Pseudoobstruction

Karamjit S. Khanduja, M.B.B.S.

Refer to Algorithm 63–1.

A. Acute colonic pseudoobstruction (ACPO) or Ogilvie's syndrome, is characterized by acute, massive dilatation of the cecum and right colon in the absence of organic obstruction. Without prompt treatment, the colonic distention may result in perforation, peritonitis, and death. This syndrome is commonly associated with nonoperative trauma including fractures and burns, obstetric and gynecologic procedures, and abdominal, pelvic, orthopaedic, and urologic surgery. Surgical trauma or pathology involving the retroperitoneum causing interruption of sacral innervation (S2–S4) has been suggested to cause atony by a disruption in normal parasympathetic innervation to the distal colon. This atony results in a functional obstruction.

B. Common symptoms include nausea, vomiting, abdominal pain, constipation and diarrhea. Abdominal distention is present in all cases; the quality of bowel sounds varies greatly. Abdominal tenderness may be present, and is worrisome as it may indicate intestinal ischemia.

C. The distension is associated with dehydration and metabolic derangements. Leukocytosis is present in approximately 27% of patients without ischemia or perforation. Complete blood cell count, fluid and electrolyte imbalances, and nutritional parameters must be assessed and monitored.

D. Plain abdominal radiographs should be obtained to assess the distention of the large bowel with particular attention to cecal diameter. If the diagnosis of mechanical obstruction is considered, a water-soluble contrast enema should be obtained.

E. If abdominal radiographs show the cecal diameter to be <12 cm, conservative therapy should be instituted. A large, retrospective review revealed no cases of perforation or ischemia when the cecal diameter was <12 cm.

Acute colonic pseudoobstruction (ACPO)

Diagnostic evaluation

Treatment

ACPO[A] → Laboratory[C] → X-rays[D] → ACPO[E] → Conservative[F] → Decompression → Observe[G]
cecal diameter   Measures
> 9-12 cm

History and
physical exam[B]

No
decompression

Consider
epidural[O]

Consider
epidural[O]

ACPO[I] → Colonoscopy±[H] → Decompression → Observe
cecal diameter   tube decompression
≥ 12 cm

No
decompression → Tube[J]
cecostomy

Miniperforation at cecum

ACPO[K] → Laparotomy[L] → Major perforation → Exteriorization[M]
Ischemia or
perforation

Ischemia → Resection ±[N]
anastomosis
± stoma

ALGORITHM 63–1

F. Conservative therapy consists of NPO, nasogastric suction, correction of fluid and electrolyte imbalances, discontinuation of narcotic medications, and treatment of associated conditions or infections. Gentle enemas and sigmoidoscopy are seldom helpful. Rectal tube placement (if distention extends into the distal colon) and bowel stimulants may be effective. Patients should be carefully monitored, and the cecal diameter should be assessed with serial, plain abdominal radiographs.

G. If therapy leads to resolution of symptoms and passage of flatus, patients should be observed for recurrence of abdominal distension.

H. If the patient is found to have a cecal diameter of ≥ 9-12 cm initially or during the course of conservative therapy, colonoscopic decompression should be performed. This procedure, although technically demanding, has minimal morbidity and mortality. It is efficacious in 80% of patients with ACPO. Repeating the procedure may be necessary for recurrences. Decompression may be aided with endoscopic placement of colonic tubes.

I. Patients presenting with a cecal diameter of ≥ 9-12 cm should undergo colonoscopic decompression and initiation of other conservative measures.

J. If colonscopic decompression is unsuccessful or unavailable, tube cecostomy should be performed. Tube cecostomy has a success rate of 100% and has the lowest mortality rate of the operative procedures. The procedure can be percutaneously performed under local anesthesia, either under radiologic guidance, or in the operating room.

K. Ischemic injury of the colon and perforation are encountered with cecal diameter ≥ 12 cm. Patients with these complications manifest fever and usually have signs of peritonitis with leukocytosis. In addition, free air may be detected on abdominal radiographs.

L. Laparotomy is required to treat patients with signs of perforation or ischemic injury of the colon. Rarely, at laparotomy a very small cecal perforation with little spillage (miniperforation) may be encountered; these injuries may be treated by tube cecostomy through the perforation. The entire colon should be carefully inspected and additional resection performed of any nonviable areas.

M. For patients found to have perforation and spillage of the colon, the injury may be exteriorized or resected.

N. Ischemic bowel encountered at laparotomy should be resected. Both resection and exteriorization are associated with high rates of morbidity and mortality because of the complication itself and the serious comorbid disease.

O. Epidural anesthesia has been advocated for pseudoobstruction based on the theory that excess sympathetic activity to the lower gastrointestinal tract is the cause of the functional obstruction. Therefore blocking this excess sympathetic nervous activity should increase colonic mobility. The technique has been reported to successfully treat Ogilvie's syndrome in 63% of cases.

BIBLIOGRAPHY

1. Lee JT, Taylor BM, Singleton BC: Epidural anesthesia for acute pseudo-obstruction of the colon (Ogilvie's syndrome) *Dis Colon Rectum* 31:686–691, 1988.

2. Nivatvongs S: Complications of colonic disease and their management. In Gordon PH, Nivatvongs S (eds): *Principles and Practice of Surgery for the Colon, Rectum and Anus.* St. Louis: Quality Medical Publishing, 1992.

3. Vanek VW, Al-Salti M: Acute pseudo-obstruction of the colon (Ogilvie's syndrome). An analysis of 400 cases. *Dis Colon Rectum* 29:203–210, 1986.

4. Wegener M, Börsch G: Acute colonic pseudo-obstruction (Ogilvie's syndrome). Presentation of 14 of our own cases and analysis of 1027 cases reported in the literature. *Surg Endosc* 1:169–174, 1987.

See also Chapters 56, 58, 62 and 76.

CHAPTER 64

Ischemic Colitis

Anthony M. Vernava, III, M.D. and Walter E. Longo, M.D.

Refer to Algorithm 64–1.

A. Ischemic colitis can occur spontaneously in the presence of a normal arterial system in a low-flow state as well as in atherosclerotic disease or can occur after a precipitating event. The disorder can involve the entire colon and rectum, or it can involve a segment or segments of the large bowel. The upper gastrointestinal tract may or may not be affected. The ischemic process may only involve the mucosa, in which case the disorder is self-limited and will resolve with supportive care, or it may involve the entire thickness of the bowel wall, in which case resection of the involved colon is required.

B. Spontaneous ischemic colitis can occur in association with the disorders listed in the algorithm, but it can also occur without any systemic disease. Most of the reported cases of truly "spontaneous" ischemic colitis have occurred in elderly patients with presumed atherosclerotic disease.

C. The prototypic patient with ischemic colitis is one with shock as the precipitating cause. Virtually any cause of shock will alter splanchnic blood flow and may result in critical ischemia to the large bowel. The degree and duration of the shock, and hence ischemia, will determine whether the insult to the colon is transient and reversible, affecting only the mucosa, or catastrophic, resulting in full-thickness gangrene.

D. The signs and symptoms of ischemic colitis are subtle, nonspecific and unreliable. They are frequently attributed to other, noncatastrophic intra-abdominal problems including postoperative pain and ileus. Minor abdominal pain, usually over the affected intestine, nausea, emesis diarrhea, melena, guaiac positive stool, fever, and leukocytosis can all be present. The lack of a reliable symptom complex frequently leads to a delay in diagnosis resulting in full-thickness gangrene and a high mortality (>50%). The key to early diagnosis is a high degree of clinical suspicion, particularly in those high-risk patients listed above.

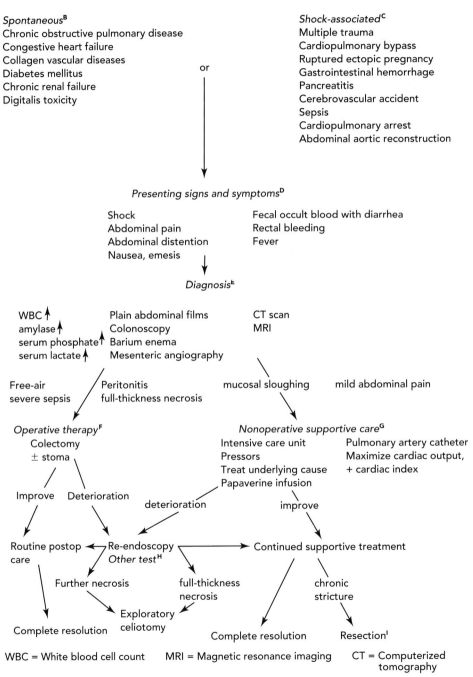

Ischemic Colitis

History
Predisposing factors[A]

Spontaneous[B]
Chronic obstructive pulmonary disease
Congestive heart failure
Collagen vascular diseases   or
Diabetes mellitus
Chronic renal failure
Digitalis toxicity

Shock-associated[C]
Multiple trauma
Cardiopulmonary bypass
Ruptured ectopic pregnancy
Gastrointestinal hemorrhage
Pancreatitis
Cerebrovascular accident
Sepsis
Cardiopulmonary arrest
Abdominal aortic reconstruction

Presenting signs and symptoms[D]

Shock   Fecal occult blood with diarrhea
Abdominal pain   Rectal bleeding
Abdominal distention   Fever
Nausea, emesis

Diagnosis[E]

WBC ↑   Plain abdominal films   CT scan
amylase ↑   Colonoscopy   MRI
serum phosphate ↑ Barium enema
serum lactate ↑   Mesenteric angiography

Free-air   Peritonitis   mucosal sloughing   mild abdominal pain
severe sepsis   full-thickness necrosis

Operative therapy[F]   *Nonoperative supportive care*[G]
  Colectomy   Intensive care unit   Pulmonary artery catheter
  ± stoma   Pressors   Maximize cardiac output,
                                      Treat underlying cause   + cardiac index
                                      Papaverine infusion

Improve   Deterioration   deterioration   improve

Routine postop ← Re-endoscopy   → Continued supportive treatment
care   *Other test*[H]

          Further necrosis   full-thickness   chronic
                               necrosis   stricture

Complete resolution Exploratory   Complete resolution   Resection[I]
                     celiotomy

WBC = White blood cell count   MRI = Magnetic resonance imaging   CT = Computerized
                                                                         tomography

ALGORITHM 64–1

E. Unfortunately, there is no reliable, reproducible method currently available to diagnose intestinal ischemia. The most commonly employed biochemical tests employed are nonspecific and include leukocytosis, elevated amylase, decreased arterial pH, and elevated serum inorganic phosphate. Other serum markers of intestinal ischemia have been described including hexosaminidase, diamine oxidase and porcine ileal peptide but these markers are unproven and not widely available. Plain abdominal roentgenograms may reveal a gasless abdomen, thumbprinting, pneumotosis, or a gas cutoff sign. A barium enema should not be performed because of the risk of perforation and barium peritonitis and because it renders angiography uninterpretable. When a barium enema is performed, it may reveal thumbprinting, edema, intramural barium or a stricture. Endoscopy, either colonoscopy or flexible sigmoidoscopy is a preferred initial diagnostic test to visualize the mucosa and obtain mucosal biopsies and to exclude other pathologies. Rectal involvement usually elimates ischemia in the differential diagnosis. Colonoscopy should not be done when peritonitis is present. In difficult cases a CT scan of the abdomen may be done and when intestinal ischemia is present may reveal: bowel edema, pneumotosis, portal gas, or vascular thrombus; a magnetic resonance imaging (MRI) may reveal the same findings. Generally, mesenteric angiography is not helpful in establishing the diagnosis of ischemic colitis since most cases occur due to nonocclusive etiologies. However, mesenteric angiography is essential in the diagnosis and management of suspected mesenteric ischemia.

F. Patients with obvious peritonitis, radiographic pneumoperitoneum or other evidence of full-thickness intestinal necrosis should undergo emergency celiotomy with resection of the involved intestine. Generally, an anastomosis is avoided and an end-diverting stoma, either a colostomy or an ileostomy, is created. The superior mesenteric artery should be assessed. Intraoperative evaluation of questionably ischemic intestine can be performed using Doppler ultrasound, intravenous fluorescein with an ultraviolet light, surface oximetry, or infrared photoplethysmography. In those difficult cases where the majority of intestine is questionably viable, the patient should undergo a planned second laparotomy within 24 hours.

G. Those patients felt to have nongangrenous, reversible colonic ischemia should be admitted to the intensive care unit and aggressively monitored and resuscitated. The underlying cause of their shock (e.g., sepsis, myocardial infarction, congestive heart failure) should be treated. To facilitate resuscitation a pulmonary artery catheter should be placed and appropriate ionotrophic and chronotrophic agents employed to maximize cardiac function. Papaverine infusion (0.6 mg/min) can be used in patients who have nonocclusive ischemia and severe vasoconstriction. Most patients aggressively managed have resolution of ischemia without operation. These patients should be monitored very closely with serial abdominal exams. Repeat colonoscopy should be performed at frequent intervals to document improvement or diagnose worsening ischemia.

H. Any patient who has been treated, operatively or nonoperatively, for ischemic colitis should be constantly assessed for clinical improvement. Those patients who fail to improve or who clinically deteriorate should undergo repeat endoscopy and/or any testing required (as during their initial presentation) to assess intestinal viability.

I. Long-term follow-up of these patients is necessary since ischemic areas of the colon may stricture and cause obstruction. The risk of significant, chronic stricture formation causing obstructive symptoms is as high as 40%. In such cases, elective resection of the involved segment is indicated.

BIBLIOGRAPHY

1. Abel ME, Russell TR: Ischemic colitis: comparison of surgical and nonoperative management. *Dis Colon Rectum* 26:113–115, 1983.
2. Bailey RW, Hamilton SR, Morris JB, et al: Pathogenesis of nonocclusive ischemic colitis. *Ann Surg* 203:590–599, 1986.
3. Boley SJ: Colonic ischemia—25 years later. *Am J Gastroenterol* 85:931–934, 1990.
4. Boley SJ, Schwartz S, Lash J, et al: Reversible vascular occlusion of the colon. *Surg Gynecol Obstet* 116:53–60, 1963.
5. Guttmorson NL, Bubrick MP: Mortality from ischemic colitis. *Dis Colon Rectum* 32:469–472, 1989.
6. Kaminski DL, Keltner RM, Willman VL: Ischemic colitis. *Arch Surg* 106:558–563, 1973.
7. Longo WE, Ballantyne GH, Busberg RJ: Ischemic colitis: patterns and prognosis. *Dis Colon Rectum* 35:726–730, 1992.
8. Sakai L, Keltner R, Kaminski DL: Spontaneous and shock-associated ischemic colitis. *Am J Surg* 140:755–760, 1980.

See also Chapters 10, 11, 12A, 12B, 13, 14, 20, 51, 52, 54, 55 and 74.

CHAPTER 65

Stricture

Alan E. Timmcke, M.D.

Refer to Algorithm 65–1.

A. Strictures are not easily identified endoscopically and are instead better diagnosed and better characterized radiographically.

B. Spasm can frequently be mistaken for a stricture or carcinoma. Current radiographic techniques such as the use of air-contrast barium enema and fluoroscopy minimize the likelihood of misinterpreting spasm as a fixed narrowing.

C. Rectal strictures can result from nearly all the same etiologies as colonic strictures except perhaps diverticulitis. The etiologies listed in Algorithm 65–1 are unique to the rectum.

D. Radiation strictures occur most frequently in the rectosigmoid or sigmoid. They generally involve a long segment, have tapering ends, and are more common in women.

E. Lymphogranuloma venereum (LGV) manifests primarily as an indolent inguinal or femoral lymphadenitis. LGV can produce strictures, most commonly of the rectum and rectosigmoid. The radiographic appearance is that of a long-segment stricture with tapering ends. Rectal stricturing occurs more commonly in women. Blind internal sinuses are common, and fistulas to skin or vagina may occur. LGV is caused by *Chlamydia trachomatis,* which is treated with tetracycline or chloramphenicol. Stricture producing obstructive symptoms can be dilated. If complete obstruction occurs, a colostomy is the treatment of choice.

F. Avoid surgery for radiation injury if at all possible. If surgery is mandatory, avoid extensive resections or multiple anastomoses. Avoid extensive lysis of adhesions whenever possible. Protect anastomoses with a proximal diverting stoma. (See also Chapter 47.)

G. Colon carcinoma typically exhibits the radiographic appearance of mucosal destruction and shouldering ("apple-core" lesion) (see also Chapter 70.)

H. Crohn's colitis may appear as multiple strictures separated by areas of more normal-appearing colon ("skip lesions"). (See also Chapter 51.)

I. Strictures of the transverse colon can be secondary to pancreatitis or gastric or pancreatic cancer.

349

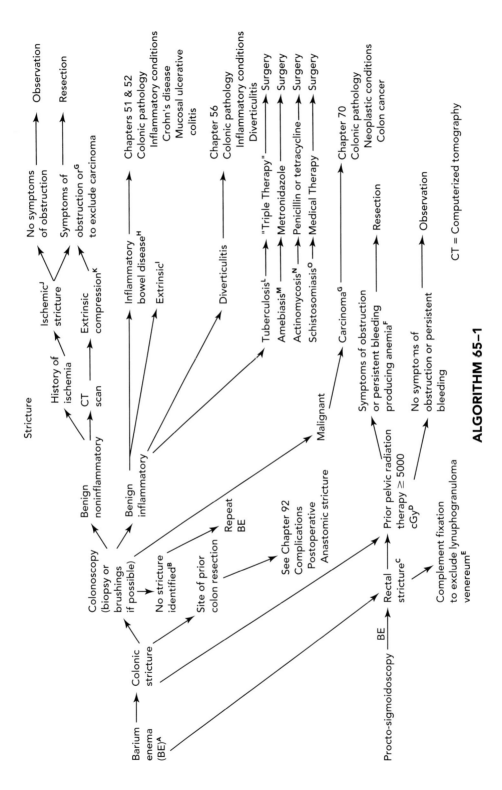

ALGORITHM 65-1

CT = Computerized tomography

J. Ischemic strictures are smooth and fibrous with tapering ends. They occur in perhaps one-third of cases in which florid ulceration is acutely exhibited.

K. Strictures resulting from compression by an extrinsic carcinoma are rare. Secondary malignancies such as carcinoid or lymphoma can also produce strictures. Endometriosis can produce narrowing, but it is generally not circumferential. Strictures of "linitis plastica"-type carcinoma can be indistinguishable from compression by an extrinsic carcinoma.

L. Tuberculosis produces nonspecific inflammatory changes most frequently of the terminal ileum and cecum that can result in stricturing that is not easily distinguishable from Crohn's disease. Triple therapy with a variety of antituberculous agents should virtually always preceed any consideration of surgery. Commonly used agents include ethambutol, rifampin, and isoniazid.

M. Amebiasis in its granulomatous form (ameboma) may produce strictures that are often multiple and most frequently of the cecum, transverse colon, and flexures simulating Crohn's disease. Occasionally "thumbprinting" occurs creating the appearance of ischemic colitis. In fact, transmural amebic colitis is a progressive, segmental, ischemic necrosis of the entire thickness of the colon wall. Diagnosis is confirmed by the identification of ameba in the stool in tissue biopsies. Treatment consists of metronidazole. Surgical management in emergency situations consists of a proximal diverting loop ileostomy and intraoperative prograde colonic lavage. Resectional surgery is reported to result in a 24% mortality rate. Occasionally strictures remain after treatment for severe acute amebic colitis, and these may require elective resection.

N. Actinomycosis of the intestinal tract has a tendency to localize in the cecum and occasionally produces fistulization in addition to stricturing. The diagnosis is confirmed by demonstration of sulfur granules or ray fungus in purulent discharge or biopsies. Penicillin and tetracycline are effective treatment. In severe cases resection may be necessary.

O. Schistosomiasis may rarely produce fibrosis and calcifications of the left colon resulting in a stricture. Drug treatment consists of a variety of agents including praziquantel, metriphonate, oxamniquine, sodium antimony dimercaptosuccinate, antimony potassium tartrate, and niridazole. Patients with longstanding schistostomal colitis are at increased risk for carcinoma. Thus prophylectic colectomy is a reasonable alternative in any patient with a schistostomal stricture.

BIBLIOGRAPHY

1. Fazio VW (ed): *Current Therapy in Colon and Rectal Surgery.* Philadelphia; Decker, 1990.

2. Fielding LP, Goldberg SM (eds): *Surgery of the Colon, Rectum and Anus,* 5th ed. London: Butterworth-Heinemann, 1993.

3. Schwartz SI, Shires GT, Spencer FC (eds): *Principles of Surgery,* 5th ed. Vol II. New York; McGraw-Hill, 1989.

4. Sutton DA, (ed): *A Textbook of Radiology and Imaging,* 4th ed. Churchill Livingstone, New York, 1987, Vol. I.

5. Teplick JG, Haskin ME (eds): *Surgical Radiology.* Philadelphia: W.B. Saunders, 1981, Vol I.

See also Chapters 37, 47, 51, 52, 55, 56, 70 and 92.

SECTION 5D

Colonic Pathology
Neoplastic Conditions

CHAPTER 66

Benign Neoplastic Conditions of the Colon

Pascal Frileux, M.D. and Anne Berger, M.D.

Refer to Algorithm 66--1.

A. *Polyps* are circumscribed formations of the surface epithelium.
B. *Nonneoplastic lesions* such as metaplastic (hyperplastic) polyps or hamartomas (juvenile polyps, Peutz--Jeghers syndrome, juvenile polyposis) are beyond the scope of this chapter.
C. *Adenomas* are the most common benign neoplasms of the colon, with an incidence of 10--50% in Western countries according to autopsy series. *Tubular adenomas* are sessile or pedunculated growths, 1--10 mm in size with a smooth surface. *Villous adenomas* are sessile growths, sometimes forming large carpet-like surfaces. The *Adenomas* may degenerate into cancer through progressive dysplasia and gene mutations. Risk of degeneration increases with size, type (villous > tubular), degree of dysplasia, age of the patient, and location with the colon (distal > proximal). It is estimated that 10--25% of adenomas can degenerate into cancer in between 3 and 10 years.
D. Screening for benign and malignant colonic neoplasms in an asymptomatic population with fecal occult blood testing significantly reduces the mortality related to colorectal cancer. The immunologic test (Hemeselect[R]) appears to be more sensitive than the guaiac test (Hemoccult[R], Hemoquant[R]). Other forms of screening such as flexible sigmoidoscopy or even colonoscopy have been proposed. Fecal occult blood testing is the most practical tool, although the positive rate (around 2%) sensitivity (50%) and positive predictive value (10% for cancer, 30% for adenomas) are very disappointing. Nonetheless, annual digital examination with fecal occult blood testing and periodic proctosigmoidoscopy remain the recommended screening guidelines.
E. *Selected Screening of high-risk groups,* such as first-degree relatives of patients with cancer or adenomas, is more productive (15--30% of screened patients harbor neoplastic lesions); in this group it is advisable to perform colonoscopy once every 5 years after the age of 40.

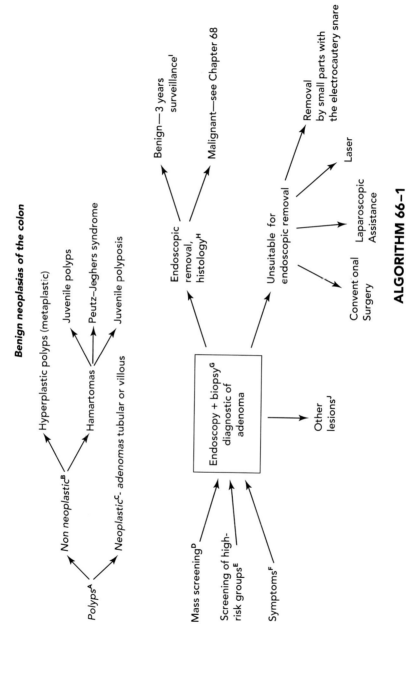

Benign neoplasias of the colon

Polyps[A]

Non neoplastic[B]

Neoplastic[C] - adenomas tubular or villous

Hyperplastic polyps (metaplastic)

Hamartomas

Juvenile polyps

Peutz–Jeghers syndrome

Juvenile polyposis

Mass screening[D]

Screening of high-risk groups[E]

Symptoms[F]

Endoscopy + biopsy[G] diagnostic of adenoma

Other lesions[J]

Endoscopic removal, histology[H]

Unsuitable for endoscopic removal

Benign— 3 years surveillance[I]

Malignant—see Chapter 68

Conventional Surgery

Laparoscopic Assistance

Laser

Removal by small parts with the electrocautery snare

ALGORITHM 66–1

356

F. Symptoms are rare but may include bleeding or even anemia in some cases.

G. *Treatment of small adenomas* is simple in principle: colonoscopic excisional biopsy. Colonoscopic polypectomy in a given group of patients, results in a lower incidence of colorectal cancer, when compared to a reference group as documented by cohort studies.

H. Controversy exists regarding treatment of larger and/or sessile adenomas. *Laser* therapy requires multiple sessions and multiple washouts for preparation and it provides no histology. The recurrence rate is 50%, and perforation or hemorrhage occur in 5% of patients. *Surgery* is the safe solution for tumor control but it obviously has a high potential morbidity. Piecemeal endoscopic excision, using the coagulating snare, is a difficult maneuver, is potentially dangerous, and gives limited information in terms of histology. The decision should be based on the age of the patient, the appearance of the growth, its location on the colon, the skills of the endoscopist, and the requests of the patient. Our position is to propose *surgery* in the fit patient and to leave endoscopic treatment--the *laser* or *snare* according to the skills available—to poor-risk patients. At surgery, the extent of resection is identical to what is realized in cancer surgery. The rationale for this approach is in case the adenomas have transformed into carcinomas, a finding in 40–50% of growths > 2 cm. Laparoscopic segmental colectomy may be a good treatment alternative in these instances as long as a formal cancer resection is performed. Laparoscopic assisted colotomy and polypectomy is always contraindicated.

I. After removal of adenomas, colonoscopic surveillance should be undertaken; the usual interval is one year, recent data suggested that it could be extended to 3 years (7).

J. Other lesions

- *Mesenchymal tumors.* Benign mesenchymal tumors such as fibroma, eosinophilic granuloma, and leiomyoma are extremely rare. Lipoma is the second most common benign neoplasia of the colon after adenoma, occurring 0.2% in autopsy series. They are situated in the cecal area, the right colon, or the sigmoid; particular features which enable diagnosis at barium enema or colonoscopy include testing and the "pillow sign." They do not require treatment except when they ulcerate or cause symptoms.

- *Tumors of neural origin,* such as neurofibromas with Von Recklinghausen disease and granular cell tumors, are exceedingly rare.

- *Vascular lesion. Hemangiomas* are congenital lesions that commonly bleed in childhood and adolescence; local excision, when possible, is the treatment of choice; giant hemangiomas may require major surgery and/or radiotherapy.

BIBLIOGRAPHY

1. Beck DE, Karulf RE: Laparoscopic assisted full-thickness endoscopic polypectomy. *Dis Colon Rectum* 36:693–695, 1993.

2. Mandel JS, Bond JH, Church TR, et al (The Minnesota Colon Cancer Control Study): Reducing mortality from colorectal cancer by screening for occult blood testing. *N Engl J Med* 328:1365–1371, 1993.

3. Morson B: The polyp-cancer sequence in the large bowel. *Proc Roy Soc Med* 67:451–457, 1974.

4. Rosen L, Abel ME, Gordon PH, et al: Practice parameters for antibiotic prophylaxis to prevent infective endocarditis or infected prosthesis during colon and rectal endoscopy. *Dis Colon Rectum* 35:277–285, 1992.

5. Ruget O, Burtin P, Ben Bouali AK, et al: Traitement par laser des tumeurs villeuses rectocoliques. Evaluation des résultats par méthode multifactorielle. *Gastroentérol Clin Biol* 17:938–943, 1993.

6. Stryker SJ, Wolff BG, Culp CE, et al: Natural history of untreated colonic polyps. *Gastroenterology* 93:1009–1012, 1987.

7. Wexner SD, Brabbee GW, Wichern WA Jr: Sensitivity of hemoccult testing in patients with colorectal carcinoma. *Dis Colon Rectum.* 27:775–776, 1984.

8. Wexner SD, Cady B (eds). The future of laparoscopy in oncology. Surg Oncol Clin NA. New York: W.B. Saunders, 1994.

9. Winawer SJ, Zauber AG, May NH, et al. (The National Polyp Study Group): Prevention of colorectal cancer by colonoscopic polypectomy. *N Engl J Med* 326:1977–1981, 1993.

10. Winawer SJ, Zauber AG, O'Brien MJ, et al. (The National Polyp Study Workgroup): Randomized comparison of surveillance interval after colonoscopic removal of newly diagnosed adenomatous polyps. *New Engl J Med* 328:903–906, 1993.

See also Chapters 2, 15, 45, 68, 69 and 70.

CHAPTER 67

Familial Adenomatous Polyposis

Robin S. McLeod, M.D. and Zane Cohen, M.D.

Refer to Algorithm 67–1.

A. *At risk subject.* Familial adenomatous polyposis (FAP) is a genetic disorder with autosomal dominant transmission. Thus, approximately 50% of the offspring of affected individuals are at risk for developing FAP. The primary manifestation is polyps in the colon and rectum. In addition, it is now recognized that other malignant and benign lesions occur with greater frequency in these individuals. These associated problems are listed in Tables 67–1 and 67–2 respectively. A distinction between FAP and Gardner's syndrome is no longer made. Registries play a major role in education of affected individuals and plotting out their family trees so that at-risk individuals can be identified, screened, and treated prior to the development of a colorectal cancer.

B. *Evaluation of at-risk subjects.* With the identification of the APC gene on the long arm of Chromosome 5, the evaluation of "at risk" subjects has changed. Previously, sigmoidoscopy was used to detect rectal polyps. Until polyps appeared, one could not be certain whether the person was affected. Now, linkage analysis can be performed soon after birth to identify subjects who are at high risk for the development of the disease. In the near future, it is likely that results of these tests will be used without other intervention necessary to accurately identify patients affected by the disease and with which manifestations. Pigmented eye lesions, so-called congenital hypertrophy of the retinal pigmented epithelium (CHRPE), have a high specificity for FAP. They are found in approximately 80% of patients with FAP. Thus, ophthalmic examinations can be performed to predict high risk for developing the disease. However, because CHRPE is not 100% sensitive, it cannot be relied on in isolation to exclude FAP.

   Thus, subjects in whom genetic studies suggest that there is a high probability of the disease and in whom there are CHRPE present, require early and

Diagnosis and management of familial adenomatous polyposis (FAP)

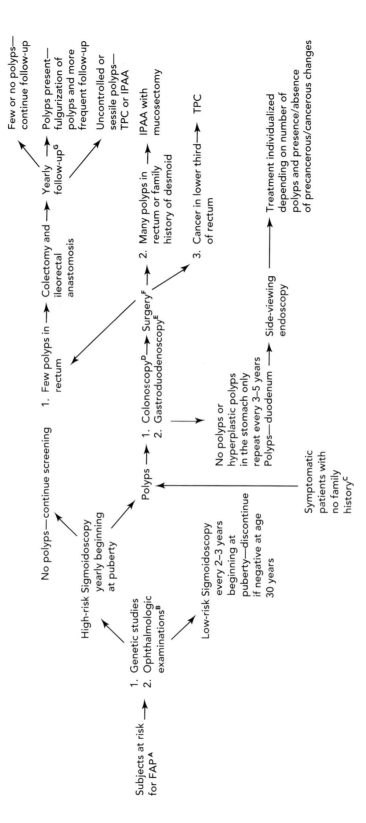

Few or no polyps—
continue follow-up

Polyps present—
fulgurization of
polyps and more
frequent follow-up

Uncontrolled or
sessile polyps—
TPC or IPAA

IPAA with
mucosectomy

1. Few polyps in → Colectomy and → Yearly → follow-up[G]
   rectum   ileorectal
                       anastomosis

2. Many polyps in
   rectum or family
   history of desmoid

3. Cancer in lower third → TPC
   of rectum

Treatment individualized
depending on number of
polyps and presence/absence
of precancerous/cancerous changes

No polyps—continue screening

High-risk Sigmoidoscopy
yearly beginning
at puberty

Polyps → 1. Colonoscopy[D] → Surgery[F]
          2. Gastroduodenoscopy[E]

Side-viewing
endoscopy

No polyps or
hyperplastic polyps
in the stomach only
repeat every 3–5 years

Polyps—duodenum

1. Genetic studies
2. Ophthalmologic
   examinations[B]

Low-risk Sigmoidoscopy
every 2–3 years
beginning at
puberty—discontinue
if negative at age
30 years

Symptomatic
patients with
no family
history[C]

Subjects at risk → FAP[A]
for FAP[A]

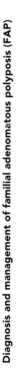

ALGORITHM 67–1

TPC = Total proctocolectomy
IPPA = Ileal pouch anal anastomosis

TABLE 67–1 MALIGNANT EXTRACOLONIC
MANIFESTATIONS

Duodenal carcinoma
Bile duct carcinoma
Gastric carcinoma
Small bowel carcinoma
Desmoid tumours
Medulloblastoma
Glioma
Adrenal carcinoma

TABLE 67–2 BENIGN EXTRACOLONIC
MANIFESTATIONS

Epidermoid cysts
Osteomas
Gastric (fundic gland) polyps
Gastric adenomas
Duodenal adenomas
Jejunal adenomas
Ileal adenomas
Retinal pigmentation
Adrenal adenomas

intensive screening. In these individuals, annual sigmoidoscopic examinations should be performed beginning at puberty and continuing until polyps are detected. For subjects whose genetic studies place them at low risk for developing FAP, screening sigmoidoscopy can be started at puberty but performed at 2–3 yearly intervals and discontinued at the age of 30 years if no polyps are present. Of course when the patient is age 40–50 years they should enter the screening protocol for the standard risk population. Either flexible or rigid sigmoidoscopy is adequate for screening these individuals in that there have been only a few reports of polyps and a cancer being present in the proximal colon without evidence of polyps in the rectum. It is essential that a biopsy be taken to confirm the adenomatous nature of the polyps, even if there is a family history of FAP. Other non-FAP polyposis syndromes can occur and their management may differ.

C. *Subjects with no family history of FAP.* Approximately 10–30% of affected individuals have no family history of FAP, and it is presumed that they are affected because of a genetic mutation. Most commonly, they present with bleeding or a change in bowel habit and the diagnosis of FAP is made on sigmoidoscopy or colonoscopy. In many of these individuals, a cancer may be present at diagnosis. Rarely, these individuals are referred for evaluation because dental abnormalities, an osteoma or a desmoid tumor has been detected and the referring physician is suspicious of FAP.

D. *Preoperative evaluation.* Once the diagnosis of FAP has been confirmed, surgery is recommended to these individuals. Timing may vary depending on the number of polyps, whether there is a cancer present, and the age of the patient. Generally, patients identified by screening are in their early teens and have relatively few polyps. Surgery in these individuals may be deferred to a convenient time, such as the next summer vacation. Colonoscopy should be performed in all individuals prior to surgery to evaluate the number of polyps and to determine whether there is a cancer present. Although FAP is defined by the presence of more than 100 polyps in the colon, in young individuals, there may not be that many. However, if a patient has a family history or positive genetic tests, the diagnosis of FAP can made even if less than 100 polyps are present.

Preoperative gastroduodenoscopy is performed (as discussed in the next section), but other diagnostic tests are unnecessary. Desmoid tumors rarely occur in patients who have not had abdominal surgery, and even if one were present, surgical removal of the colon would probably be indicated.

E. *Evaluation of the upper gastrointestinal tract.* Because of the high prevalence of gastroduodenal polyps and the greatly increased incidence of periampullary carcinoma, gastroduodenoscoy is indicated in these individuals. Most polyps in the proximal stomach are hyperplastic polyps, whereas adenomas occur in the antrum and duodenum. It is the latter which have malignant potential. If there are duodenal polyps identified, side-viewing endoscopy should be performed to further evaluate the ampulla of Vater. Treatment of these polyps may be difficult because they tend to be sessile and are not easily removed endoscopically. Treatment, which may include duodenal mucosectomy, duodenectomy, or a Whipple procedure, must be individualized depending on the number of polyps present and whether there is any dysplasia or invasive cancer in the polyps. Evaluation of the stomach and duodenum should be performed at regular intervals throughout the patient's life, the frequency varying depending on the findings.

F. *Surgery.* There is controversy as to whether colectomy and ileorectal anastomosis or ileal-pouch anal anastomosis (IPAA) is the preferred procedure in patients with FAP. It is our preference to perform a colectomy and ileorectal anastomosis in patients in whom there are <10 polyps in the rectum. It is an easier procedure associated with fewer complications, and more consistent functional results than those following the IPAA procedure. The risk of cancer and further surgery are low although patients require regular postoperative follow-up. However, follow-up is needed no matter what procedure is performed, because of the risk of developing extracolonic manifestations. In our practice, initial IPAA is reserved for patients who have multiple polyps in the rectum or for those who have a family history of desmoid tumors. The latter indication is because subsequent surgery in these people, should they require proctectomy, might be difficult if they were to develop a desmoid tumor. A mucosectomy is always performed. Total proctocolectomy is rarely indicated except in individuals with cancers in the lower third of the rectum in whom a cancer operation would be compromised by an IPAA operation.

G. *Follow-up of patients postoperatively.* Patients who have had a colectomy and ileorectal anastomosis are evaluated annually with sigmoidoscopy. If polyps are present, they are cauterized. If there are multiple polyps or confluent, sessile polyps, one must be concerned that a cancer may develop and excision of the rectum is recommended with conversion to an IPAA or total proctocolectomy. Screening for extracolonic manifestations, other than for gastroduodenal lesions, is generally not advocated because although there is an increased incidence, the risk still is low.

BIBLIOGRAPHY

1. Bapat BV, Parker JA, Berk T, et al: Combined Use of molecular and biomarkers for presymptomatic carrier risk assessment in familial adenomatous polyposis: implications for screening guidelines. *Dis Colon Rectum* 37(2):165–71, 1994.
2. Berk T, Cohen Z, McLeod RS, et al: Congenital hypertrophy of the retinal pigment epithelium as a marker for familial adenomatous polyposis. *Dis Colon Rectum* 31:253–257, 1988.
3. Bodmer WF, Bailey CJ, Bodmer J, et al: Localization of the gene for familial polyposis coli on Chromosome 5. *Nature* 328:614–616, 1987.
4. Sarre RG, Jagelman DG, Beck GJ, et al: Colectomy with ileorectal anastomosis for familial adenomatous polyposis. The risk of rectal cancer. *Surgery* 101:20–26, 1987.
5. Tsunoda A, Talbot RC, Nicholls RJ: Incidence of dysplasia in the anorectal mucosa in patients having restorative proctocolectomy. *Br J Surg* 77:506–508, 1990.
6. Wexner SD, Jagelman DG: Familial adenomatous polyposis. In: Timmcke A, Veidenheimer MC (eds). *Seminars in Colon Rectal Surg.* Philadelphia: W.B. Saunders 26:269–276, 1991.

See also Chapters 45, 66 and 70.

CHAPTER 68

Management of Cancer in a Polyp

Leif Hulten, M.D., Ph.D.

Refer to Algorithm 68–1.

A. The endoscopist (gastroenterologist or surgeon) should be familiar with the pathologist's terminology. Terms such as *adenoma with atypia, cancer in situ, superficial carcinoma, focal carcinoma,* and *intramucosal carcinoma* applied to an adenomatous polyp are of little clinical significance. They often cause confusion or misunderstanding, and their inclusion in a pathology report may be seriously questioned. Polyps to which these terms are applied lack malignant potentials—there is no invasion through the lamina muscularis mucosae. Further surgery is not justified provided that such a lesion has been completely excised. If there is even slight doubt of radical endoscopic removal of a polyp, however, the target should be controlled with a repeated endoscopy. This is particularly important for sessile tubulovillous or villous adenoma in the rectum as these adenomas frequently recur and may contain foci of malignancy.
B. For a proper management of the malignant polyp the pathologist's report should include depth of invasion, grade of malignancy, and information on whether the excision is considered complete. To allow for a proper pathology analysis, the excised polyp should be carefully mounted (the transection site marked; the stalk should be identifiable, with a sessile polyp preferably pressed on a piece of filter paper before immersing in formalin). If the pathologist nevertheless is unable to make a clear and firm statement on these essentials, bowel resection should be done. Polyps should be resected and not biopsied. Piecemeal resection of large polyps presents special problems for the pathologist. Haggitt's classification of malignant polyps is excellent for evaluating the depth of invasion in pedunculated and sessile polyps (Fig. 68–1).

Management of cancer in a polyp

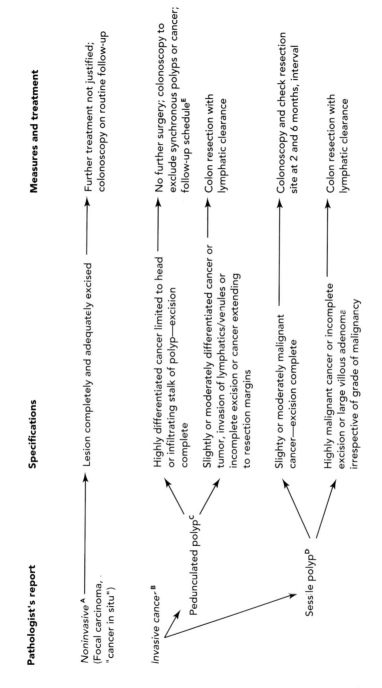

Pathologist's report	Specifications	Measures and treatment
Noninvasive [A] (Focal carcinoma, "cancer in situ")	Lesion completely and adequately excised ⟶	Further treatment not justified; colonoscopy on routine follow-up
Invasive cancer [B]		
Pedunculated polyp [C]	Highly differentiated cancer limited to head or infiltrating stalk of polyp—excision complete ⟶	No further surgery; colonoscopy to exclude synchronous polyps or cancer; follow-up schedule [E]
	Slightly or moderately differentiated cancer or tumor, invasion of lymphatics/venules or incomplete excision or cancer extending to resection margins ⟶	Colon resection with lymphatic clearance
Sessile polyp [D]	Slighty or moderately malignant cancer—excision complete ⟶	Colonoscopy and check resection site at 2 and 6 months, interval
	Highly malignant cancer or incomplete excision or large villous adenoma irrespective of grade of malignancy ⟶	Colon resection with lymphatic clearance

ALGORITHM 68–1

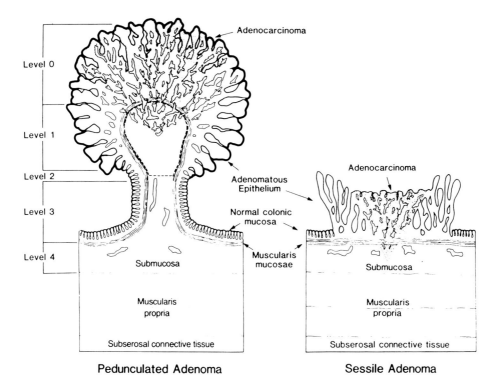

FIGURE 68-1 Levels of invasion in a pedunculated adenoma (*left*) and a sessile adenoma (*right*). The *stippled areas* represent zones of carcinoma. Note that any invasion below the muscularis mucosae in a sessile lesion represents level 4 invasion, i.e., invasion into the submucosa of the bowel wall. In contrast, invasive carcinoma in a pedunculated adenoma (*left*) must traverse a considerable distance before it reaches the submucosa of the underlying bowel wall. The *dotted line* in the head of the pedunculated adenoma represents the zone of level 1 invasion. Although more pedunculated adenomas have a tubular pattern and most sessile adenomas are villous, exceptions to this generalization occur. With author's permission [Haggitt 1985 (Ref. 3)].

Level	Depth of Invasion
0	Lamina muscularis mucosae not invaded
1	Invasive into head of the pedunculated polyp
2	Invasive into neck of the pedunculated polyp
3	Invasive into stalk of the pedunculated polyp
4	Invasive into submucosa of bowel wall

Note that all sessile invasive lesions are level 4 according to this classification.

C. Controversy exists as to whether a pedunculated polyp with invasive carcinoma should be treated differently from a sessile polyp. The presence or absence of a stalk may well influence the potential for deep penetration of a carcinoma in a polyp, but its presence must not be the sole determining factor in the decision making for treatment. Collective results imply that the overall incidence of lymph node metastasis and residual tumor after bowel resections for pedunculated polyps with invasive carcinoma is 7.8% and 2.3% respectively. Snaring of these polyps would mean a 10% failure rate. With cancer restricted to the head of the polyp (level 1), the incidence of lymph node metastasis was only 3% compared with an incidence of 20% when invasion into neck or polyp stalk (levels 2–3) was present. Cancer of the cut margin or near the margin, high-grade malignancy with invasion into the submucosa or into the neck or stalk, or in lymphatic or vascular vessels constitute high-risk factors, and bowel resection should be recommended.

D. The incidence of lymph note metastasis and residual tumor in bowel resections for sessile polyps amounts to 15% and 6%, respectively, implying a failure rate of 20% should endoscopic snaring have been done instead. In general, a sessile polyp with cancer should therefore be seriously considered for colonic resection with lymph node clearance. Only provided that the margin of transection is free of tumor cells, if the malignancy is well differentiated, and if follow-up endoscopic examination reveals no residual tumor at the polypectomy site, the malignant sessile polyp might be considered adequately removed. The risk of malignancy in an adenoma is strongly correlated with the type (highest in the villous adenoma) and the size of the adenoma. While 46% of large adenomas (≥2 cm) contain foci of malignancy, the risk is less than 1% in smaller adenomas (<1 cm). While many adenomas with carcinoma should be best treated with colon resection and lymphatic clearance, the risk of surgery in elderly patients and poor-risk patients have to be balanced against the benefit of surgery. A close cooperation between the physician and pathologist (physician–pathologist joint management) is a prerequisite for correct management of patients with cancer in a polyp.

E. Follow-up schedule even for patients in whom polypectomy is considered adequate may be justified to exclude the presence of synchronous cancer (5%) and/or synchronous polyps (8%).

BIBLIOGRAPHY

1. Christie JP: Polypectomy or colectomy? Management of 106 consecutively encountered colorectal polyps. *Am Surg* 54:93–99, 1988.
2. Coverlizza S, Risio M, Ferrari A, et al: Colorectal adenomas containing invasive carcinoma: pathologic assessment of lymph node metastatic potential. *Cancer* 64:1937–1947, 1989.
3. Haggitt RC, Glotzbach RE, Soffer EE, et al: Prognostic factors in colorectal carcinomas arising in adenomas: implications for lesions removed by endoscopic polypectomy. *Gastroenteorlogy* 89:328–336, 1985.
4. Morson BC, Whiteway JE, Jones EA, et al: Histopathology and prognosis of malignant colorectal polyps treated by endoscopic polypectomy. *Gut* 25:437–444, 1984.
5. Muto T, Sawada T, Sugihara K: Treatment of carcinoma in adenomas. *World J Surg* 15:35–40, 1991.

6. Nivatvongs S, Rojanasakul A, Reiman HM, et al: The risk of lymph node metastasis in colorectal polyps with invasive adenocarcinoma. *Dis Colon Rectum* 34:323–328, 1991.

7. Pollard CW, Nivatvongs S, Rojanasakul A, et al: The fate of patients following polypectomy alone for polyps containing invasive carcinoma. *Dis Colon Rectum* 35:933–937, 1992.

8. Riddell RH: Hands off "cancerous" large bowel polyps. *Gastroenterology* 89:432–441, 1985.

9. Wexner SD: Management of the malignant polyp. In: Fazio VW, Veidenheimer M (eds). *Seminars in Colon Rectal Surg.* Philadelphia: W.B. Saunders, 2:22–27, 1991.

See also Chapters 2, 45, 66, 67, 69 and 70.

CHAPTER 69

Follow-up of Adenomatous Polyps

Jonathan E. Jensen, M.D.

Refer to Algorithm 69-1.

A. During the past 3 years a series of studies regarding follow-up of adenomatous polyps have been published from a large database developed by the National Polyp Study Group. This consortium of independent centers have reviewed an extensive number of adenomas and published a series of papers that have allowed insight into appropriate management of adenomatous polyps.

B. Despite vigorous efforts to evaluate and identify environmental and genetic factors producing colorectal cancer, the primary effort at the present time is to produce a "clean colon" by removal of all adenomatous polyps identified at colonoscopy.

C. Both size and histology are statistically significant independent risk factors.

D. Patients with multiple adenomas are much more likely to have a high-grade dysplastic adenoma than are patients with single adenomas. Villous adenomas are also more likely to develop high-grade dysplastic pathology than are tubular adenomas. Advanced age (>60 years), but not sex, is an independent risk factor for the development of high-grade dysplasia.

E. On the basis of the national polyp study, current recommendation for single adenomatous polyps is follow-up colonoscopy in 3 years.

F. Since the percentage of high-grade dysplasia increased markedly in patients with three or more adenomas, the recommendation is for follow-up colonoscopy in 1 year with subsequent follow-up reverting to 3 years if less than three adenomatous polyps were identified. These recommendations are strictly for average-risk patients with adenomatous polyps.

G. The recommendations do not encompass patients with advanced pathologic features or have potential risk factors such as colon cancer or positive family history of colon cancer.

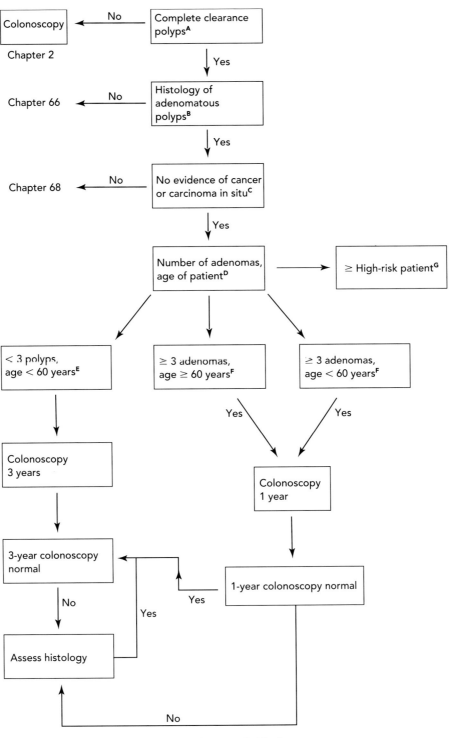

ALGORITHM 69–1

BIBLIOGRAPHY

1. O'Brien MJ, Winawer SJ, Zauber AG, et al: The National Polyp Study. Patient and polyp characteristics associated with high grade dysplasia in colorectal adenomas. *Gastroenterology* 98:371–379, 1990.

2. Ransohoff DF, Lang CA, Kuo HS: Colonoscopic surveillance after polypectomy: considerations of cost effectiveness. *Ann Int Med* 114:177–182, 1991.

3. Winawer SJ, Zauber AG, O'Brien MJ, et al: The National Polyp Study. *Cancer* 70:1236–1245, 1992.

4. Winawer SJ, Zauber AG, O'Brien MJ, et al: Randomized comparison of surveillance intervals after colonoscopic removal of newly diagnosed adenomatous polyps. *N Engl J Med* 328:901–906, 1993.

5. Winawer SJ, Zauber AG, Ho MN, et al: Prevention of colorectal cancer by colonoscopic polypectomy. *N Engl J Med* 329:1977–1981, 1993.

See also Chapters 2, 45, 49, 67, 68 and 70.

CHAPTER 70

Colon Cancer

Robert W. Beart, Jr., M.D. and Gary J. Anthone, M.D.

Refer to Algorithm 7–1.

A. *Diagnosis and evaluation.* The annual incidence of colon carcinoma in the United States is approximately 110,000, accounting for 50,000 deaths. Unexplained abdominal pain or weight loss, hemoccult positive stools, a change in bowel habits, anemia, or a palpable abdominal mass are signs of colon cancer and demand prompt evaluation with a thorough history and physical examination including a detailed family history for prior malignancies. A colonoscopy or sigmoidoscopy and barium enema are then performed to confirm the diagnosis. Synchronous tumors are present in 5–7% of patients with colon cancer.

B. *Preoperative workup.* The routine use of computed tomography (CT), magnetic resonance imaging (MRI), or ultrasonography is costly, usually not helpful, and therefore, reserved only for those patients with elevated liver function tests. Cystoscopy and intravenous pyelography are valuable tools in staging patients with urinary symptoms when an extended surgical resection is planned. Preoperative chest radiography and electrocardiography are mandatory in patients over the age of 40. The risk of postoperative wound infection is minimized by mechanical and oral antibiotic bowel preparation and perioperative systemic antibiotics.

C. *Treatment.* If colon cancer is detected in patients with ulcerative colitis or familial polyposis, a total proctocolectomy with ileal pouch anal anastomosis is performed. In patients <30 years of age colon cancer is best treated with a subtotal abdominal colectomy and ileorectostomy because of their higher risk for subsequent metachronous colon cancers and for ease of endoscopic follow-up. In patients >30 years of age, the appropriate colon cancer operation is performed depending on the primary site of the lesion. Adjacent contiguous structures involved by cancer should be resected in continuity en bloc with the colon cancer. Survival rates in these patients approach those of the colon cancer population as a whole. In patients found to have hepatic metastasis, the

Colon cancer

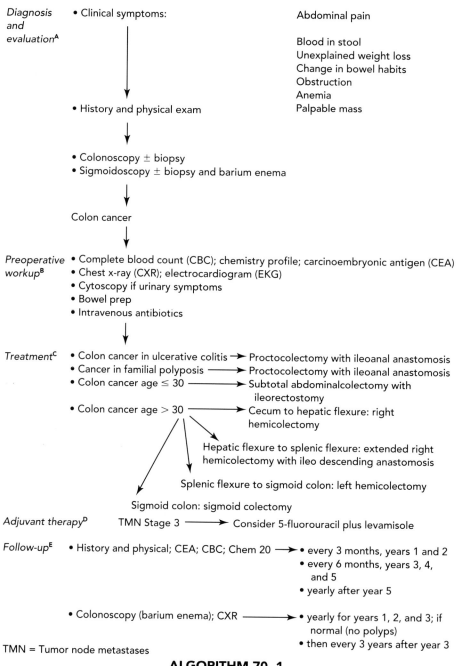

Diagnosis and evaluation[A] • Clinical symptoms: Abdominal pain

Blood in stool
Unexplained weight loss
Change in bowel habits
Obstruction
Anemia
Palpable mass

• History and physical exam

• Colonoscopy ± biopsy
• Sigmoidoscopy ± biopsy and barium enema

Colon cancer

Preoperative workup[B] • Complete blood count (CBC); chemistry profile; carcinoembryonic antigen (CEA)
• Chest x-ray (CXR); electrocardiogram (EKG)
• Cytoscopy if urinary symptoms
• Bowel prep
• Intravenous antibiotics

Treatment[C] • Colon cancer in ulcerative colitis → Proctocolectomy with ileoanal anastomosis
• Cancer in familial polyposis ⟶ Proctocolectomy with ileoanal anastomosis
• Colon cancer age ≤ 30 ⟶ Subtotal abdominalcolectomy with ileorectostomy
• Colon cancer age > 30 ⟶ Cecum to hepatic flexure: right hemicolectomy

Hepatic flexure to splenic flexure: extended right hemicolectomy with ileo descending anastomosis

Splenic flexure to sigmoid colon: left hemicolectomy

Sigmoid colon: sigmoid colectomy

Adjuvant therapy[D] TMN Stage 3 ⟶ Consider 5-fluorouracil plus levamisole

Follow-up[E] • History and physical; CEA; CBC; Chem 20 ⟶ • every 3 months, years 1 and 2
• every 6 months, years 3, 4, and 5
• yearly after year 5

• Colonoscopy (barium enema); CXR ⟶ • yearly for years 1, 2, and 3; if normal (no polyps)
• then every 3 years after year 3

TMN = Tumor node metastases

ALGORITHM 70–1

following guidelines generally apply: (1) isolated lesions of the left lateral segment or lesions removed safely by wedge resection may be resected synchronously at the time of primary colorectal resection. (2) major hepatic lobar resections should be done later at a second operation, and (3) patients found to have unresectable metastasic disease should undergo limited resection and anastomosis for local disease control. In patients with perforated or obstructing cancers who are unsuitable for primary resection, an end colostomy and drainage is appropriate. Primary resection with end colostomy is preferable in patients of appropriate operative risk. Primary resection with anastomosis is associated with a higher mortality rate and is generally reserved for patients where an ileo-colonic anastomosis is performed.

D. *Adjuvant therapy.* In the absence of distant metastases, prognosis is determined by the depth of tumor invasion through the intestinal wall and by the presence of regional lymph node metastases. Patients with colonic wall penetration or with metastatic carcinoma in regional lymph nodes may have improved survival with adjuvant systemic 5-fluorouracil and levamisole.

E. *Follow-up.* Cancer recurs in approximately 40% of patients who undergo resection for cure, half of these recurrences are diagnosed within the first 18 months. Follow-up evaluation is important since some patients with recurrent disease can be cured by surgical resection. Metachronous cancers occur on a 0.35% per year rate with a peak incidence of 8–5 years after the initial diagnosis supporting the need for lifelong follow-up in these patients.

BIBLIOGRAPHY

1. Bruinvels DJ, Stiggelbout AM, Kievit J, et al: Follow-up of patients with colorectal cancer. *Ann Surg* 219:174–182, 1994.

2. Corman ML, Beart RW, Pena A: Carcinoma of the colon. In *Colon and Rectal Surgery,* 3rd ed. Philadelphia: Lippincott, 1993.

3. Cozart DT, Lang NP, Hauer-Jensen M: Colorectal cancer in patients under 30 years of age. *Am J Surg* 166:764–767, 1993.

4. McGregor JR, O'Dwyer JO: The surgical management of obstruction and perforation of the left colon. *SG&O* 177:203–208, 1993.

5. NIH Consensus Conference: Adjuvant therapy for patients with colon and rectal cancer. *JAMA* 264:1444–1450, 1990.

6. Talamonti MS, Shumate CR, Carlson GW, et al: Locally advanced carcinoma of the colon and rectum involving the urinary bladder. *SG&O,* 481–87, 1993.

7. Wexner SD, Nogueras JJ: Malignant diseases of the colon and rectum. In: Rakel RE (ed): *Conn's Current Therapy.* Philadelphia: W.B. Saunders 1994, pp476–479.

8. Zeng Z, Cohn AM, Urmacher C: Usefulness of carcinoembryonic antigen monitoring despite normal preoperative values in node-positive colon cancer patients. *Dis Colon Rectum* 36:1063–1068, 1993.

See also Chapters 46, 47, 48, 71, 72 and 73.

CHAPTER 71

Metastatic Disease Therapy

Anthony M. Vernava, III, M.D. and Walter E. Longo, M.D.

Refer to Algorithm 71–1.

A. The liver is the most frequent site of metastatic disease for patients with colon cancer. In fact, as many as 30% of patients who undergo "curative" resection have occult hepatic metastases at the time of their resection. According to Finlay et al., the mean doubling time for clinically apparent liver metastases was 155±34 days, whereas the mean doubling time for occult liver metastases was 86±12 days. The average survival of untreated hepatic metastases is 6–12 months but survival averages only 4.5 months for patients who have hepatic metastases discovered during their "curative" resection. Ultimately, as many as 45% of patients with colon cancer develop hepatic metastasis. The only known effective therapy for hepatic metastases is resection but, unfortunately, only 10% of patients are candidates for resection. Systemic chemotherapy may prolong survival in both resectable and nonresectable metastatic disease. There is no proven benefit for hepatic arterial infusion of chemotherapy with 5-fluouracil or 5-fluorouracil deoxyribonucleoside (5-FU or FUDR).

B. Small synchronous hepatic metastases should be resected at the time of colectomy if there is no extrahepatic disease. If the lesion is potentialy curable but is large and requires a major hepatectomy (trisegmentectomy, right hepatic lobectomy, extended left lobectomy), then resection of the metastasis should be delayed until after recovery from colectomy. Prior to resection, evaluation should be done to exclude other intra and extrahepatic disease.

C. Treatment of hepatic metastases has evolved from nihilism in the past to one of selective resection. Currently, only approximately 10% of patients who develop liver metastases are candidates for resection. Prior to resection, recurrence at the resected primary site and extrahepatic metastases must be excluded. Occasionally, recurrence at the primary site can be re-resected and the hepatic metastasis can then be resected.

D. Patients with concomitant extrahepatic metastases are not curable by hepatic resection and are not usually candidates for hepatic resection. Palliation should be the aim of therapy. Systemic chemotherapy (5-fluoruracil with leukovorin) that may prolong survival should be considered.

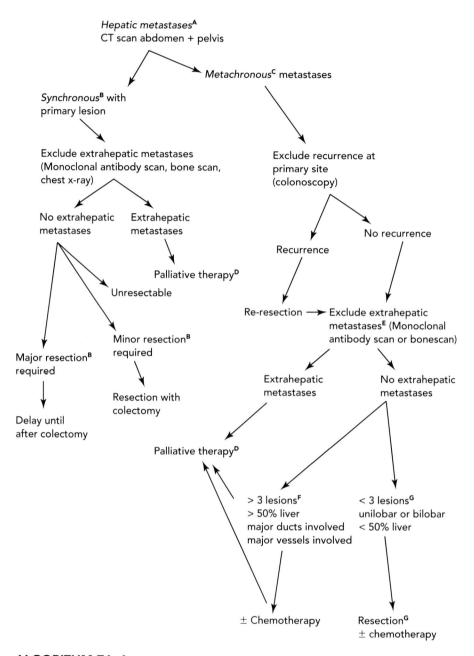

ALGORITHM 71–1

ALGORITHM 71–1,
Continued

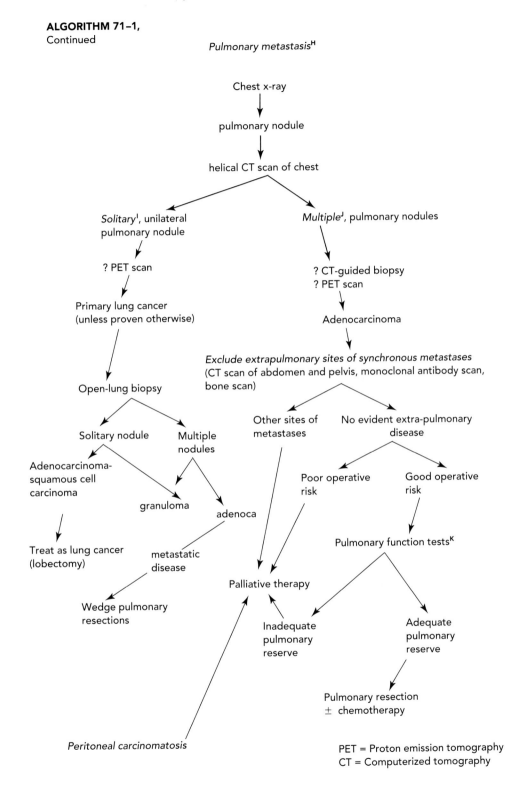

Pulmonary metastasis[H]

Chest x-ray

pulmonary nodule

helical CT scan of chest

Solitary[I], unilateral
pulmonary nodule

Multiple[J], pulmonary nodules

? PET scan

? CT-guided biopsy
? PET scan

Primary lung cancer
(unless proven otherwise)

Adenocarcinoma

Exclude extrapulmonary sites of synchronous metastases
(CT scan of abdomen and pelvis, monoclonal antibody scan,
bone scan)

Open-lung biopsy

Other sites of
metastases

No evident extra-pulmonary
disease

Solitary nodule

Multiple
nodules

Poor operative
risk

Good operative
risk

Adenocarcinoma-
squamous cell
carcinoma

granuloma

adenoca

Treat as lung cancer
(lobectomy)

metastatic
disease

Pulmonary function tests[K]

Palliative therapy

Wedge pulmonary
resections

Inadequate
pulmonary
reserve

Adequate
pulmonary
reserve

Pulmonary resection
± chemotherapy

Peritoneal carcinomatosis

PET = Proton emission tomography
CT = Computerized tomography

E. Once widespread extrahepatic metastases have been excluded the selection criteria for resection are controversial. Generally, patients are not candidates for resection if they have more than three metastases, if the metastases involve more than 50% of the liver parenchyma, or if the major hepatic veins, portal vein or vena cava are involved with disease. The number of metastases is a relative contraindication and some patients may be considered operative candidates with four to six bilobar metastatic lesions.

F. Patients are generally considered surgical candidates if they have three or fewer metastases involving less than 50% of the liver parenchyma without major vessel or hepatic duct involvement.

G. Resection of the metastasis with a margin of ≥10 mm is required. The presence of lymph node metastasis at the time of liver resection is a poor prognostic indicator. Although there are no definitive data regarding the utility of chemotherapy after hepatic resection for metastatic disease, many surgeons believe that systemic 5-FU with leukovorin prolongs the disease-free interval. There is no advantage to delivery of the drugs directly into the hepatic artery or the portal vein, and the morbidity is much higher.

H. Pulmonary metastases occur in up to 10% of patients with colon cancer. Untreated, survival is poor, with 44% of patients dead within 6 months and 91 % dead within 2 years. In properly selected patients, median survival increases to 24–44 months and 5 year survival of 21–47%. The following recommendations represent the minimum preconditions for attempted curative pulmonary resection for colorectal metastases: complete control of the primary tumor without extrapulmonary metastatic disease. Furthermore the patient must be a good operative risk with adequate pulmonary reserve. A rapid sequence, helical computerized tomography (CT) scan should be done to determine whether the pulmonary nodule is indeed solitary or whether there are multiple nodules. This type of CT is more sensitive than were the earlier generation CT scans in detecting metastases.

I. A suspicious solitary pulmonary nodule which occurs in a patient with a past history of colon cancer has a 50% chance of being a primary lung cancer and should be treated as such unless proved otherwise. Most thoracic surgeons do not require a tissue diagnosis prior to operation. Instead, an open-lung biopsy with a frozen section is performed. If the diagnosis is granuloma, then the operation is terminated. If there is, indeed, only one nodule and the frozen section diagnosis is squamous cell carcinoma or adenocarcinoma, then the lesion is treated as primary lung cancer and a lobectomy is performed. If multiple lesions are identified and the tissue diagnosis is adenocarcinoma, then the lesions are presumed to be metastatic colon cancer and wedge resections are performed.

J. As in the case of solitary pulmonary nodule, a tissue diagnosis is not required prior to operation. However, in some instances a tissue diagnosis is helpful and CT directed needle biopsy can be performed. Proton emission tomography (PET) scan holds some promise for being able to discriminate between benign and malignant pulmonary nodules. The presence of extrapulmonary metastases should be evaluated since they are a contraindication to pulmonary resection.

K. Pulmonary function tests should be done to evaluate whether the patient will tolerate resection. A FEV_1 [(forced expiratory volume) s^{-1}] <0.8 liter/s, a FVC <1.5 liter, a p_{CO_2} >45 mmHg, or a p_{O_2} <60 mmHg constitute a prohibitive operative risk, and these patients should not undergo resection. Patients with an FEV_1 of 1.01 s^{-1}, or an FVC <2.01 require additional pulmonary evaluation and medical therapy prior to resection.

BIBLIOGRAPHY

1. Adson MA: Resection of liver metastases—when is it worthwhile? *World J Surg* 11:511–20, 1987.
2. Brister SJ, Varennes BD, Gordon PH, et al: Contemporary operative management of pulmonary metastases of colorectal origin. *Dis Colon Rectum* 31:786–92, 1988.
3. Finlay IG, Mcardle CS: Occult hepatic metastases in colorectal carcinoma. *Br J Surg* 73:732–735, 1986.
4. Finlay IG, Meek D, Branton F, et al: Growth rate of hepatic metastases in colorectal carcinoma. *Br J Surg* 75:641–644, 1988.
5. Leveson SH, Wiggins PS, Giles GR, et al: Deranged liver blood flow patterns in the detection of liver metastases. *Br J Surg* 72:128–130, 1985.
6. Machi J, Isomoto H, Kurohiji T, et al: Detection of unrecognized liver metastases from colorectal cancer by routine use of operative ultrasonography. *Dis Colon Rectum* 29:405–409, 1986.
7. Saclarides TJ, Krueger BL, Szeluga DJ, et al: Thoracotomy for colon and rectal cancer metastases. *Dis Colon Rectum* 36:425–429, 1993.

See also Chapters 49, 50, 70, 71 and 72.

CHAPTER 72

Postoperative Follow-up of Colon Cancer

Martin A. Luchtefeld, M.D.

Refer to Algorithm 72-1.

A. The follow-up after a potentially curative resection for colon cancer is designed with two goals in mind: (1) to detect recurrent and metastatic cancer at a potentially curable stage and (2) to detect metachronous lesions at an early stage. Approximately 50% of patients with colon cancer will have a recurrence of their disease and even with close follow-up salvage rates are low (2–3%). In colon cancer, the pattern of recurrent disease is primarily distant metastasis with local recurrence being much less of a concern than in rectal cancer.

B. Although many different schedules of follow-up exist, Table 72-1 illustrates a suggested timetable of testing. Since most recurrences are found in the first 2 years, this interval is the period of most intensive follow-up activity. This protocol is notable for the exclusion of CT scan, which is not indicated in the asymptomatic patient with normal laboratory values.

C. At each designated interval and patient contact, a pertinent history should be elicited and a physical examination done. Constitutional symptoms are very important as are any specific symptoms relating to gastrointestinal function. As part of the physical examination, rigid or flexible sigmoidoscopy should be included if the anastomosis is within reach of this instrumentation.

D. Carcinoembryonic antigen (CEA) is one of the mainstays of follow-up for colon cancer. Although imperfect, it is often the first sign of recurrent or metastatic disease. A single elevation of CEA should not cause alarm, but instead a pattern of rising CEAs should elicit full evaluation for recurrent disease. Liver function tests (LFTs) are not included as the CEA almost always rises prior to or simultaneous with any elevation of the LFTs.

E. Chest x-ray (CXR) is also included on a yearly basis. CXRs will be invaluable in picking up those patients who have pulmonary metastases (~10–20%), of which approximately 10% are resectable.

F. Colonoscopy is of most value in detecting metachronous polyps (10–30%) and cancers (3–8%). It can also be used to evaluate for local recurrence at the

385

Postoperative follow-up of colon cancer

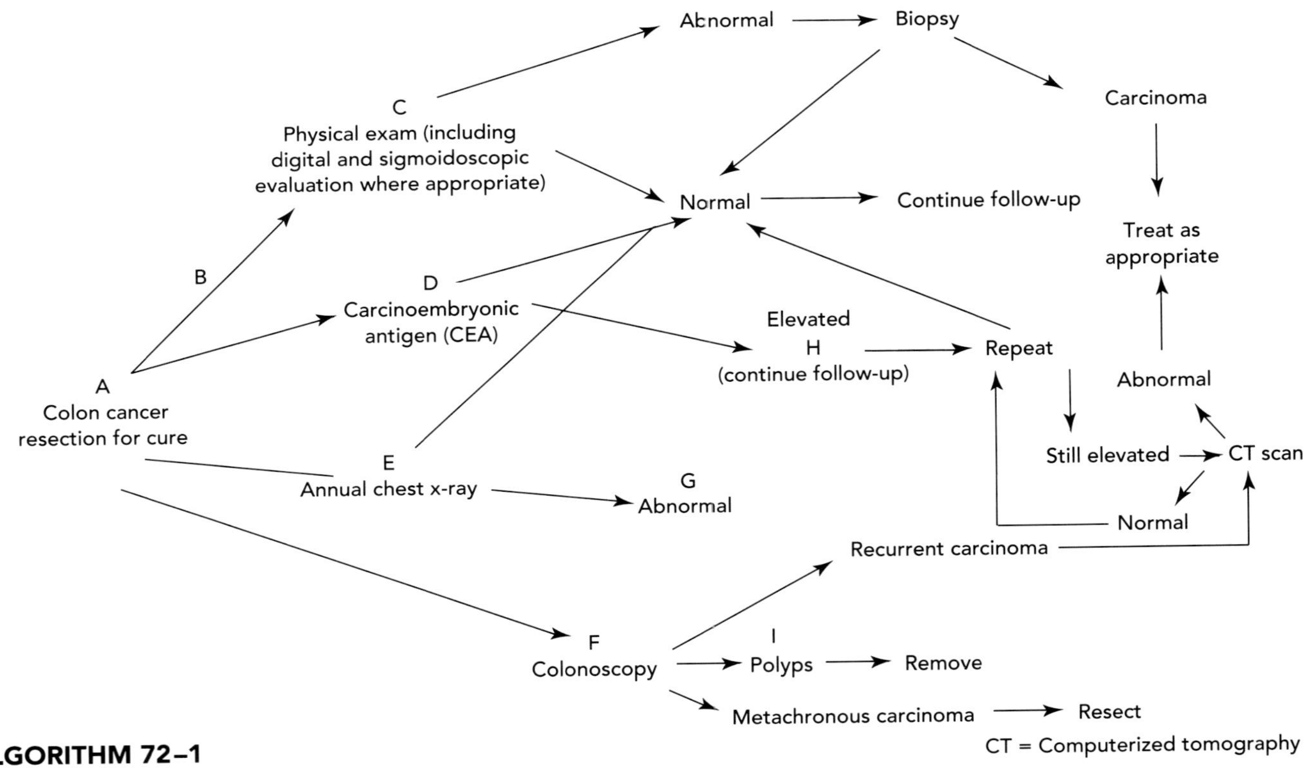

ALGORITHM 72–1

TABLE 72–1 SCHEDULE FOR FOLLOW-UP OF COLON CANCER: RESECTION FOR CURE

Months	3	6	9	12	15	18	21	24	30	36	42	48	54	60
CEA	x	x	x	x	x	x	x	x	x	x	x	x	x	x
PE	x	x	x	x	x	x	x	x	x	x	x	x	x	x
CXR				x				x		x		x		x
CE				x								x		

CEA = carcinoembryonic antigen, PE = physical exam, CXR = chest x-ray, CE = colonoscopy

anastomotic site, but this circumstance is relatively unusual and carries a dismal prognosis when it does occur.

G. If physical exam, CEA, or chest x-ray is positive, a full evaluation for recurrent disease and its extent is initiated. The evaluation and treatment of recurrent colon cancer is dealt with in Chapter 73.

H. If these same evaluations are all negative, follow-up should continue as outlined in Table 72-1. Once the patient has survived for 5 years, evaluations can be spaced at 1-year intervals.

I. All polyps identified at colonoscopy are removed. If there is a metachronous cancer, an appropriate resection is carried out. If colonoscopy detects locally recurrent disease, further evaluation for widespread cancer should also be undertaken. This topic is further discussed in Chapter 73.

BIBLIOGRAPHY

1. Corman ML: Colon carcinoma. *Colon and Rectal Surgery*. Philadelphia: Lippincott, 1993, pp 487–595.

2. Minton JP, Hoehn JL, Gerber DM, et al: Results of a 400 patient carcinoembryonic antigen second-look colorectal cancer study. *Cancer* 55:1284–1290, 1985.

3. Moertel CG, Fleming TR, Macdonald JS, et al: An evaluation of the carcinoembryonic antigen (CEA)—test for monitoring patients with resected colon cancer. *JAMA* 270:943–947, 1993.

4. Rocklin MS, Senagore AJ, Talbott TM: Role of carcinoembryonic antigen and liver function tests in the detection of recurrent colorectal carcinoma. *Dis Colon Rectum* 34:794–797, 1991.

5. Sugarbaker PH, Gianola FJ, Dwyer A, et al: A simplified plan for follow-up of patients with colon and rectal cancer supported by prospective studies of laboratory and radiologic test results. *Surgery* 102:79–87, 1987.

6. Törnqvist A, Ekelund G, Leandoer L: The value of intensive follow-up after curative resection for colorectal carcinoma. *Br J Surg* 69:725–728, 1982.

7. Woolfson K. Tumor markers in cancer of the colon and rectum. *Dis Colon Rectum* 34:506–511, 1991.

See also Chapters 49, 50, 71 and 73.

CHAPTER 73

Recurrent Colon Cancer

Francis A. Frizelle, M.B.Ch.B., M.Med. Sci.
and Heidi Nelson, M.D.

Refer to Algorithm 73–1.

A. *Recurrent colon cancer.* Despite improvements in perioperative mortality and in overall survival for patients undergoing curative resection for colorectal cancer, recurrence can still be anticipated in 25–50% of patients. Risk of recurrence is stage- and site-dependent with Dukes' "A," 0–13%, "B," 11–16%, and "C," 32–88%, and right and sigmoid colon cancers, 24–34% and transverse and left colon cancers 10–12%, respectively. Additional risk factors for recurrent disease include obstruction, perforation, adjacent organ involvement, aneuploidy, and histologic features of poor differentiation, mucin production, and venous or perineural invasion. Most recurrences occur within 2–3 years and involve the liver, 26%; locoregional, 10–25%; lung, 10%; bone, 7%; ovaries, 3–5%; anastomosis, 3%; and brain, 2%. Isolated locoregional, or focal metastatic disease can be treated for cure with surgical resection. When a cancer recurs as a diffuse metastatic process, systematic and focal palliative therapies may prolong life and improve quality of life, respectively. To differentiate local, regional, focal, and diffuse metastatic disease requires a focused history, complemented with a focused physical exam including inspection for icterus, jaundice, general physical status and weight, as well as palpatation for abdominal masses, adenopathy, hepatomegaly, splenomegaly, and pleural effusions. A complete blood count (CBC), chemistry panel, chest x-ray, colonoscopy, and computerized tomography (CT) will identify most recurrences. Additional studies as guided by presenting symptoms will localize bone and brain metastases. Peritoneal tumor implants frequently remain elusive until an obstructive process requires laparotomy. The role of CEA in detecting and monitoring recurrent disease remains controversial.

B. *Local and regional (locoregional) recurrence.* Although stage most accurately predicts local recurrence, other important factors include blood and lymphatic invasion, tumor perforation, surgical expertise, and tumor grade and fixation. En-bloc resection of adjacent organs is associated with acceptable morbidity and superior cancer outcomes and is, therefore, recommended when adherence is identified at the time of primary resection.

389

Recurrent colon cancer[A]

Local regional[B]
Anastomosis[C] → Resection
Regional/tumor bed[D] → Resection ± Radiation therapy

Focal Metastases[E]

Liver[F]
- Surgical resection[G]
- Cryotherapy[H]
- Hepatic artery ligation[I]
- Medical therapy[J]
  - Hepatic artery infusion
  - Systemic chemotherapy
  - Immune therapy
  - Direct injections
  - Alcohol
  - Gene therapy

Lung[K] → Pulmonary resection[L]

Ovarian[N] → Medical therapy[M]

Peritoneal (carcinomatosis)[O]

Bone[P]

Brain[Q]

Diffuse metastases[R]
- Palliative chemotherapy[S]
- Immunotherapy[T]
- Focal palliation[U]

ALGORITHM 73–1

C. *Anastomotic recurrence.* Anastomotic recurrence may be asymptomatic, discovered during surveillance colonoscopy, or may present as a symptom complex including gastrointestinal and systemic symptoms. Endoscopic biopsies will generally confirm the diagnosis and CT scan will establish whether an extraluminal component is present. Differentiating between an anastomotic recurrence and metachronous lesion is important since it influences the extent of resection, with the former generally requiring wider lateral or radial margins for clearance and the latter often requiring a subtotal colectomy to minimize future risk in a genetically predisposed colon. *Re-resection:* 20–26% of patients will be amenable to re-resection. The absence of symptoms is associated with a greater chance of re-resection (66%) and a longer survival (12–72 months), compared to symptomatic patients (1–24 months). At reoperation consideration should be given to the use of ureteral stents, and intraoperative radiotherapy, discussed below.

D. *Regional tumor bed.* Only 15–25% of asymptomatic recurrences are detected by clinical examination. Colonoscopy may be normal, as local recurrence may be entirely extraluminal. CT scan may detect local recurrence in only 41–88%, as the appearance of early local recurrence may be indistinguishable from posttreatment changes. Surgery, if feasible, remains the treatment of choice as in some cases it may be curative. Intraoperative radiotherapy (IORT) has been used with good results to sterilize sites of local recurrence after resection. IORT can achieve biologic effects equivalent to 2–3 times the biologic equivalent delivered as external beam. For local recurrences treated with external beam, surgery, and IORT, 5-year actuarial disease-free survival rates of 54% for complete resection and 6% for partial resection can be anticipated. Since the majority of regional recurrences occur alongside disseminated disease, palliative radiotherapy and chemotherapy will frequently be indicated.

E. *Focal metastases.* Although the spread of cancer cells to other organs indicates a metastatic process, it is at times possible to offer surgical approaches with 20% cure rates. For management purposes the diagnostic evaluation should differentiate between focal metastatic disease and diffuse disease.

F. *Liver metastases.* The mean survival with untreated hepatic metastases, the most common site of recurrence, is 6–12 months. In contrast, 5-year survival rates as high as 20–34% have been reported for hepatic resection.

G. *Hepatic resection.* Surgical therapy, despite being the most effective therapeutic alternative, is indicated in only 10% of patients with hepatic metastases. Even though restaging is performed preoperatively, with a scan, as many as 26% of patients will have intraabdominal extrahepatic disease, usually metastasizing via portal and celiac lymph nodes. Liver ultrasound, arteriography, and more recently CT–portography can be useful in delineating the extent of disease and its relationship to key anatomic structures. Test selection is determined by institutional resources and expertise. Hepatic resection for colorectal metastatic disease is indicated when (1) there are fewer than four lesions, (2) extrahepatic disease is not present, and (3) a resection margin of ≥10 mm can be achieved. A favorable prognosis can be anticipated if (1) the primary cancer is of limited locoregional extent, (2) a long interval has elapsed between primary resection and detection of metastases, (3) fewer than four lesions are detected and removed, (4) wide margins are accomplished, and (5) no extrahepatic disease is detected. Operative mortality ranges form 0% to 11.8%, and morbidities range from 10% to 28%. Median survival at 2 years range from 23% to 90%; at 3 years, from 36% to 58%; and at 5 years, from 25% to 34%.

H. *Cryotherapy*. Cryotherapy is generally reserved for patients who are not surgical resection candidates, based on distribution of disease. At laparotomy a cryoprobe with circulating liquid nitrogen is introduced into the metastasis. A spherical iceball is produced around each lesion. Using this focal treatment, the surgical team can treat multiple sites of disease without affecting large vessels or other vital structures. Complications such as hemorrhage and abscess formation can occur. Mean post operative survival is 21.4 months.

I. *Hepatic artery ligation*. Hepatic artery ligation is a last-effort option. As liver metastases derive most of their blood supply from the hepatic artery, ligation can be followed by tumor regression. As many as 97% of patients respond and have a mean survival time of 23 months. After ligation, tumor liquefaction, hepatic necrosis or abscess may occur.

J. *Medical treatment*. Chemotherapeutic regimes, including systemic and direct intraportal and intraarterial administration, have limited impact. Refer to paragraph S for discussion of palliative chemotherapy. For practical purposes, the most common therapies offered include hepatic artery infusions because (1) the liver has a dual blood supply, but normal hepatocytes gain most of the blood supply from the portal vein, and metastases >1 mm derive most of their blood supply from the hepatic artery; and (2) when fluorodeoxyuridine (5FUDR) is infused intraarterially, tumor cell uptake is about 15 times higher as compared with portal vein infusion. Additional approaches, including hepatic artery embolization, chemoembolization, hepatic artery ligation, and irradiation, are of questionable benefit. The complications of intraarterial infusion include, sepsis, sclerosing cholangitis, chemical hepatitis, peptic ulcer, and diarrhea. Mean survival ranging from 8 to 14 months. Percutaneous injections of alcohol directly into tumors has been reported and although the technique is safe and has few side effects, the effectiveness is questionable. The use of monoclonal antibodies and gene therapy remains experimental.

K. *Lung metastases*. Of the 10% of metastases that occur in the lungs, 10% of those (1% total) will be amenable to surgical resection. Consideration should be given to whether the lesion is in fact a primary lung neoplasm rather than a metastases. The diagnostic and staging evaluation for these patients should include confirmation of the diagnosis, which may include tomograms, CT scans, bronchoscopy and biopsy, and sputum cytology.

L. *Pulmonary resection*. Criteria favoring resection include (1) solitary metastases or metastases confined to one lung, (2) locally controlled primary colon carcinoma, (3) no extrapulmonic metastatic disease, and (4) a medically fit patient with sufficient reserve to tolerate a pulmonary resection. Disease-free interval, number of metastases, locoregional stage, and type of pulmonary resection, do not reliably predict outcome. Lobectomy or wedge resection are associated with low operative mortality (0–4%), and morbidities (0–12%) with 2- and 5-year survival rates of 70% and 30%, respectively.

M. *Medical treatment*. For nonresectable disease see paragraph S, on palliative chemotherapy.

N. *Ovarian metastases*. Since the chance of cure at reoperation for metastatic disease to the ovaries is low, bilateral oophorectomy has been recommended on a prophylactic basis. The value of this procedure has not been established.

O. *Peritoneal carcinomatosis.* Peritoneal carcinomatosis is not curable by any means available at present. Cytoreduction surgery with interperitoneal chemotherapy is useful for cystoadenocarcinoma, but has doubtful impact on patients with recurrent adenocarcinoma of the colon.

P. *Bone metastases.* Bone metastases are most often associated with widespread metastatic disease and occur in 5.1%; isolated skeletal metastases are rare, (1.8%). Useful investigations include site-specific skeletal x-rays, bone scan, CT scan, or MRI, with needle biopsy under radiologic guidance as an option. Treatment is directed at pain control and the avoidance of pathologic fractures. This can be achieved with radiotherapy and at times internal fixation of areas of pending fractures. The mean life expectancy of patients with bone metastases is 10–13 months.

Q. *Cerebral metastases.* Cerebral metastatic disease is uncommon, and usually associated with diffuse metastatic disease. Rarely, the brain is the only site of metastatic disease, and in this circumstance a craniotomy and resection is indicated. Radiotherapy and steroids may accomplish palliation.

R. *Diffuse metastatic disease.* Even though diffuse metastatic disease is not curable, palliation and improved quality of life can be achieved with appropriate management. Symptoms are usually managed nonoperatively, with attention focused on pain relief, palliative chemotherapy, and at times radiotherapy for focal symptoms.

S. *Palliative chemotherapy.* Systemic 5-FU/leukovorin or 5-FU via a protracted infusion offers optimal efficacy with acceptable toxicity. The reported response rate of 5-FU is approximately 20% (range 7–43%), while that of 5FU/leukovorin is approximately 35% (range 19–48%). Side effects include anorexia, nausea, vomiting, mucositis, diarrhea, weakness, ataxia, alopecia, and hand–foot syndrome.

T. *Immunotherapy.* Experimental immune therapy strategies include the use of genetically altered tumor infiltrating lymphocytes, biologic response modifiers, tumor cell gene transfers, and conjugate antibodies, to name only a few. The rapidly advancing knowledge regarding the genetic basis of colonic cancers promises that new approaches are on the horizon.

U. *Focal palliation.* Treatment of symptomatic metastatic deposits can frequently provide important palliation for patients who face limited life expectancy. Site-specific therapies are identical to those described according to anatomic location in the "focal metastases" (Section 5).

BIBLIOGRAPHY

1. Abulafi AM, Williams NS: Local recurrence of colorectal cancer; the problem, mechanisms, management and adjuvant therapy. *Br J Surg* 81:7–19, 1994.

2. Gunderson LL, Tepper JE, Dosoretez DE, et al: Patterns of failure after treatment of gastrointestinal cancer. In Cox JD (ed): *Proceedings of CROS-NCI Conference on Patterns of Failure after Treatment of Cancer, Cancer Treatment Symposium,* Vol 2, 1983.

3. Karp JE, Broder S: New directions in molecular medicine. *Cancer Res* 54:653–665, 1994.

4. McAfee M, Allen MS, Trastek VF, et al: Colorectal lung metastases; results of surgical excision. *Ann Thorac Surg* 53:780–786, 1992.

5. Registery of Hepatic Metastases: Resections of the liver for colorectal carcinoma metastases; a multi-institutional study of indications for resection. *Surgery* 103:278–288, 1988.

6. Willett CG, Shellito PC, Tepper JE, et al: Intraoperative electron beam radiation therapy for recurrent locally advanced rectal or rectosigmoid carcinoma. *Cancer* 67:1504–1508, 1991.

See also Chapters 50 and 71.

Small Bowel Conditions
Nonneoplastic

CHAPTER 74

Mesenteric Ischemia

Anthony M. Vernava, III, M.D, and Walter E. Longo, M.D.

Refer to Algorithm 74–1.

A. The causes of intestinal ischemia vary but can be divided into occlusive and nonocclusive categories. Atherosclerotic disease and embolic events are the occlusive causes. Hence, an antecedent history of peripheral vascular disease (PVD), atherosclerotic heart disease (ASHD) and cardiac arrythmias should be evaluated. Catastrophic nonocclusive ischemia can also occur whenever severely compromised cardiac output or severe splanchnic arterial vaso-constriction is present.

B. The symptoms of intestinal ischemia vary depending on whether the decrease in blood flow is chronic or acute and even then these symptoms are non-specific. Acute intestinal ischemia is characterized by severe abdominal pain out of proportion to the physical findings. In the absence of intestinal infarc-tion and gangrene with peritonitis, the abdomen may be soft or nondistended and there may be normoactive bowel sounds. A high index of suspicion is required for early angiography because even a slight time delay can result in intestinal infarction and significantly higher morbidity and mortality. Chronic intestinal ischemia is characterized by postprandial intestinal angina, weight loss, diarrhea and occult fecal blood.

C. Patients with peritonitis should undergo emergency celiotomy. Those with suspected ischemia, in the absence of peritonitis, should undergo routine laboratory testing and a plain abdominal x-ray.

D. Those patients who undergo exploratory celiotomy for peritonitis prior to angiography should have their superior mesenteric artery evaluated and if necessary embolectomy or superior mesenteric artery (SMA) bypass per-formed. Gangrenous intestine should be resected. Clinically equivocal intestine should be evaluated using Doppler ultrasound, fluorescein dye, surface oxime-try, or infrared photoplethysmography. In circumstances where the entire small intestine appears compromised after restoration of adequate blood flow, the intestine should be left in place and not resected, and the patient should undergo a second-look laparotomy within the next 24 hours.

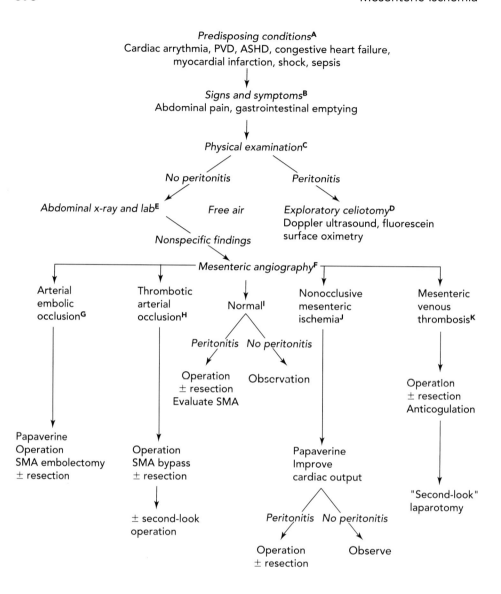

Predisposing conditions^A
Cardiac arrythmia, PVD, ASHD, congestive heart failure,
myocardial infarction, shock, sepsis

Signs and symptoms^B
Abdominal pain, gastrointestinal emptying

Physical examination^C

No peritonitis   Peritonitis

Abdominal x-ray and lab^E   Free air   Exploratory celiotomy^D
                                                  Doppler ultrasound, fluorescein
                     Nonspecific findings   surface oximetry

Mesenteric angiography^F

Arterial   Thrombotic   Nonocclusive   Mesenteric
embolic   arterial   Normal^I   mesenteric   venous
occlusion^G   occlusion^H   ischemia^J   thrombosis^K

                              Peritonitis No peritonitis

                          Operation   Observation
                          ± resection
                          Evaluate SMA

Papaverine   Operation   Papaverine   Operation
Operation   SMA bypass   Improve   ± resection
SMA embolectomy   ± resection   cardiac output   Anticogulation
± resection

                    ± second-look
                    operation   Peritonitis No peritonitis   "Second-look"
                                                                                laparotomy
                                            Operation   Observe
                                            ± resection

SMA = Superior mesenteric artery
PVD = Peripheral vascular disease
ASHD = Atherosclerotic heart disease

ALGORITHM 74–1

E. Patients with free air on the abdominal x-ray should undergo emergency laparotomy. In the absence of free air most patients will have a nonspecific gas pattern. Unfortunately, there is no single, reproducible serum marker that indicates intestinal ischemia. The laboratory findings are nonspecific and may indicate any of a number of pathologic conditions. Common laboratory findings include leukocytosis, elevated amylase, acidosis, and an elevated serum inorganic phosphate.

F. Early mesenteric angiography in patients with suspected mesenteric ischemia is essential if patients with the disorder are to be salvaged. If ischemia is in the differential diagnosis, then angiography should be performed.

G. The most common cause of acute mesenteric ischemia is embolism to the superior mesenteric artery. The majority of these emboli originate in the heart and one third of cases have an antecedent history of cerebral or extremity emboli. Fluid resuscitation and emergency SMA embolectomy should be done with a bypass if necessary. Intraarterial papaverine (0.6 mg/min) should be used to ameliorate any associated arterial spasm. Anticoagulation with intravenous heparin or dextran should be employed during and after operation but is not recommended as a substitute for operation. Those patients with questionably viable intestine after revascularization should undergo a routine second-look laparotomy within 24 hours.

H. Thrombosis of the superior mesenteric artery has a more insidious onset than does embolism, and >50% of patients so affected have an antecedent history of postprandial intestinal angina, weight loss, diarrhea, and blood in the stool. Early angiography is the key to diagnosis and management. Once the diagnosis is made, aortomesenteric bypass should be performed. Frankly gangrenous intestine should be resected. Second-look laparotomy should be performed in patients with equivocally viable intestine.

I. Patients with a normal angiogram should be closely observed, and a decision regarding operation should be based on evolving clinical findings.

J. The angiographic appearance of nonocclusive mesenteric ischemia is one of severe arterial vasoconstriction. Characteristically, the condition occurs in patients with diminished cardiac function such as after a myocardial infarction or shock. Numerous causes of shock have been associated with nonocclusive ischemia. The hallmark of therapy is the intraarterial infusion (into the SMA) of papaverine (0.6 mg/min); therapy may be instituted in the angiography suite as soon as the condition is recognized. The underlying cause of shock should be aggressively treated; the patient should be cared for in the intensive care unit with a pulmonary artery catheter in place and cardiac output maximized. Operation should be reserved for those individuals with evidence of full-thickness gangrene.

K. Venous intestinal infarction, also known as *mesenteric venous thrombosis,* was first recognized as a cause of intestinal infarction by Warren and Eberhard in 1935. The condition accounts for approximated 5–15% of all cases of mesenteric ischemia. The superior mesenteric vein is primarily involved in 95% of cases and leads to bowel ischemia and infarction. Its incidence is highest in the sixth and seventh decades of life but can occur at any age. Associated conditions include thrombophlebitis, intraabdominal infection, postabdominal surgical state, cirrhosis, congestive heart failure, trauma, polycythemia vera, malignancy, and sickle cell disease. The disorder is characterized by the gradual, rather than acute, onset of symptoms including colicky, nonlocalizing, abdominal pain. Diagnosis is very difficult, and laboratory and roentgenographic findings are variable. Angiography may demonstrate border blush, arterial spasm, aortic reflux of contrast, and decreased or absent venous return of contrast. Resection with systemic anticoagulation is the treatment of choice and has an associated mortality of 15%. Operation alone, without anticoagulation, has a mortality of 65%. Most authors advocate routine second-look laparotomy within 24 hours.

BIBLIOGRAPHY

1. Brandt, LJ, Boley SJ: Nonocclusive mesenteric ischemia. *Ann Rev Med* 42:107–117, 1991.
2. Clarke RA, Gallant TE: Acute mesenteric ischemia: angiographic spectrum. *Am J Roentgenol* 142:555–562, 1984.
3. Kitchens CS: Evolution of our understanding of the pathophysiology of primary mesenteric veonous thrombosis. *Am J Surg* 163:346–388, 1992.
4. Prasad CN, Wade TP: Mesenteric venous thrombosis. In Vernava AM, Longo WE (eds): Vascular disorders: ischemia. *Seminars Colon Rectal Surgery.* 4:218–221, 1993.
5. Renius JF, Brandt LJ, Boley SJ: Ischemic diseases of the bowel. *Gastroenterol Clin Am* 19:319–343, 1990.
6. Vernava AM, Longo WE (eds): Vascular disorders: ischemia. *Seminars Colon Rectal Surg* 4:181–266, 1993.
7. Vernava AM, Longo WE (eds): Vascular disorders: hemorrhage. *Seminars Colon Rectal Surg,* 1994.

See also Chapters 10, 11, 12A, 12B, 13, 14, 64 and 75.

CHAPTER 75

Small Intestinal Hemorrhage

Anthony M. Vernava, III, M.D. and Walter E. Longo, M.D.

Refer to Algorithm 75–1.

A. Gastrointestinal (GI) hemorrhage from the small intestine is unusual and accounts for 3–5% of all GI hemorrhage. Patients who continue to hemorrhage and who do not have an identifiable bleeding site after esophagogastroduoden-oscopy (EGD) and colonoscopy should be evaluated for a small intestinal source. There are many causes of hemorrhage from the small intestine but angiodysplasias account for 70–80% of bleeding episodes. Small intestinal tumors are the second most common cause of bleeding from the small intestine and account for 5–10% of cases; most of the tumors are benign. Other causes include jejunoileal diverticula, Meckel's diverticulum, duplication cyst, aortoenteric fistula, and ulcerating diseases of the small intestine such as Crohn's disease, radiation enteritis, infectious enteritis, and drug induced ulceration.

B. Upper gastrointestinal series (UGI) with small bowel follow-through (SBFT) barium x-rays can be done in the elective setting, when hemorrhage is not severe. If bleeding is rapid, an UGI with SBFT should not be done since it will compromise the performance of an angiogram. The test is a gross evaluation of the small intestine. It can detect mucosol abnormalities such as in active Crohn's disease, but many small bowel tumors are missed. The test has no ability to detect angiodysplasias and most jejuno-ileal diverticulae are missed.

C. A small bowel enema or enteroclysis, is more sensitive than is the small bowel series alone in detecting tumors, diverticulae and mucosal abnormalities. However, the test cannot detect angiodysplasias.

D. Small bowel enteroscopy can be performed and is an excellent method of evaluating the presence or absence of angiodysplasias, and tumors. The limitations to the test are that it is very time-consuming and cumbersome, is very expensive, and is not widely available.

E. Technetium-labeled red blood cell scintigraphy can be performed to try to localize occult gastrointestinal hemorrhage. The test is very sensitive and can detect bleeding at a rate of 0.15–0.5 cc/min. Also, repeated scans can be done over time to try to precisely identify the bleeding origin since the ^{99m}Tc-labeled

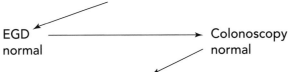

Gastrointestinal hemorrhage

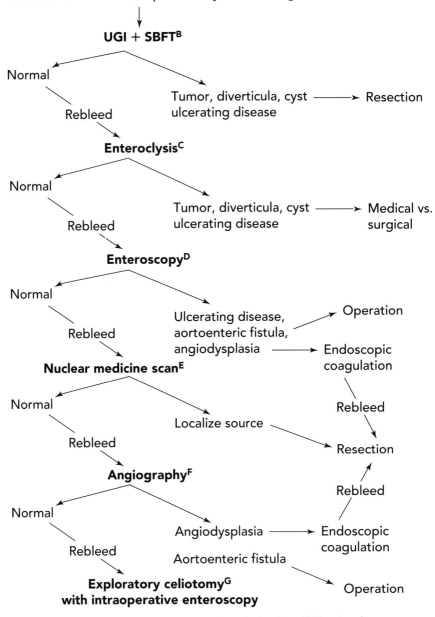

EGD normal → Colonoscopy normal

Evaluate small intestinal etiologies[A]
angiodysplasia, tumors, aortoenteric fistula, jejunoileal diverticula,
Mechel's diverticulum, duplication cyst, ulcerating diseases

UGI + SBFT[B]

Normal

Rebleed

Tumor, diverticula, cyst ulcerating disease → Resection

Enteroclysis[C]

Normal

Rebleed

Tumor, diverticula, cyst ulcerating disease → Medical vs. surgical

Enteroscopy[D]

Normal

Rebleed

Ulcerating disease, aortoenteric fistula, angiodysplasia → Operation

→ Endoscopic coagulation

Nuclear medicine scan[E]

Normal

Rebleed

Localize source

Rebleed

→ Resection

Angiography[F]

Normal

Rebleed

Angiodysplasia → Endoscopic coagulation

Aortoenteric fistula

Rebleed

→ Operation

**Exploratory celiotomy[G]
with intraoperative enteroscopy**

ALGORITHM 75–1

UGI = Upper gastrointestinal series
SBFT = Small bowel follow through
EGD = Esophagogastro-duodenoscopy

red blood cells remain in the circulation for up to 24 hours. Investigators differ on the ultimate utility of the test, but because it is noninvasive and easily obtainable, it is almost universally performed in such cases. In fact, many institutions require the nuclear scan be done prior to angiography.

F. Angiography should be done to localize hemorrhage when the previous tests have been equivocal or in cases of massive bleeding it can detect bleeding at a rate of 0.5 cc/min.

G. When all else fails to identify the source of hemorrhage, exploratory laparotomy with intraoperative endoscopy, including enteroscopy, can be performed.

BIBLIOGRAPHY

1. Gilmore PR: Angiodysplasia of the upper gastrointestinal tract. *J Clin Gastroenterol* 10:386–394, 1988.

2. Hunter JM, Pezim ME: Limited value of technetium 99m-labelled red cell scintigraphy in localization of lower gastrointestinal bleeding. *Am J Surg* 159:504–506, 1990.

3. Lewis BS, Waye JD: Bleeding from the small intestine. In Sugawa C, Schuman BM, Lucas CE (ed): *Gastrointestinal Bleeding.* Igaku-Shoin, New York, 1992, pp 178–188.

4. Lewis B, Wenger J. Wayne J: Small bowel enteroscopy and intraoperative enteroscopy for obscure gastrointestinal bleeding. *Am J Gastroenterol* 86:171–174, 1991.

5. Longo WE, Vernava AM: Clinical implications of jejunoileal diverticular disease. *Dis Colon Rectum* 35:381–388, 1992.

6. Markisz JA, Front D, Royal HD, et al: An evaluation of [99m]TC-labelled red blood cell scintigraphy for the detection and localization of gastrointestinal bleeding sites. *Gastroenterology* 83:394–398, 1982.

7. Rollins ES, Picus D, Hicks ME, et al: Angiography is useful in detecting the source of chronic gastrointestinal bleeding of obscure origin. *Am J Radiol* 156:385–388, 1991.

See also Chapters 10, 11, 12A, 12B, 13, 14, 64 and 74.

CHAPTER 76

Small Bowel Obstruction

Guillermo O. Rosato, M.D.

Refer to Algorithm 76-1.

In performing a clinical evaluation, the physician should be able to determine the possible cause and site of obstruction. Therefore, an adequate history with evaluation of signs and symptoms, and physical exam, together with lab tests and imaging will help in the management.

A. Chest x-ray must be obtained in order to look for pneumoperitoneum. When pneumoperitoneum is confirmed, laparotomy should be performed as an emergency.
B. Preoperative stoma marking should include, whenever possible, one site in each of the four quadrants. Stomas should be sited away from prior scars, planned incisions, hernias, and bony prominences.
C. Abdominal x-ray may show *air in small bowel.*
D. If localized to right iliac quadrant with leukocytosis and peritoneal rebound tenderness to compression, the possibility of appendicitis should be considered.
E. Appendectomy must be performed. In young women, laparoscopy might be an alternative diagnostic and/or therapeutic procedure.
F. If localized to the right epigastrium, with fever and leukocytosis, increased amylasemia and vomiting, an abdominal ultrasound or computerized tomography (CT) scan should be performed. If the pancreatic area is normal and gallstones are shown, cholecystitis should be considered.
G. Laparoscopy with cholecystectomy may be appropriate after diagnostic confirmation.
H. If the pancreas shows edema, pancreatitis can be the cause.
I. Medical treatment should be instituted, including intravenous hydration, bowel rest, and possibly antibiotics. Serum leukocytes, amylase, and lipase should be monitored.
J. If amylasemia worsens, amylasuria increases, leukocytosis increases, and hemoglobin diminishes, then hemorrhagic pancreatitis must be suspected.
K. If the patient has a history of previous abdominal surgery and regional ileus is found, adhesions must be considered.

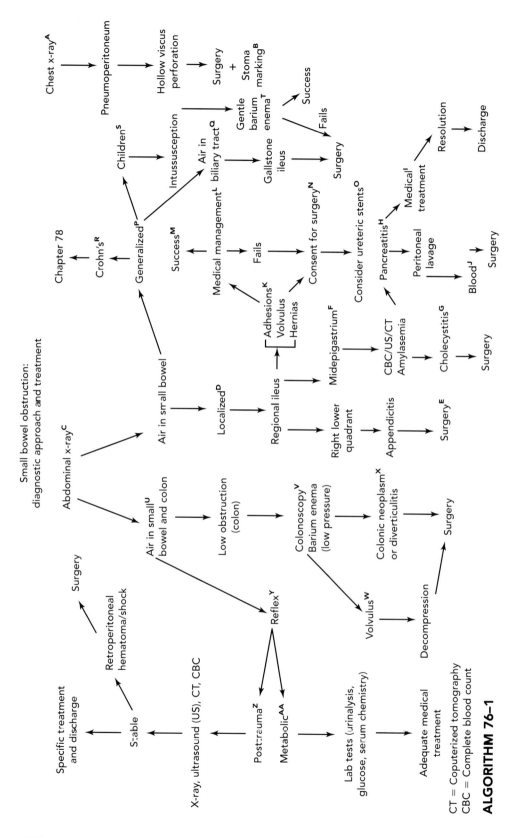

Small bowel obstruction:
diagnostic approach and treatment

Chest x-ray^A → Pneumoperitoneum → Hollow viscus perforation → Surgery + Stoma marking^B

Abdominal x-ray^C

Air in small bowel → Localized^D → Regional ileus → Midepigastrium^F → CBC/US/CT Amylasemia → Cholecystitis^G → Surgery

Generalized^P → Children^S → Intussusception → Gentle barium enema^T → Success
Generalized^P → Crohn's^R → Chapter 78
Air in biliary tract^Q → Gallstone ileus → Surgery

Success^M ← Medical management^L → Fails → Consent for surgery^N → Consider ureteric stents^O → Pancreatitis^I → Medical treatment → Resolution → Discharge
Pancreatitis^I → Peritoneal lavage → Blood^J → Surgery

Adhesions^K Volvulus Hernias → Medical management^L

Right lower quadrant → Appendicitis → Surgery^E

Air in small^U bowel and colon → Low obstruction (colon) → Colonoscopy^V Barium enema (low pressure) → Colonic neoplasm^X or diverticulitis → Surgery
Volvulus^W → Decompression → Surgery

Reflex^Y → Posttrauma^Z
Reflex^Y → Metabolic^{AA}

Retroperitoneal hematoma/shock → Surgery
Stable → Specific treatment and discharge

X-ray, ultrasound (US), CT, CBC

Lab tests (urinalysis, glucose, serum chemistry) → Adequate medical treatment

CT = Computerized tomography
CBC = Complete blood count

ALGORITHM 76–1

406

L. In the absence of peritonitis, fever, leukocytosis, or hyperamylasemia, conservative management can be instituted. Such therapy includes nasogastric decompression, intravenous hydration, correction of any electrolyte abnormalities, and close observation. There is no proven role for a "long tube."

M. If medical management is successful (usually within 24-72 hours), then a small bowel series or enteroclysis should be planned for soon after hospital discharge. This exam should help exclude any stenotic areas likely to cause recurrence. If such areas are found, elective laparotomy and enteroclysis may be worthwhile. Such a situation is very rare.

N. If the patient has peritonitis, or pyrexia, leukocytosis, or hyperamylasemia, or fails to improve after 24-72 hours of conservative therapy, laparotomy should be undertaken. Preoperative consent must include the possibility of a stoma. Enterostomal consultation should be sought. Bowel resection should be done when blood supply compromises vitality of the bowel wall. This is more likely to happen in volvulus and crural or internal hernias. Primary small bowel anastomosis is generally possible. After enteroclysis, the bowel must be carefully inspected. Any myotomies or enterotomies should be repaired.

O. If previous pelvic radiotherapy has been employed, consideration should be given to intraoperative ureteric catheters.

P. If air is generalized to the small bowel and extends into the biliary tract, gallstone ileus is to be considered. Sometimes the gallstone can be seen on a plain abdominal x-ray.

Q. In the case of gallstone ileus, a laparotomy should be undertaken and an enterotomy performed proximal to the obstruction to remove the stone.

R. Another cause of small bowel obstruction is Crohn's disease due to a segmental stenosis. In general, obstructions secondary to Crohn's disease do not require emergency laparotomy. Instead, these patients usually require nutritional supplementation, hydration, steroid supplementation, and thorough enterocolonic evaluation. After these measures, elective or semielective surgery can be undertaken.

S. Generalized air in the small bowel can be found in children with no previous abdominal surgery if an ileocolonic intussusception is the cause.

T. If barium enema fails to reduce the intussusception, laparotomy should be performed. If vascular compromise is present, resection should be undertaken. One must be sure to exclude the presence of any small bowel polyp that could have been the cause of intussusception. In these cases, either colotomy and polypectomy or resection are indicated.

U. If air is shown in the small bowel and colon, a distal colonic obstruction should be considered.

V. Colonoscopy or low-pressure barium enema can demonstrate colonic stenosis due to a neoplasm, diverticulosis, or a volvulus.

W. In the latter setting, colonoscopic compression is attempted. If successful, elective sigmoidectomy is recommended. If colonoscopic decompression fails or the volvulus recurs, surgery should be undertaken.

X. When a tumor is the cause of obstruction, surgery is indicated. Therapeutic alternatives include resection with stoma resection with intraoperative lavage and anastomosis, resection with anastomosis and proximal fecal diversion, or diversion alone. The alternative should be individualized to both the patient and the pathology.

Y. Reflex ileus can be due to trauma.

Z. If a retroperitoneal hematoma is diagnosed, the patient should be treated by a vascular surgeon.

AA. When metabolic ileus is diagnosed, medical treatment is indicated.

BIBLIOGRAPHY

1. Uriburu J, in: Michans JR, *Patología Quirúrgica*. Cap. 31. Tomo 3. Ileo-Obstrucción Intestinal. El Ateneo (Ed.) Buenos Aires. 1968.

2. Welch JP: *Bowel Obstruction. Differential Diagnosis and Clinical Management.* W.B. Saunders Company, Philadelphia, 1990.

3. Yamada T, Alpers D, Owyang C, Powell D, Silverstein F. *Textbook of Gastroenterology.* J.B. Lippincott (Ed.). Philadelphia, 1991.

See also Chapters 14, 58, 62, 63, 65, 77 and 78.

CHAPTER 77

Radiation Enteritis

Lars Påhlman, M.D., Ph.D.

Refer to Algorithm 77-1.

A. The exact incidence of complications to radiation, both acute and late, is difficult to estimate due to the lack of large prospective studies; furthermore most reports are from surgical series. Severe complication rates after abdominal and pelvic radiation have been estimated to range from <3% to as much as 20%. Using modern radiation techniques and dose planning systems, it can be estimated that severe complication rates will be below 5%. No definite correlations between acute and late effects have been found.

B. In cancer of the bladder, prostate, cervix, uterus, rectum, and anus, external, with or without internal radiotherapy has been used either alone or in combination with surgery. A dose level of >45 Gy (gray) is essential to reach to elicit an observable effect on subclinical disease in the above mentioned tumors. Higher dose levels must be given if control of macroscopic disease is required. Table 77-1 shows the tolerance for the small bowel.

C. In the acute phase, radiation causes an edematous and hyperemic mucosa. Small ulcerations may be seen. Late intestinal complications are seen as hyaline thickening of small vessel walls, hyperthrophy of the smooth muscle cells, and different degrees of fibrosis, not only in the bowel wall but also in the mesentery which can be thick and shortened.

D. Symptoms of acute toxicity include nausea, vomiting, diarrhea, abdominal pain, and tenesmus. Late symptoms to radiation complications include adhesions, stricture, obstruction, ischemia, fistulas, and malabsorption.

E. It must be emphasized that late adverse effects can be difficult to distinguish from generalized or recurrent cancer. Obvious findings such as obstruction or fistulation can easily be diagnosed. In more diffuse cases conventional x-ray of the bowel can disclose typical "thumbprint signs" indicating a damaged area. The most frequently involved part is the distal ileum. Malabsorption tests are a good complement to other diagnostic procedures.

F. In order to minimize radiation damage, it is essential to avoid irradiation to tissue not at risk of tumor. If this goal cannot be reached without compromising the dose to tumor-containing tissues, the dose to the organs at risk should

409

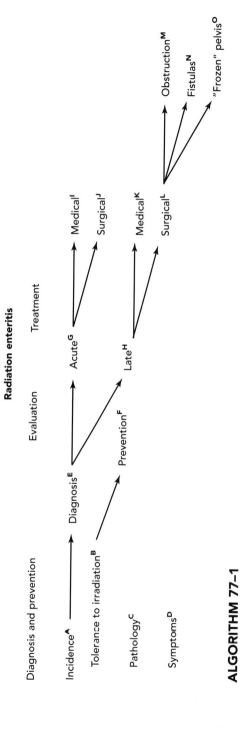

Radiation enteritis

Diagnosis and prevention   Evaluation   Treatment

Incidence^A ———→ Diagnosis^E ———→ Acute^G ———→ Medical^I

Tolerance to irradiation^B   ↗ Surgical^J

Prevention^F

Pathology^C   Late^H ———→ Medical^K

Symptoms^D ———————————→ Surgical^L ———→ Obstruction^M

                                                    ↗ Fistulas^N

                                                    ↗ "Frozen" pelvis^O

ALGORITHM 77–1

TABLE 77–1 UPPER NORMAL TOLERANCE LEVEL (< 5% SEVERE ADVERSE EFFECTS)

Organ	Dose Level (Gy)[a]
Kidney	<30
Liver	35
Parts of the Liver	45–50
Entire small bowel, no previous surgery	45–50
Entire small bowel, previous surgery	40–45
Fixed small bowel loop	45–50
Large bowel	60

[a] Provided the irradiation is given with 1.8–2 Gy daily, 5 times per week.

be as low as possible using appropriate dose planning and radiation techniques. Ideally, preoperative as opposed to postoperative radiation is preferred. If postoperative radiation is planned, different techniques with artificial mesh or an omental pedicle have been described to avoid small bowel radiation.

G. Acute injury is dependent on daily radiation dose and usually starts within 2–4 weeks from the start of treatment. The proportion of patients who will have symptoms is dependent on the radiated volume, ranging from virtually none to 100%.

H. Late injury can appear many years after treatment, but the first symptoms usually occur within the first 2 years.

I. The most prominent symptoms are nausea and diarrhea. They can be successfully treated with antiemetics and/or antidiarrheal drugs and rarely require hospitalization. The symptoms usually resolve completely within a few weeks.

J. Emergency surgery is rarely indicated, and in the acute phase of irradiation reaction, surgery should be avoided. If surgery is performed, tissue edema is often found and the risk of anastomotic dehiscense is great. A diverting stoma should be strongly considered.

K. Symptomatic treatment including antidiarrheals, opiates, and antispasmodics, can improve function as can low-fat and low-lactose diet. In severe cases, complete bowel rest with total parenteral nutrition is the only option.

L. Surgery must be carefully considered as high morbidity and mortality are legion. When resection is necessary, nonirradiated bowel should be used to create the anastomosis. If colon is used as one part, the risk of anastomotic complications is substantially reduced. Perioperative laser–Doppler measurements can be helpful in evaluation of blood supply. Enteroclysis must be cautiously undertaken due to poor blood supply and hence the risk for postoperative fistulas.

M. It is controversial whether a resection or a bypass should be performed. Less complications have generally been reported if bypass is used, but more recent studies favor resection.

N. If surgery is considered, resection is advocated. Fistulas to the urogenitalial tract must be operated upon because of bandaging problems, whereas fistulas to the abdominal wall can be conservatively managed. If a distal obstruction is present, the fistulas will never heal and surgery must be considered.

O. The frozen pelvis is a dangerous setting as enteroclysis and dissection in this area can have catastrophic sequelae. Instead, a bypass operation is often advisable. However, one must ensure that the bypass is between an afferent and an efferent loop of bowel. Furthermore, some surgeons create mucous fistulas of both the afferent and efferent loops.

BIBLIOGRAPHY

1. DeLuca FR, Ragins H: Construction of an omental envelope as a method of excluding the small intestine from the field of postoperative irradiation to the pelvis. *Surg Gynecol Obstet* 160:365–372, 1985.

2. Fletcher GH: Subclinical disease. *Cancer* 53:1274–1284, 1984.

3. Galland RB, Spencer J: Surgical aspects of radiation injury to the intestine. *Br J Surg* 66:135–139, 1979.

4. Harling H, Balslev I: Radical surgical approach to radiation injury of the small bowel. *Dis Colon Rectum* 29:371–375, 1986.

5. Jagelman DG, Rothenberger DA, Wexner SD: Irradiation injuries to the intestine. In Schrock T (ed): *Perspectives in Colon and Rectal Surgery*. St. Louis: Quality Medical Publishing 3:275–296, 1990.

See also Chapters 48, 65, 73 and 76.

CHAPTER 78

Small Bowel Crohn's Disease

Joe J. Tjandra, M.D. and Findlay A. MaCrae, M.D.

Refer to Algorithm 78–1.

A. Crohn's disease can involve any part of the gastrointestinal tract and the perianal region. Common sites of disease are in the ileocolic region and the small bowel.

B. Crohn's disease is often segmental with sections of intervening grossly normal bowel. Symptoms relate to the ulcerated mucosa, to strictures, to intraabdominal sepsis, and to a variety of extraintestinal manifestations.

C. Crohn's disease is a diffuse and chronic inflammatory condition that tends to affect the full thickness of the bowel wall. Extent of involvement may vary in different sites of the bowel. Aphthous ulceration is generally believed to be the first macroscopically recognizable sign of Crohn's disease. In chronic disease, the bowel wall becomes thickened and rigid, with wrapping of fat on the serosa. Deep linear ulcers are characteristic, giving rise to a cobblestone appearance. There are no specific histologic features of Crohn's disease; diagnosis depends on pattern recognition. Noncaseating granulomata are present in only 60% of patients.

D. Extent of disease is established by clinical assessment, upper intestinal and small bowel follow-through barium studies, and colonoscopy or barium enema. Indium-111-labeled granulocyte scan may delineate the anatomic extent of disease in both the large and the small intestines. This test requires no bowel preparation but is less accurate than the other tests.

E. There is no specific therapy for Crohn's disease. Control rather than cure of the disease is the aim of treatment.

F. Sulfasalazine is composed of a sulfa moiety, sulfapyridine (the "carrier"), which is covalently bonded to an aspirin analog, mesalamine (the active moiety). While sulfasalazine is effective for the treatment of mild to moderately active Crohn's colitis, it has no effect on small intestinal disease. Adverse reactions to the sulfapyridine portion of sulfasalazine occurred in 15% of patients. Sulfasalazine does not have corticosteroid-sparing effect.

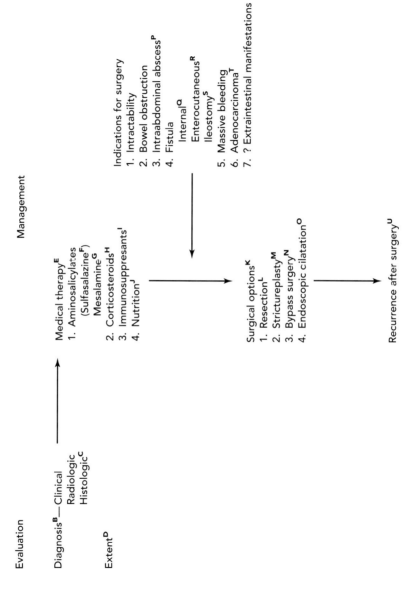

Small bowel Crohn's disease[A]

Evaluation

Diagnosis[B]—Clinical
Radiologic
Histologic[C]

Extent[D]

Management

Medical therapy[E]
1. Aminosalicylates
   (Sulfasalazine[F])
   Mesalamine[G]
2. Corticosteroids[H]
3. Immunosuppressants[I]
4. Nutrition[J]

Indications for surgery
1. Intractability
2. Bowel obstruction
3. Intraabdominal abscess[P]
4. Fistula
   Internal[Q]
   Enterocutaneous[R]
   Ileostomy[S]
5. Massive bleeding
6. Adenocarcinoma[T]
7. ? Extraintestinal manifestations

Surgical options[K]
1. Resection[L]
2. Strictureplasty[M]
3. Bypass surgery[N]
4. Endoscopic cilatation[O]

Recurrence after surgery[U]

ALGORITHM 78–1

G. Delayed-release mesalamine preparations (asacol, pentasa, mesasal) are better tolerated and are effective at high doses in ileocolonic Crohn's disease. Their use in the maintenance of disease remission remains controversial.

H. Corticosteroids are efficacious for the treatment of active Crohn's disease, regardless of the disease distribution. Good initial symptomatic response occurs in 75–90% of patients. They are not indicated as maintenance therapy for disease in complete remission.

 I. The main indications for 6-mercaptopurine or azathioprine are (1) steroid toxicity or dependence, (2) fistulization (enterocutaneous, symptomatic internal fistula) and (3) recurrent Crohn's disease with multiple prior small bowel resections with the aim of avoiding short bowel syndrome from further resection(s). The onset of action may require 3–6 months. Preliminary data have indicated a more rapid onset of efficacious action (about 2 weeks) with Cyclosporin A in ileocecal and fistulous Crohn's disease. All these medications have significant toxicity.

J. Nutritional support is an important part of the overall management. In severe cases, parenteral nutrition and bowel rest may be necessary. Specific dietary associations with Crohn's disease have been investigated but not clearly identified.

K. The timing of operation on a patient with Crohn's disease is controversial. Surgery is commonly indicated for complications rather than for intractability to medical therapy. Although Crohn's disease is a chronic, relapsing, and potentially panintestinal disease, the specific site of severe disease itself may be a more important factor in malnutrition and poor health than is the loss of that diseased segment of bowel.

L. For most patients, resection is the procedure of choice. A conservative resection margin of 2–5 cm of bowel is adequate. More radical margins are not associated with fewer recurrences. Enlarged mesenteric lymph nodes are resected only if they compromise the blood supply of the remaining small bowel. Anastomoses in bowel with aphthous ulceration or microscopic evidence of Crohn's disease heal as well as those in normal bowel.

M. The nomenclature (Heineke–Mikulicz; Finney) and principles of strictureplasty are analogous to those of phyloroplasty. It increases the diameter of the bowel and relieves the obstruction without sacrificing any bowel. This lessens the risk of short bowel syndrome associated with repeated bowel resections. The procedure is safe and effective in selected strictures of the small bowel and an anastomosis (small bowel, ileocolic, or ileorectal). There has been no mortality. Major septic complications were 6%. The rate of symptomatic restricture of the strictureplasty sites was 2.8% after a median interval of 3 years. Strictureplasty is ideal for short fibrotic strictures but has been safely performed in longer and softer strictures, so long as the bowel edges retain the sutures well. Bowel conservation should be particularly considered in the presence of diffuse disease and if there is a shortage of small bowel because of previous resection(s). Strictureplasty is contraindicated in acute inflammatory phlegmon, sites of overt perforation, a short segment of bowel containing multiple strictures, and when the serum albumin level is less than 20 g per liter.

N. An example is a side-to-side ileotransverse anastomosis for inflammatory or obstructive ileocolic Crohn's disease. This is now rarely performed because of the risk of persistent inflammation and adenocarcinomas in the bypassed segment. Occasionally, bypass surgery is performed when the patient is very ill or if the inflammatory mass firmly adheres to other organs, precluding a safe excision. The bypassed segment is resected several months later.

O. Strictures that are related endoscopically 7 or 8 years after resection tend to stay open, while those in areas of actual disease tend to recur. There is a small risk of perforation and the long-term benefit is not clear. The technique should be restricted to short strictures affecting ileocolic or ileorectal anastomoses.

P. With localized abscess, a preliminary CT-guided percutaneous drainage of the abscess, followed by definitive resection several weeks later, is helpful. In the presence of occult abscess during a planned laparotomy, the site is drained and quarantined with omental interposition, and the diseased bowel is resected. In most cases, a primary anastomosis is still possible. With free perforation and generalized peritonitis, emergency operation with resection of the perforated bowel is performed. In very ill patients with severe sepsis, a diverting ileostomy may be prudent.

Q. Internal fistulas are not always symptomatic and do not always demand surgical treatment. The primary fistulizing disease is usually in the distal ileum. At surgery, the diseased small bowel is resected. Secondarily affected sites, such as duodenum, small bowel, sigmoid colon, and bladder, seldom are afflicted with Crohn's disease and can be managed by wedge excision and primary closure. In the presence of significant phlegmonous reaction, more formal resection of the secondary sites, such as sigmoid resection and anastomosis or wider duodenal excision with side-to-side duodenojenunal anastomosis, may be necessary.

R. Once a enterocutaneous fistula has developed, the fistula rarely heals without resection. The operation is seldom urgent. Patients who have had multiple recurrences and who have a low-output "pouchable" fistula are best treated nonoperatively with hyperalimentation, bowel rest, sandostatin, and sometimes 6-mercaptopurine (or azathioprine). Those fistulas that arise within the first week after surgery are usually due to technical problems rather than residual Crohn's disease.

S. Ileostomy fistula is treated by resection and neoileostomy, unless the fistula is superficial to the skin level and easily pouchable. Relocation of the stoma may be necessary if there is significant sepsis at the original stoma site.

T. Diagnosis of adenocarcinoma of the small bowel is often delayed at an advanced stage, resulting in a poor prognosis. It tends to affect more distal small bowel than in patients with non-Crohn's adenocarcinoma of the small bowel. About one-third of the reported cases have occurred in excluded small bowel segments.

U. Recurrence rates vary with the length of follow-up, the definition of "recurrence," and the site(s) of disease. Endoscopic evidence of recurrent disease may develop early and is often asymptomatic. Overall, when followed at 5 years, approximately one-quarter of patients with either small bowel resection or strictureplasty require treatment (operative and nonoperative) of recurrent disease at the sites of previous surgery or at new sites. There is a predilection of recurrence in certain sites after surgery—in the terminal ileum immediately proximal to the ileostomy; in the preanastomotic ileum after ileocolic or ileorectal anastomosis. Late (after more than 10 years) recurrences are more often successfully managed nonoperatively than those that occur early. Preliminary data on adjuvant therapy with small bowel released mesalamine preparations after resection are encouraging. A short-term study of adjuvant metronidazole also seems to lessen the severity of recurrence.

BIBLIOGRAPHY

1. Lichtenstein GR: Medical therapies for inflammatory bowel disease. In Donaldson RM Jr (ed): *Current Opinion in Gastroenterology*. Philadelphia: Current Science, 1993, Vol 9 (4).

2. Nivatvongs S. Crohn's disease. In Gordon PH, Nivatvongs S (eds): *Principles and Practice of Surgery for the Colon, Rectum and Anus*. St. Louis: Quality Medical Publishing, 1992.

3. Tjandra JJ, Fazio VW. Techniques of strictureplasty. In Schrock TR (ed): *Perspectives in Colon and Rectal Surgery*. St. Louis: Quality Medical Publishing, 1992, Vol 5 (2).

4. Tjandra JJ, Fazio VW: Crohn's disease: surgical management. In Bayless TM (ed): *Current therapy in Gastroenterolgy and Liver Disease,* 4th ed. Philadelphia: Mosby Year Book, 1994.

5. Wexner SD: Elective surgical options in the treatment of mucosal ulcerative colitis and Crohn's disease. In Sleissinger M, Sachor DB (eds): *Seminars in Gastroenterology*. Philadelphia: W.B. Saunders 2:90–106, 1991.

See also Chapters 51, 76, 79 and 80.

CHAPTER 79

Enterocutaneous Fistulas

Michael R. B. Keighley, M.S., F.R.C.S.

Refer to Algorithm 79–1.

A. A *fistula* is an abnormal communication between two epithelial surfaces. Fistulas may be specific or postoperative. Specific fistulas, with examples, are classified as follows; some factors that are starred (*) may be responsible for postoperative fistulas.

Congenital:	Persistent vitellointestinal duct; anorectal agenesis and rectourinary or rectovaginal fistula
Acquired:	
*Traumatic	Iatrogenic injuries; penetrating and visceral injuries
*Ischemic	Small bowel disease such as polyarteritis nodosa
*Inflammatory	Crohn's disease and diverticular disease
*Infective	Acute (e.g., pyogenic infections)
	Chronic (e.g., tuberculosis, actinomycosis, amebiases)
*Radiation damage	
*Neoplastic disease	Benign disease
	Malignant disease

Primary   Adenocarcinoma of the colorectum; transitional cell carcinoma of the uroepithelium

Secondary   Squamous cell carcinoma of the cervix, uterus, or vagina

Fistulas may be further classified as simple or complex. Simple fistulas are short, direct tracks that run between two epithelial surfaces with no coexisting sepsis. Complex fistulas are often long tracks, usually with an intervening abscess cavity between the two epithelial surfaces. There may be a communication between more than one site; for instance, an enterocutaneous fistula may communicate with other loops of bowel (enteroenteric fistula), with the bladder (enterovesicle fistula), with the vagina (enterovaginal fistula), or with the perineum (enteroperineal fistula).

Enterocutaneous fistulas

420

Classify:
Biopsy
Culture
Radiology
Endoscopy

A Origin:
Small bowel
Large bowel

B Specific

Simple

Complex
± Enteroenteric
Enterovaginal
Enterovesical
Enteroperineal

Congenital
Acquired

C Infective

Trauma

D Inflammatory

E Crohn's

F Diverticular

G Neoplastic

H Radiation

Acute — Drain

Chronic — Specific: tuberculosis, actinomycosis, amebiasis → Specific therapy

Resect + close communicating fistula + drain ± divert

Sigmoid resection

Primary—adenocarcinoma]
—transitional] → Radical resection
—squamous]

Secondary

Resection and anastomosis to bowel outside radiation field + divert

I Post-operative

Factors: Anastomosis
Iatrogenic damage
Ischemia
Infection
Neoplastic
Radiation

J Resuscitate

K Protect skin

L Drain sepsis
± Divert

M Total parenteral nutrition

6 weeks

Healed

N Persistent

Exclude persistent disease and distal obstruction

O Resect ± divert

ALGORITHM 79–1

B. *In established fistula* the first consideration is to make a diagnosis by percutaneous or ultrasound-directed biopsy, endoscopic biopsy, or radiology. Infective causes will require culture of pus or tissue.

C. *Specific infective fistulas* require specific treatment such as antituberculous chemotherapy or penicillin for actinomycosis.

D. *Specific noninfective fistula* should be treated by resection where possible and adjuvant therapy if necessary.

E. *In Crohn's disease* the aim is to identify the principal site of disease and to resect it. There may be multiple communications with uninvolved bowel, in which case these connections to bladder, bowel, or vagina are merely disconnected and the uninvolved communications are closed. A primary anastomosis is usually advised unless there is gross sepsis, leaving open the option to defunction the anastomosis if there are high-risk factors such as malnutrition or steroids anemia.

F. *In diverticular disease,* the sigmoid colon is resected and communications to the skin and any other viscera are disconnected and closed. An unprotected anastomosis is usually performed provided there is no overt sepsis.

G. *In malignancy,* the aim is to perform a radical resection of the primary neoplasm and any fistulous communications that may have developed. Preoperative radiotherapy may be necessary in advanced local disease. The extent of the resection will depend on local involvement of adjacent structures. Where possible, a monoblock excision is desirable with any other involved organ such as small bowel, bladder, or vagina, followed by primary anastomosis. In extensive disease partial or total cystectomy, with or without total abdominal hysterectomy, may be necessary. If radiotherapy has been performed preoperatively, or if there is sepsis, proximal decompression may be necessary.

H. *Fistulas complicating long-standing radiotherapy* will require resection and anastomosis outside the field of radiation. For pelvic fistulas this will often require anastomosis of the transverse colon to the anus.

I. *Postoperative fistulas* usually result from iatrogenic damage to bowel at operation, or a leak from a stoma closure site, but principally from the breakdown of an intestinal anastomosis. Factors implicated in postoperative fistulas are malnutrition, sepsis, steroid medication, and bowel ischemia as well as persistent, undisclosed Crohn's disease, previous radiation, and advanced malignancy.

J. Resuscitation is the first consideration in the management of postoperative fistula. These patients are generally septic, acidotic, dehydrated, malnourished, hypercatabolic, and electrolyte-depleted. Good venous access is essential, replacement of fluids and electrolytes needs to be carefully monitored by regular blood chemistry, and urine output and central venous monitoring may be necessary in patients with associated cardiovascular disease.

K. Skin protection is next on the list of priorities. A drainage bag with a wide baseplate is usually adequate but some high fistulas discharging into the depths of an open wound may require a suction catheter, preferably incorporated into a drainage bag.

L. The third urgent consideration in postoperative fistulas is to drain any associated sepsis. This may simply involve opening a part of the incision. More frequently it involves ultrasound-, computerized tomography (CT)-, or magnetic resonance imaging (MRI)-guided percutaneous drainage of intraabdominal or retroperitoneal sepsis. In exceptional cases, early laparotomy with open drainage and proximal fecal diversion may be necessary if the fistula simply cannot be managed by drainage or if there is uncontrollable sepsis.

M. Only when sepsis is properly under control is it safe to start total parenteral nutrition. In our experience, only total parenteral nutrition adequately corrects the negative nitrogen balance and achieves a substantial reduction in the volume output of the fistula. The only exception is a low-output large bowel fistula, and under these circumstances enteral feeding may have a role. There is a high risk of line sepsis if total parenteral nutrition is started when the patient is still septic. Once total parenteral nutrition has been established, patients must be mobilized to restore morale. They should not take fluids or food by mouth as this tends to increase the fistula output. Rehabilitation in the physiotherapy gym and occupational therapy is desirable.

N. If the fistula is still present after 6 weeks, or if the output at 4 weeks has not fallen substantially, the possible causes of persistent fistula should be sought. These are as follows: distal bowel obstruction, persistent sepsis, or unresolved underlying disease, particularly Crohn's disease or malignancy. Thus, the patients require contrast radiology, particularly fistulography, small bowel enema, and in some cases a barium enema as well. Establishing a tissue diagnosis of persistent underlying disease may be possible by endoscopic biopsy or by fine-needle aspiration cytopathology.

O. If the fistula is still present after 6 weeks, it rarely heals by further total parenteral nutrition. At this stage, provided there is no coexisting sepsis, the patient should have gained weight with improvement of muscle function and no longer present an anesthetic risk. Thus, a full laparotomy is now indicated, requiring meticulous dissection of the entire small bowel, resection of the fistula, and any distal obstruction or persistent disease if present. If there is any technical difficulty with the anastomosis or if there is coexisting sepsis, a proximal diverting ileostomy would be advised.

BIBLIOGRAPHY

1. Alexander-Williams J and Irving M: *Intestinal fistula.* Bristol: Wright, 1982.

2. Chapman R, Foran R, and Duaphy JE: Management of intestinal fistulas. *Am J Surg* 108:157–164, 1964.

3. Cousoftides T and Fazio VW: Small intestinal cutaneous fistulas. *Surg Gynecol Obstet* 149:333–336, 1979.

4. Fazio VW, Cousoftides T, and Steiger E: Factors influencing the outcome of treatment of small bowel cutaneous fistula. *World J Surg* 7:481–488, 1983.

5. Galland RB & Spencer J: Radiation-induced gastrointestinal fistulae. *Ann R Coll Surg Engl* 68:5–7, 1986.

6. Hill GL: Operative strategy in the treatment of enterocutaneous fistulas. *World J Surg* 7:495–501, 1983.

7. Hollender LD, Meyer C, Avet D, and Zeyer B: Post-operative fistulas of the small intestine: therapeutic principles. *World J Surg* 7:474–480, 1983.

8. Stiges-Serra A, Jaurrieta E, and Stiges-Crows A: Management of post-operative enterecutaneous fistulas: the roles of parenteral nutrition and surgery. *Br J Surg* 69:147–150, 1982.

See also Chapters 78 and 80.

CHAPTER 80

Enterovaginal Fistulas

Michael R. B. Keighley, M.S., F.R.S.C.

Refer to Algorithm 80–1.

A. *Classification* (see enterocutaneous). Enterovaginal fistula may be specific or postoperative. An anatomic classification, as well as the etiologic one used in enterocutaneous fistula is helpful:

Ileovaginal	These fistulas are usually due to a loop of small bowel adherent to the posterior fornix. They are more common after a previous hysterectomy. The most common causes are Crohn's disease, radiation damage, or postoperative complications.
Colovaginal	Usually these are from the sigmoid colon to the posterior vaginal vault. Common causes are diverticular disease, advanced malignancy, and postoperative fistulas.
Rectovaginal	These are subdivided as follows:
Septal	Usually this is a direct communication from the rectum to the middle of the vagina. These fistulas may be due to Crohn's disease or rectal or cervical malignancy, or they may occur as a result of obstructed labor due to ischemic necrosis of the rectovaginal septum.
Extrasphincteric	These fistulas lie just above the external sphincter; they may occur after pouch surgery or from obstetric tears.
Transphincteric	These are usually cryptoglandular in origin, but they may occur after pouch surgery.

The first task is to establish a diagnosis to ascertain the cause of a fistula. A careful examination under anesthetic is essential with sigmoidoscopy, speculum examination of the vagina, and possibly laparoscopy if there is disease in the pouch of Douglas. Any abnormality should be biopsied; contrast radiology may also be indicated.

B. *Congenital.* In children anorectal agenesis is often associated with a rectovaginal fistula, which is now commonly treated by posterior saggital rectoplasty.

Enterovaginal fistula

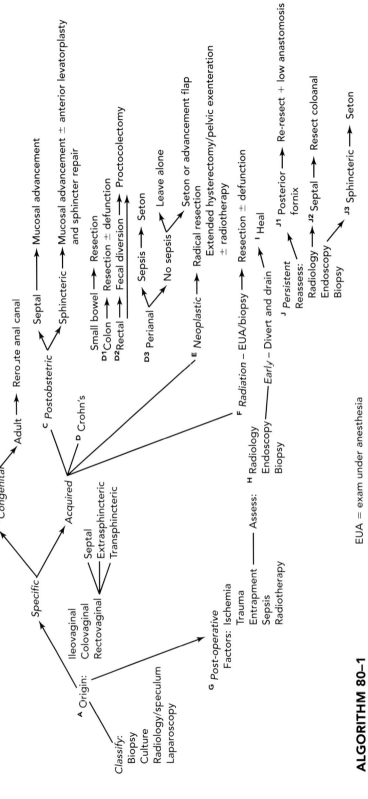

ALGORITHM 80–1

EUA = exam under anesthesia

In adults, rerouting of an anteriorly placed anus with closure of any rectovaginal fistula is usually the preferred management.

C. *Postobstetric fistulas.* Careful evaluation of the fistula may necessitate anal ultrasonography, magnetic resonance imaging (MRI) scans, and a functional assessment of the anorectum, since pudendal neuropathy may be associated with compromised sphincter function, even if the fistula is successfully repaired. Today the usual approach for postobstetric fistulas is an endoanal advancement flap, but repair of the perineal body by anterior levatorplasty and even sphincter repair may be necessary if there is coexisting sphincter damage.

D. *Crohn's fistula.* The management of Crohn's enterovaginal fistula depends largely on the site of the fistula and the presence of rectal disease. Hence, the first step is to establish the anatomy of the fistula by careful clinical assessment, imaging, and sigmoidoscopy for rectovaginal fistula and by contrast radiology for fistulous disease in the pouch of Douglas.

D1. Fistulas from bowel in the pouch of Douglas to the posterior fornix usually arise from a loop of involved small bowel or from the sigmoid colon. The treatment is either by ileal resection if the fistula is from the small bowel or by subtotal colectomy if the fistula is from the large bowel. Proximal fecal diversion may be necessary if a primary anastomosis is undertaken particularly in the presence of sepsis.

D2. If the fistula is rectovaginal and if the rectum is involved, repair is doomed to failure. These patients are usually hopelessly incontinent with perianal soiling; hence urgent defunction is frequently necessary by loop ileostomy. In a few patients no further procedure is required, but in the majority a proctocolectomy is eventually accepted by the patient. Indeed, proctocolectomy may be advised as an elective procedure for a rectovaginal fistula in Crohn's disease.

D3. Low anorectal fistulas to the vagina may give rise to few symptoms; if so, they should be left alone since surgical treatment may result in poor healing and cause more trouble than was experienced by the original fistula. If the fistula is symptomatic and the rectum is uninvolved, a mucosal advancement flap may be successful but healing is often slow, recurrent fistulas are not uncommon, and many surgeons now advise a proximal loop ileostomy to minimize the risk of sepsis and breakdown of the repair. For very low fistulas, seton division may be an alternative method of treatment.

E. *Neoplastic rectovaginal fistulas* usually represent advanced disease. If the fistula is due to gynecological malignancy, preoperative radiotherapy and radical extended hysterectomy with proctectomy is the only prospect of cure. Sphincter-saving resection may be possible, but primary anastomosis may be ill advised in advanced disease or after previous radiotherapy. A similar approach is used in adenocarcinoma of the rectum, but in some cases primary protected coloanal anastomosis with radical extended hysterectomy is feasible.

F. *Radiation of rectovaginal fistulas* requires very careful assessment. The first priority is to ensure that there is no recurrence of the original malignancy; thus, careful examinations under anesthetic (EUA) and biopsy are absolutely vital. Assessment of the anatomy of the fistula is again crucial since fistulas complicating long-standing radiotherapy are complex, often involving the small bowel as well as the rectovaginal septum. Detailed radiologic evaluation is essential. The principles of operation are to resect the damaged bowel causing the fistula and to anastomose bowel outside the field of radiation. For irradiation of rectovaginal fistula the best treatment option is a sleeve colo-anal anastomosis with a covering loop ileostomy.

G. *Postoperative rectovaginal fistula* usually arise from an anastomotic break-down. Factors implicated in these are pelvis sepsis, ischemia of the bowel or vagina, operative trauma to the vagina, entrapment of the vagina in staple instruments, and previous radiotherapy.

H. Postoperative rectovaginal fistulas need careful evaluation to define their anatomy. Hence, contrast radiology and endoscopy are generally essential. However, if the fistula is due to an early anastomotic breakdown, it may be prudent to divert the fecal stream first and to drain any coexisting sepsis.

I. In many early postoperative rectovaginal fistulas, drainage and diversion alone may achieve complete healing. Hence, no further therapy is necessary.

J. If the fistula persists, radiology, endoscopy, and biopsy will be essential to define the anatomy of the track, exclude any persistent underlying disease, as well as to define the anatomy of the tract and any involvement of other viscera in the pelvis.

J1. For postoperative fistulas from bowel in the pouch of Douglas, treatment will involve resecting the leaking anastomosis, clearing any pelvic sepsis, and constructing a new anastomosis with the rectum at a lower level; almost always a covering stoma will be necessary.

J2. For postoperative fistulas through the rectovaginal septum, resection and coloanal anastomosis with a covering stoma is advised.

J3. For postoperative fistulas above or through the sphincters, as may be encountered in pouch vaginal fistula, seton fistulotomy or advancement flap offers the best prospect of cure.

BIBLIOGRAPHY

1. Cuthbertson AM: Resection and pull-through for rectovaginal fistula. *World J Surg* 10:228–236, 1986.

2. Givel JC, Hawker P, Allan RN, and Alexander-Williams J: Enterovaginal fistulas associated with Crohn's disease. *Surg Gynecol Obstet* 155:494–496, 1982.

3. Heyen F, Winsler MC, Andrews H, Alexander-Williams J, and Keighley MRB: Vaginal fistulas in Crohn's disease. *Dis Colon Rectum* 32:379–383, 1989.

4. Hoexter B, Kabow SB, and Moseson MD: Transanal rectovaginal fistula repair. *Dis Colon Rectum* 28:572–575, 1985.

5. Hudson CN: Acquired fistulae between the intestine and the vagina. *Ann R Coll Surg Engl* 46:20–40, 1970.

6. Rex JC Jr, Khubchandani IT: Rectovaginal fistula: complication of low anterior resection. *Dis Colon Rectum* 35:354–356, 1992.

7. Rothenberger DA and Goldberg SM: The management of rectovaginal fistulae. *Surg Clin North Am* 63:61–79, 1983.

8. Scott NA, Nair A, and Hughes LE: Anovaginal and rectovaginal fistula in patients with Crohn's disease. *Br J Surg* 79:1379–1380, 1992.

See also Chapters 25, 26, 27, 78 and 79.

SECTION 6B

Small Bowel Conditions
Neoplastic

CHAPTER 81

Small Bowel Polyps

Witold A. Kmiot, M.S., F.R.C.S.

Refer to Algorithm 81–1

A. A polyp is a macroscopic description used for any circumscribed tumor or elevation, irrespective of its nature, that projects above the surface of flat, normal mucous membrane as either a raised mass or a pedunculated swelling.

B. Patients may present with intermittent abdominal pain, abdominal distension, and blood loss per rectum.

C. Radiologic imaging of the small intestine using contrast media such as barium may be useful. However, early tumors may be submucosal, and thus detection may be difficult until the lesion is large. Overlapping small bowel loops may also present diagnostic difficulties.

D. A harmartoma is a tumor-like but primarily nonneoplastic malformation of congenital maldevelopment characterized by an abnormal mixture of tissues indigenous to the area. An excess of one of more of these lesions may be evidence of an underlying developmental abnormality that may manifest at birth or by excessive growth in the postnatal period. The developmental area may involve epithelial and connective tissue or both.

E. Hyperplastic polyps are rare. However, in the duodenum they may be associated with inflammation due to peptic ulcer, while in the distal small bowel, they occur with *Campylobacter enteritis*.

F. Inflammatory polyps are usually associated with Crohn's disease but have also been associated with bacterial overgrowth in blind loops of small intestine.

G. Small bowel polyps are microscopically the same as colonic polyps. They tend to be rare in the small bowel, but most are found around the ampulla of Vater.

H. The classic Peutz–Jehgers syndrome has three components: gastrointestinal polyps, oral pigmentation, and autosomal dominant inheritance. However, penetrance can be variable and various forms of the syndrome exist. Polyps can develop anywhere in the gut but the duodenum predominates.

I. Hyperplastic polyps are usually multiple and may range from 1 to 10 mm in diameter.

J. Polyps in Crohn's disease may be associated with either disease activity or quiescence. Associated histologic features such as small bowel ulceration and

429

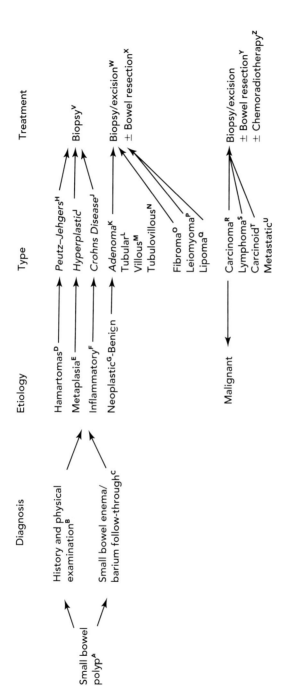

Small bowel polyps

Diagnosis

History and physical examination[B]

Small bowel enema/barium follow-through[C]

Small bowel polyp[A]

Etiology

Hamartomas[D]

Metaplasia[E]

Inflammatory[F]

Neoplastic[G]-Benign

Malignant

Type

Peutz–Jehgers[H]

Hyperplastic[I]

Crohns Disease[J]

Adenoma[K]
Tubular[L]
Villous[M]
Tubulovillous[N]

Fibroma[O]
Leiomyoma[P]
Lipoma[Q]

Carcinoma[R]
Lymphoma[S]
Carcinoid[T]
Metastatic[U]

Treatment

Biopsy[V]

Biopsy/excision[W]
± Bowel resection[X]

Biopsy/excision
± Bowel resection[Y]
± Chemoradiotherapy[Z]

ALGORITHM 81–1

narrowing are invariably present. Alternative diagnoses are polyps associated with rare conditions such as eosinophilic granulomatosis and histiocytosis-x syndrome.

K. Most small bowel adenomas are single (solitary). They may be pedunculated and cause bleeding or obstruction.

L. Tubular adenomas consist of epithelial tubules separated by lamina propria. The overlying mucosa and submucosa are normal.

M. The macroscopic appearance results from marked folding of the mucosal surface. Each fold consists of a core of lamina propria and epithelial cells.

N. Tubulovillous polyps are a mixed pattern of polyp. Malignant potential and dysplasia are related to the size rather than individual histologic type of polyp.

O. Fibromas may occur as a single inflammatory fibroid polyp. They are macroscopically sessile and often pedunculated in appearance. There may be associations with neurogenic tumors such as ganglioneuromas and neurofibromas. However, these lesions are extremely rare.

P. Leiomyomas are associated much more often with cavitation rather than polyp formation.

Q. Lipomas are fairly uniformly distributed in the small bowel. Macroscopically they can arise from submucosal adipose tissue or serosal fat.

R. Adenocarcinomas from small bowel form <1% of all gastrointestinal carcinomas. They are slightly more common than are small intestinal endocrine cell tumors and are distributed more or less evenly throughout the small bowel. Macroscopically most of the growths are annular and constricting, but a few are polypoid or fungating. Prognosis is poor, with a mean 20% 5-year survival.

S. Lymphomas, although rare in Western populations, account for about 20% of all small bowel malignancies. Macroscopically tumors often protrude into the bowel lumen. Bulky polypoid masses are often associated with secondary mucosal ulceration. (See Algorithm 82–1 on lymphoma.)

T. Carcinoid is the most common tumor of the endocrine cell type. There may well be systemic symptoms in the presence of liver metastases such as diarrhea, facial flushing, and right-sided heart lesions. Malignant potential is usually low in these slow-growing tumors.

U. Metastatic deposits of carcinoma in the small bowel are uncommon. However, they have been reported from primary tumors in bronchus, adrenal, ovary, stomach, and large bowel. The majority of these deposits are multiple, discrete, and localized to the submucosa.

V. Histologic diagnosis is usually all that is necessary for hamartomas, metaplasias, and inflammatory polyps.

W. Depending on the size and site, small tumors that are entirely benign can be adequately treated by simple biopsy with histological diagnosis.

X. Large polyps, especially adenomas associated with dysplasia, should be excised either in toto or associated with bowel resection.

Y. Biopsy of carcinoma, lymphomas, and carcinoids may be all that is possible in the presence of disseminated disease. Bowel resection with radical local lymph node clearance is preferable if the tumor is curable.

Z. Chemoradiotherapy is primarily the treatment for small bowel lymphoma after the establishment of tissue diagnosis, especially in the presence of widespread small bowel involvement.

BIBLIOGRAPHY

1. Bouchier IAD, Allan RN, Hodgson HJ, et al: The small intestine. Bouchier IAD, et al (eds). In *Textbook of Gastroenterology*. London: Bailliere Tindall, 1984, pp 615–633.

2. Harding Rains AJ, Mann CV: Small and large intestines. In Mann CV, Russell RCG (eds). *Bailey & Love's Short Practice of Surgery*. London: Chapman & Hall, 1992, pp 1027–1064.

3. Morson BC, Dawson IMP (eds). Small intestine. In *Gastrointestinal Pathology*. London: Blackwell Scientific Publications, 1979, pp 211–448.

See also Chapters 45, 66, 67, 76 and 82.

CHAPTER 82

Intestinal Lymphoma

Michael M. Krausz, M.D. and Petachia Reissman, M.D.

Refer to Algorithm 82-1.

A. Lymphoma of the gastrointestinal tract is the most common type of primary extranodal lymphoma, accounting for 4–12% of all non-Hodgkin's lymphoma. Gastrointestinal (GI) lymphomas are a heterogenous group of tumors with variable clinical and pathologic features. In the Western population, the majority (50–60%) of GI lymphomas occur in the stomach and 20–30% arise in the small bowel. This finding is in contrast to GI lymphomas in the Middle East, where the small bowel is the site of origin in more than half of the patients. In general, malignant tumors of the small bowel are far less common than are those affecting the colon and stomach. Primary small bowel lymphomas currently constitute less than 2% of all GI malignancies. In adults, lymphomas represent 10–40% of all the small bowel malignant tumors, and are third in frequency after adenocarcinoma and carcinoid. Conversely, in children < 10 years of age, lymphoma is the most common small bowel tumor. On the basis of clinical findings, small bowel lymphoma may be classified as either Western-type primary small intestinal lymphoma (PSIL) or immunoproliferative small intestinal disease (IPSID), Mediterranean type. Several features are in sharp contrast between these two types of intestinal lymphomas. The most important difference is the pattern of involvement of the small bowel. The Western-type PSIL is usually localized and most frequently involves short segments of ileum. Consequently, patients commonly present with abdominal pain and obstructive symptoms. Conversely, in IPSID related disorders, long loops of proximal small bowel are involved by diffuse mucosal infiltrate, clinically manifested by the triad of abdominal pain, diarrhea, and malabsorption. The histologic appearance of the tumor and its pathogenesis and pattern of involvement in the small bowel are also in sharp contrast. In IPSID, a spectrum of conditions can be observed. At one end is an innocent-looking plasma cell hyperplasia of the small bowel mucosa; and at the other end of the spectrum, a highly malignant lymphoma. The tumor is usually confined to the bowel and its mesentery and adjacent organs. Systemic involvement of the liver, spleen, and peripheral lymph nodes is extremely rare. In Western-type

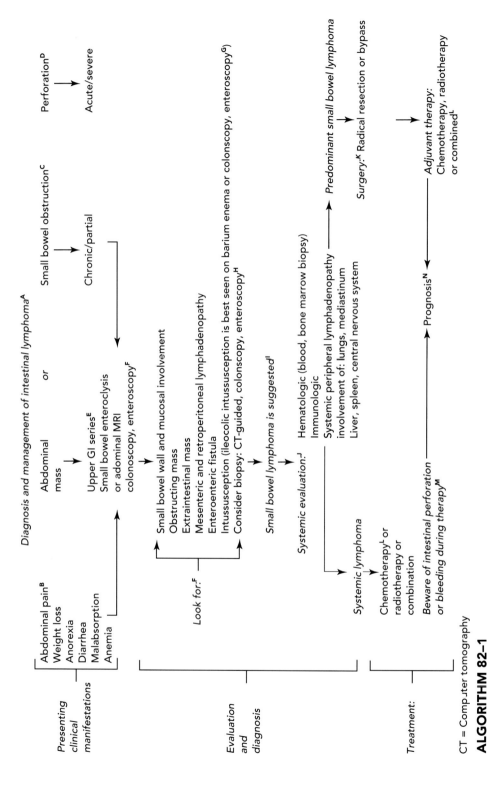

Diagnosis and management of intestinal lymphoma[A]

Presenting clinical manifestations
- Abdominal pain[B]
- Weight loss
- Anorexia
- Diarrhea
- Malabsorption
- Anemia

Abdominal mass → or → Small bowel obstruction[C] → Chronic/partial

Perforation[D] → Acute/severe

Evaluation and diagnosis

Upper GI series[E]
Small bowel enteroclysis or abdominal MRI
colonoscopy, enteroscopy[F]

Look for:[F]
- Small bowel wall and mucosal involvement
- Obstructing mass
- Extraintestinal mass
- Mesenteric and retroperitoneal lymphadenopathy
- Enteroenteric fistula
- Intussusception (ileocolic intussusception is best seen on barium enema or colonscopy, enteroscopy[G])
- Consider biopsy: CT-guided, colonscopy, enteroscopy[H]

Small bowel lymphoma is suggested[I]

Systemic evaluation:[J]
- Hematologic (blood, bone marrow biopsy)
- Immunologic
- Systemic peripheral lymphadenopathy
- Systemic involvement of: lungs, mediastinum
  Liver, spleen, central nervous system

Systemic lymphoma → Predominant small bowel lymphoma

Treatment:

Chemotherapy[L] or radiotherapy or combination

Surgery:[K] Radical resection or bypass

Prognosis[N]

Adjuvant therapy:
Chemotherapy, radiotherapy or combined[L]

Beware of intestinal perforation or bleeding during therapy[M]

CT = Computer tomography

ALGORITHM 82–1

434

lymphoma, secondary involvement of the spleen, liver, and extraabdominal lymph nodes is common. A marked contrast between the clinical, epidemiologic, and pathologic features of IPSID and the Western types of PSIL was also demonstrated. IPSID is highly prevalent in low socioeconomical segments of the population in third-world countries, implicating environmental factors in the pathogenesis. Peak incidence of IPSID is in the second and third decades of life, while in the Western-type PSIL, there is no specific type of socioeconomic distribution, and the age distribution is bimodal: below the age of 10 years and in the fifth and sixth decades. No environmental or constitutional risk factors have been identified, except for the congenital occurrence of the disease and its occurrence in immunodeficient patients such as those with celiac disease or AIDS.

B. *Malignant lymphoma of the rectum* is extremely rare and is usually secondary to disseminated disease. Only a few cases of primary lymphoma of the rectum have been reported so far. On the basis of the limited experience, the evaluation and management should be similar to that of small bowel lymphoma with surgery (abdominoperineal or anterior resection) reserved for localized lesions, followed by chemotherapy and radiotherapy. The overall *presenting clinical manifestations* may include various gastrointestinal symptoms including abdominal pain, anorexia, diarrhea, malabsorption, anemia, and weight loss.

C. Other, more specific, manifestations include an abdominal mass or acute small bowel obstruction.

D. Rarely, in some patients with high-grade T-cell lymphoma, tumor perforation, and peritonitis have been observed.

E. In the majority of cases, however, *initial evaluation* is possible and should consist of: upper GI series, small bowel enteroclysis, abdominal computerized tomography (CT), or magnetic resonant imaging (MRI). Colonoscopy and/or enteroscopy may also be considered.

F. Suggestive findings of small bowel lymphoma include bowel wall and mucosal tumor involvement, obstructing lesion, extraintestinal mass, enteroenteric fistula, intussusception (small bowel into small bowel or ileocolic), and mesenteric or retroperitoneal lymphadenopathy.

G. Is cases of suspected ileocolic intussusception, a barium enema or colonoscopy are the procedures of choice.

H. The diagnosis may be confirmed by CT-guided biopsies of mesenteric or retroperitoneal mass or by biopsies during colonoscopy/enteroscopy.

I. When small bowel lymphoma is diagnosed or highly suspected, a *systemic evaluation* to exclude systemic disease with secondary intestinal involvement is undertaken.

J. This evaluation should focus on potential involvement of peripheral lymph nodes, liver, spleen, lungs, mediastinum, central nervous system (CNS), and bone marrow. Thus the additional evaluation should include chest and brain CT or MRI, lumbar puncture, and hematologic evaluation of bone marrow (BM) and peripheral blood. Other tissue biopsies may be indicated according to the findings. Immunohistochemical analysis with a panel of antibodies may be used for classification of intestinal lymphoma according to the updated Kiel European Association of Hematology schema, to B-cell or T-cell origin with high- or low-grade malignancy (Table 82–1). HIV testing should also be performed at this stage.

TABLE 82–1 CLASSIFICATION OF GUT LYMPHOMA BY THE UPDATED KIEL
SCHEME

B Cell	T Cell

Low-grade
  Low-grade lymphoma of MALT[a]
    including immunocytoma
  Alpha-chain disease
  Centroblastic/centrocytic
  Centrocytic with MLP[b]
  Plasmacytic
	Low-grade
	  Pleomorphic small cell

High-grade
  Centroblastic
  Burkitt's lymphoma
  Lymphoblastic
  Immunoblastic
  Large cell anoplastic
  Unclassifiable
	High-grade
	  Pleomorphic medium cell and
	  large cell
	
	  Immunoblastic
	  Large cell anoplastic
	  Unclassifiable

[a] MALT: mucosa-associated lymphoid tissue.
[b] MLP: malignant lymphomatous polyposis.

K. *Treatment options* depend on the evaluation findings. If the lymphoma is confined to the intestine or has only local lymphadenopathy, radical surgical resection should be performed. In advanced tumors, palliative surgery such as intestinal bypass, debulking, or stoma creation may be indicated. Debulking resection in advanced tumors may enhance the response to chemotherapy and/or radiotherapy and decrease the risk of bowel perforation or bleeding due to tumor necrosis during the treatment. Surgery may also be performed as a diagnostic procedure if previous evaluation failed to reveal accurate diagnosis. The recently introduced laparoscopic technique for exploration and biopsies may become an increasingly performed diagnostic procedure for selected cases. Although it may offer several advantages such as decreased postoperative pain, improved cosmesis, shorter hospitalization, and faster return to normal activity, the role of laparoscopic resection for intestinal lymphoma has not yet been established. Obviously, in cases of acute intestinal obstruction, perforation or bleeding surgery is performed without delay, and the final diagnosis of intestinal lymphoma is made intra or postoperatively. If systemic lymphoma is diagnosed, initial chemotherapy or combination of chemo and radiotherapy are indicated.

L. Surgery, either curative or palliative, should be followed by chemotherapy or combination chemoradiotherapy. Several series have shown an advantage of the combination modality.

M. However, in the presence of a symptomatic enteric fistula or intussusception secondary to systemic lymphoma, surgery is indicated prior to treatment. During the adjuvant treatment, complications such as bowel perforation or bleeding, which demand immediate surgery, should be anticipated in 10–30% of the patients.

N. The prognosis of intestinal lymphoma depends on the stage, histologic grading, and localization of the disease. Terminal ileal lesions are associated with better prognosis than are proximal jejunal lesions. Advanced-stage, high-grade, multiple intestinal tumors and perforation are all considered poor prognostic factors. Cell type (B or T) and tumor size do not have a role in long-term survival. Overall, 10-year survival in patients who underwent radical surgery for localized disease followed by adjuvant chemotherapy may reach 75%, whereas a 20–50% 5-year survival may be expected in more advanced cases after palliative debulking.

BIBLIOGRAPHY

1. Al-Mondhiry H: Primary lymphomas of the small intestine: East–West contrast. *Am J Hematol* 22:89–105, 1986.
2. Devine RM, Beart RW Jr, Wolff BG: Malignant lymphoma of the rectum. *Dis Colon Rectum* 29:821–824, 1986.
3. Domizio P, Owen RA, Sheperd NA, et al: Primary lymphoma of the small intestine. A clinicopathological study of 119 cases. *Am J Surg Pathol* 17:429–442, 1993.
4. Gospodarowicz MK, Sutcliffe SB, Clark RM, et al: Outcome analysis of localized gastrointestinal lymphoma treated with surgery and postoperative irradiation. *Int J Radiat Oncol Biol Phys* 19:1351–1355, 1990.
5. Lymphomas of the small intestine. In Bouchier IAD, Allan RN, Hodgson HJF, et al (eds): *Textbook of Gastroenterology*. Philadelphia: Bailliere Tindall, 1984; p 465.
6. Rambaud JC: Small intestinal lymphomas and alpha-chain disease. *Clin Gastroenterol* 12:743–766, 1983.
7. ReMine SG, Braasch JW: Gastric and small bowel lymphoma. *Surg Clin NAM* 66:713–722, 1986.
8. Stanofeld AG, Diebold J, Kafanci Y, et al: Updated Kiel classification for lymphomas. *Lancet* 1:292–293, 1988.
9. Stewart AK, Shepherd FA, Goss PE, et al: Gastrointestinal non-Hodgkin's lymphoma. *Leuk Lymph* 4:167–176, 1991.
10. Tedeschi L, Romanelli A, Dallavalle G, et al: Stages I and II non-Hodgkin's lymphoma of the gastrointestinal tract. *J Clin Gastroenterol* 18:99–104, 1994.
11. Weingrad DN, Decosse JJ, Scherlock P, et al: Primary gastrointestinal lymphoma: a 30 year review. *Cancer* 49:1258–1265, 1982.
12. Wexner SD, Cohen SM, Johansen OB, et al: Laparoscopic colorectal surgery: a prospective assessment and current perspective. *Br. J. Surg* 80:1602–1605, 1993.

See also Chapters 14 and 38.

CHAPTER 83

Carcinoma

Graham L. Newstead, M.D.

Refer to Algorithm 83–1.

A. Small intestinal cancers constitute less than 5% of gastrointestinal cancers; 90% occur within 20 cm of either side of the ligament of Treitz. Adult celiac disease demonstrates an increased risk of adenocarcinoma, as well as lymphoma, which tends to occur in the jejunum. There may be a (rare) genetic predisposition. Gardner's syndrome carries a significant risk of dysplasia becoming invasive in the small intestine as well as the duodenum. Crohn's disease may develop malignant change in excluded segments, adjacent to or in chronic fistulas and at stricture sites in long-standing disease. Cancers are more prevalent in the terminal ileum but may be remote from overtly active disease. Bypassed loops make recognition difficult; symptoms of malignancy and continuing inflammatory activity may be similar. Careful inspection of mucosa at strictureplasty sites is essential and frozen section may be necessary. Peutz–Jegher syndrome has a low risk (2–3%) of malignancy in what are otherwise regarded as harmartomata.

B. Adenocarcinoma of the small intestine may be associated with other gastrointestinal carcinomas and may be multicentric. Most are of primary epithelial origin but may be metastatic. Variations in cell type include adenosquamous, squamous, and adenocarcinoid. Tumors of all the mural histologic elements are reported.

C. Symptoms may be absent. Patients with chronic disease carrying known predisposition should be regarded as at risk.

D. Symptoms may be nonspecific and thus delay diagnosis, resulting in anemia, poor nutrition, and weight loss.

E. A mass may be present without obstruction. It may be part of an associated process such as Crohn's disease.

F. Melena or occasionally bright rectal bleeding may occur, although rapid hemorrhage is uncommon and chronic anemia is most likely.

G. Obstruction (or obstructive symptoms) is (are) the most frequent acute presentation.

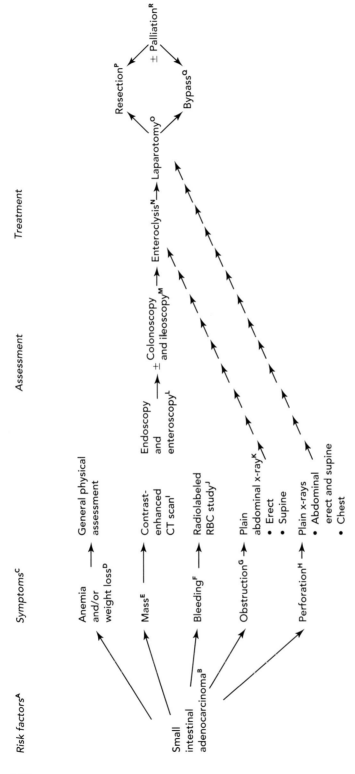

Risk factors[A]

Symptoms[C]

Assessment

Treatment

Small intestinal adenocarcinoma[B]

Anemia and/or weight loss[D] → General physical assessment

Mass[E] → Contrast-enhanced CT scan[I]

Bleeding[F] → Radiolabeled RBC study[J]

Obstruction[G] → Plain abdominal x-ray[K]
- Erect
- Supine

Perforation[H] → Plain x-rays
- Abdominal erect and supine
- Chest

Endoscopy and enteroscopy[L] → ± Colonoscopy and ileoscopy[M] → Enteroclysis[N] → Laparotomy[O]

Resection[P]

Bypass[Q]

± Palliation[R]

CT = Computer tomography
RBC = Red blood cell

ALGORITHM 83–1

H. Perforation is uncommon, the diagnosis is unsuspected, and identification is made at laparotomy immediately after resuscitation.

I. A computerized tomography (CT) scan may identify the organ of origin, associated lymphadenopathy, and the possibility of distant metastasis. Contrast enhancement may aid delineation, particularly in the absence of other known intestinal disease.

J. Bleeding > 0.5 mL/min may be assessed by ^{99}Tc-labeled red cells. Blood loss is usually slower, however.

K. High jejunal obstruction may produce no fluid levels. The absence of previous abdominal surgery should arouse suspicion.

L. Gastroscopy will exclude gastroduodenal pathology as far as the third part of the duodenum. Enteroscopy may be available and allow more distal assessment.

M. Similarly, colonoscopy will exclude colonic pathology and allow terminal ileoscopy.

N. Enteroclysis (or small bowel enema) via a nasoduodenal tube allows measured barium instillations to provide high-quality air-contrast studies of the small intestine, which are preferable to single contrast follow-through studies and much more accurate.

O. Demonstration of a tumor or a high index of suspicion warrants laparotomy. Laparoscopy is, at present, an imperfect technique of complete small intestinal assessment due to its length and mobility and to the lack of tactile sensation.

P. Resection is usually possible and should involve full mesenteric clearance to include lymph nodes. Mobilization may be required for the third and fourth parts of duodenum and ileocolic resection for tumors of the terminal ileum. End-to-end anastomosis is usual. Late presentation has a poor prognosis, but wide nodal clearance provides good staging information.

Q. Bypass may be necessary for a fixed obstructing tumor, but resection is generally preferable both for local tumor control and to prevent anemia.

R. There is no proven benefit from adjuvant chemotherapy, and radiotherapy is contraindicated in the treatment of adenocarcinoma of the small intestine except for bypassed duodenal disease. Palliative chemotherapy may have an empirical place in selected patients.

BIBLIOGRAPHY

1. Greenstein AJ, Sachar DB: Surveillance of Crohn's disease for carcinoma. In Seitz HK, Simanowski VA, Wright NA (eds): *Colorectal Cancer, from Pathogenesis to Prevention.* New York: Springer-Verlag, 1989.

2. Lillemoe KD, Cameron JL: Small bowel tumour. In Fazio VW (ed): *Current Therapy in Colon and Rectal Surgery.* Philadelphia: Decker, 1990.

3. Martin RG; Malignant tumours of the small intestine. *Surg Clin N Am* 66:779–785, 1986.

4. Stemmerman GN, Goodman MT, Nomura AM: Adenocarcinoma of the proximal small intestine. A marker for familial and multicentric cancer? *Cancer* 70:2766–2771, 1992.

See also Chapters 10, 11, 12A, 12B, 13, 14, 15, 67 and 76.

SECTION 7

Stomas

CHAPTER 84

Stomal Prolapse

John M. MacKeigan, M.D.

Refer to Algorithm 84–1.

A. Prolapse occurs in all forms of stomas including ileostomies, colostomies, urostomies, and continent urostomies. The incidence varies from 1% to 16%, and there seems to be little difference between colostomies and ileostomies in incidence, symptoms, or presentation.

B. Stomal prolapse may occur with or without parastomal hernias. While almost all hernias are external, some may be entirely subcutaneous with a normal fascial opening and no external prolapse evident.

C. The prolapse may be fixed or sliding or a combination of the two types with increasing prolapse with sitting or standing. The length and frequency of prolapse increases with obesity, obstructive pulmonary disease, ascites, and pregnancy.

D. Nonreducible prolapse may be asymptomatic or become progressive and painful, especially if the prolapse is more sudden, rather than the usual insidious process.

E. Most stomal prolapses cause cosmetic or pouch application problems as the bulging or prolapse increase. The enlarging stoma may lead to congestion, weeping of serous fluid, ulceration of the mucosa, or bleeding.

F. Incarceration may lead to some degree of obstruction or progress to ischemia. This usually leads to surgical therapy.

G. Nonoperative treatment includes reassurance and readjustment of the stoma equipment when it is asymptomatic. When congested and impending ischemia is evident, bed rest and close observation may be appropriate.

H. Operative therapy may include local or intraabdominal procedures and varies according to whether the stoma is an end or loop. An associated hernia requires repair either directly with relocation or insertion of a mesh to support the abdominal wall.

I. Local surgical therapy at the stoma site for end stomas includes circumscribing the stoma with advancement of the bowel and resection of the redundant bowel and reformation of the stoma.

445

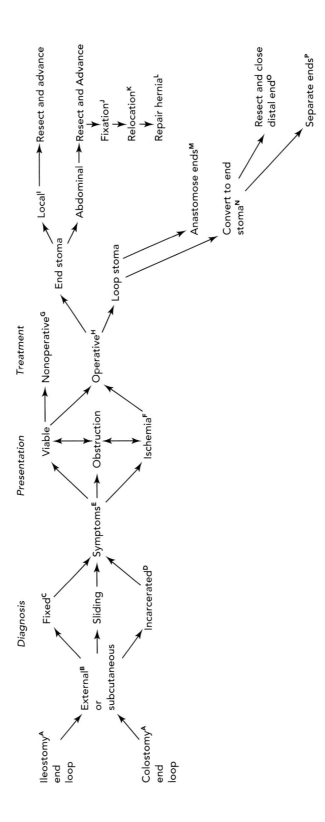

Stomal prolapse

Diagnosis *Presentation* *Treatment*

Ileostomy[A]
end
loop

Colostomy[A]
end
loop

External[B]
or
subcutaneous

Fixed[C]

Sliding

Incarcerated[D]

Symptoms[E]

Viable

Obstruction

Ischemia[F]

Nonoperative[G]

Operative[H]

End stoma

Loop stoma

Local[I] → Resect and advance

Abdominal → Resect and Advance

Fixation[J]

Relocation[K]

Repair hernia[L]

Anastomose ends[M]

Convert to end stoma[N]

Resect and close distal end[O]

Separate ends[P]

ALGORITHM 84–1

TABLE 84-1 PREVENTION OF STOMA PROLAPSE

Select proper site preoperatively
Select site through rectus muscle
Create opening admitting two fingers
Resect redundancy proximally
Fixate long portion of mesentery
Retroperitoneal placement (?)
Create proper stoma size
Utilize end or end-loop stoma for diversion
Minimize obesity

J. Internal fixation and resection of the redundant intestine with re-creation of the stoma is appropriate when relocation is not possible or when there is no associated hernia. Retroperitoneal placement of the distal intestine may have some advantage to reduce prolapse, as advocated by Goligher.
K. Relocation of the stoma to an appropriate alternate premarked site may be the best therapy for most significant prolapses. In general prolapse is better prevented than treated (Table 84-1).
L. Mesh closure of the associated hernia at the time of resection and reformation of the stoma may be necessary if an alternate site is inappropriate.
M. Loop stomas should be placed in continuity where possible.
N. Converting the loop stoma to an end stoma with resection and re-formation of the stoma is the treatment of choice.
O. Most loop stomas can be converted to end stomas by closing the distal end, introducing it into the abdomen, and developing an end stoma from the proximal limb.
P. Separating the limbs completely and developing an end stoma with a separated distal mucous fistula may be required when there is distal obstruction.

BIBLIOGRAPHY

1. Fazio VW: Complications of intestinal stomas. In Ferrari BT, Ray JE, Gathright JB (eds): *Complications of Colon and Rectal Prevention and Management*. Philadelphia: Saunders: 1985, pp 227–250.
2. Gordon PH, Nivatvongs S (eds): *Principles and Practice of Surgery for the Colon, Rectum, and Anus*. St. Louis: Quality Medical Publishing, 1992. p 873.
3. Nogueras JJ, Wexner SD: Stoma prolapse. In MacKeigan JM, Cataldo PA (eds): *Intestinal Stomas—Principles, Techniques and Management*. St. Louis: Quality Medical Publishing, 1993, pp 268–277.
4. Rubin MS, Bailey HR: Parastomal hernias. In MacKeigan JM, Cataldo PA (eds): *Intestinal Stomas—Principles, Techniques and Management*. St. Louis: Quality Medical Publishing, 1993, pp 245–267.
5. Wexner SD, Jagelman DG: J-ileostomy and split (loop end) ileostomy. In: Bauer JJ, Gorfine SR, Kroel I, Gelernt IM, Rubin P (eds): Colorectal surgery illustrated: A focused approach. New York: Mosby-Yearbook 1993, pp 289–294.
See also Chapters 14 and 38.

CHAPTER 85

Peristomal Hernias

Herand Abcarian, M.D.

Refer to Algorithm 85–1.

A. *Incidence.* Peristomal hernia is an incisional hernia that occurs at the site of an intestinal stoma. The true incidence is unclear, reflecting variations in types of stomas fashioned and length of follow-up. It is safe to say that if all stomas were followed up for at least 10 years, peristomal hernia would occur in 5–15% of the cases. Some authors suggest that the incidence approaches 50%. *Contributing factors* include systemic, intraoperative, and postoperative factors. In the former category are systemic factors, including obesity, advanced age, malignancy and malnutrition, steroid use, an increased intraabdominal pressure from ascites, obstructing uropathy and chronic obstructive pulmonary disease. The middle category are intraoperative factors including colonic stoma, large stomal incision, unplanned (urgent or emergent stomas), placement of stoma at or near present or previous laparatomy incision, and, most importantly, placement of stoma lateral to the rectus muscle. This latter factor accounts for higher incidence of peristomal hernia in end or loop colostomy as compared with end ileostomy or urostomy. In the latter category are postoperative factors including peristomal, incisional or intraabdominal infections, significant weight gain or loss, ascites, stomal prolapse, radiation therapy, and long-term survival of patients. Any bulge at the stoma site during standing, straining, or after a large meal should arouse suspicion. Any difficulty with management of the stoma such as irrigation, or appliance seal may indicate presence of hernia.

B. Physical examination should be undertaken after removing the appliance and with the patient supine, upright, and performing the Valsalva maneuver. Digital examination of the stoma with the patient changing or coughing allows the examiner to evaluate the fascial opening and peristomal subcutaneous tissues. The quality of peristomal skin and potential alternative stoma sites should also be assessed.

C. When the history suggests, but the physical examination does not reveal, a hernia, abdominal ultrasound and especially CT scan with oral contrast may be helpful. Up to 20% of paraileostomy hernias in one series were diagnosed only by CT scan of the abdomen.

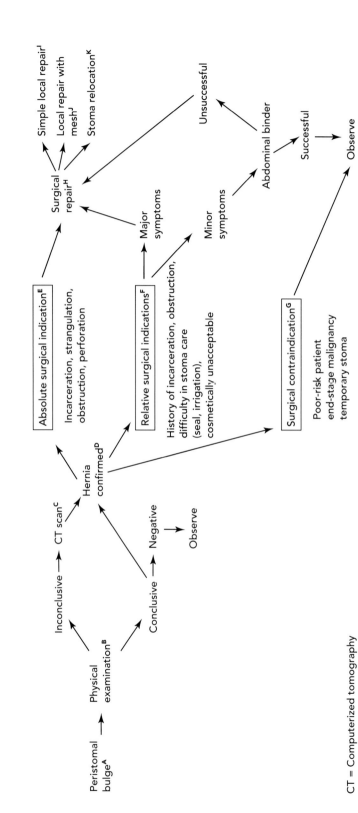

CT = Computerized tomography

ALGORITHM 85–1

D. *Conservative management.* All peristomal hernias need not be surgically repaired. Most hernias are well tolerated, and any asymptomatic or mildly symptomatic hernias are best left alone. A surgically designed abdominal binder fitted with a plastic ring over the stoma device may help keep the hernia reduced and the patient comfortable. Even in cases where surgical repair is indicated, the magnitude of the operation and its potential risk to the patient should be carefully evaluated. The overall incidence of surgical repair is 10–20% of paracolostomy and 50–70% for paraileostomy or paraurostomy hernias. *Operative indications* must be divided into absolute and relative.

E. *Absolute* surgical indications include incarceration, strangulation, obstruction, perforation, or irrigation-related fistulization. *Relative* surgical indications include a history of obstructive symptoms or incarceration, management problems with either the appliance seal or with irrigation, peristomal pain or ulceration, associated prolapse, stricture, retraction, or a cosmetically unacceptable appearance.

G. *Operative contraindications* include *absolute* contraindications such as a very-poor-risk patient or a patient with end-stage malignancy. *Relative* contraindications include severe associated disorders and recurrent or inoperable cancer associated with peritoneal spread, and ascites. In addition, it is seldom worthwhile to surgically correct a prolapsed temporary stoma. In this instance early stoma closure with concomitant defect repair is generally a superior option.

H. *Preoperative preparation* includes standard mechanical and antibiotic bowel preparation, perioperative intravenous antibiotics, and evaluation of patient by enterostomal therapist including marking alternative sites. It is generally best to have at least two alternative sites available. The *choice of operation* can be either a local repair, a local repair with mesh, or a stoma relocation.

I. Simple local repair can be effected with nonabsorbable fascial suture.

J. If a local repair is to be undertaken, mesh can also be placed either extrafascially, extraperitoneally, or intraperitoneally. In general, however, the best option in most patients who have failed conservative management is not local repair as the recurrence rates are very high.

K. Stoma relocation has the lowest recurrence rates than do either of the local repairs (with or without mesh). However, the technique requires a more extensive operation. In all cases of relocation a parastomal incision is made. Often enough redundancy exists that the bowel can then be tunnelled either blindly, or with laparoscopic assistance, to the new site. In some instances, however a formal laparatomy is required. Therefore all patients scheduled for stoma relocation should consent in advance to a possible laparotomy.

BIBLIOGRAPHY

1. Leslie D: The parastomal hernia. *Austral NZ J Surg* 51:485–486, 1981.
2. Marshall FF, Leadbetter WF, Dretler JP: Ileal conduit parastomal hernias. *J Urol* 114:40–42, 1975.

3. Rosin JD, Bonardi RA: Paracolostomy hernia repair with Marlex mesh: a new technique. *Dis Colon Rectum* 20:299–302, 1977.

4. Rubin MS, Bailey HR: Parastomal hernias. In McKeigan JM, Catalo PA (eds): *Intestinal Stomas: Principles, Techniques and Management*. St. Louis: Quality Medical Publishing, 1995, pp 245–267.

5. Sugerbaker PH: Peritoneal approach to prosthetic mesh repair of paracolostomy hernia. *Am Surg* 201:344–346, 1985.

6. Williams JG, Etherington R, Hayward MWJ, et al: Paraileostomy hernia: a clinical and radiological study. *Br J Surg* 77:1355–1357, 1990.

See also Chapters 76, 84 and 87.

CHAPTER 86

Stoma Retraction

Indru T. Khubchandani, M.D.

Refer to Algorithm 86–1.

A. Stoma retraction is secondary to either a poorly placed stoma or to tension. Ischemia, due to compromised blood supply in the mesentery or trimming the fat and appendices epiploica from the extruded bowel, will result in necrosis with subsequent retraction at the site of demarcation.

B. Excessive devascularization of the mesentery of the small bowel to facilitate eversion in preparation for ileostomy maturation will result in ischemia and retraction. The situation is common in obese patients with a thick abdominal wall and a short fat mesentery. In surgery following radiation, the combination of shortened mesentery and endarteritis predisposes to future complications.

C. The incidence of stoma retraction has been stated to be 1–6% in most series. In a review by Pearl et al. of a series of 197 complications in 610 patients with stoma construction, 26 (13.2%) patients were diagnosed with stoma retraction.

D. This complication is largely avoidable with careful surgical technique and preoperative planning.

E. Location of the stoma by an enterostomal therapist or a trained physician is of paramount importance. Avoidance of skin fold creases, bony prominences, scars, and location at a flat, smooth surface is important.

F. The bowel should be adequately mobilized, and its vascularity must be preserved. The opening in the abdominal wall should be wide enough to accommodate the intended prolapsing bowel. It is a good practice to have several centimeters of bowel left protruding through the opening for subsequent excision and primary maturation *after closure of the abdomen.* Trimming of fat and appendices epiploica is unnecessary and detrimental to blood supply. A good, healthy, pink bowel *beyond the skin level* is mandatory. Suturing of the seromuscular layer to the fascia or elsewhere does not prevent retraction and should be avoided.

G. *Diagnosis and treatment.* Early retraction may be noticed in the immediate postoperative period. In this setting the colostomy retracts into the subcutaneous layer. If primary maturation is not performed or the tension is excessive, then the bowel may retract into the peritoneal cavity, necessitating

453

Stoma retraction

Prevention	Diagnosis	Evaluation	Treatment

Prevention

Avoid tension[A]

Don't excise fat or epiploic appendages[B]

Ensure adequate blood supply[C]

Mature stoma[F]

Select proper site: avoid skin folds, scars, bony prominences[E]

Preoperative consultation with enterostomal therapist[D]

Diagnosis

Early[G]
- Ischemia; determine level: full thickness?
- Early postoperative[D] retraction

Late[H]
- Dimpled recessed stoma with
- Associated stenosis
- Severe retraction
- With Parastomal Hernia

Evaluation
- Digital exam; endoscopy: Doppler?
- Retracted colostomy
- Obesity
- Unable to perform digital exam
- Invisible colostomy between skin folds

Treatment
- Partial thickness above fascia → Observe
- Full thickness below peritoneum → Operative and refashion or relocate stoma → Success
- Reduce weight; appliance with convex faceplate[I]
- Revision (office local anesthetic)[J] | Failure
- Laparotomy relocation[K] | Failure → Success

ALGORITHM 86–1

454

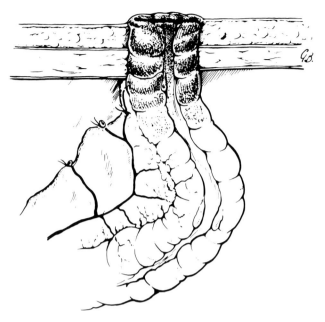

FIGURE 86–1 Pathogenesis of ishemia.

immediate laparotomy. More commonly, the retraction is due to the slough of the terminal portion of the gut (Fig. 86–1). When ischemia is suspected in a dusky looking bowel, it is important to differentiate mucosal partial ischemia from full-thickness devascularization; the level of demarcation is important. Necrosis extending proximal to the fascia obviously has much more serious consequences. The diagnosis may be made by digital rectal examination or insertion of a test tube. Endoscopy, Doppler evaluation, or vital dye study such as fluorescein may also be of help. The ischemia is mostly submucosal requiring observation unless early black necrotic bowel is recognized.

H. Late retraction presents as dimpled or recessed stoma, usually in an obese patient. It is often associated with stenosis, and the examiner is generally unable to insert the index finger into the stoma.

I. Use of an appropriate appliance with convex faceplate and a tight belt will make the stoma more manageable. Cohesive seals (Eakin®) provide further padding to the appliance.

J. When the stenotic element is more pronounced, a simple office procedure with local anesthesia (Fig. 86–2) may help alleviate the problem. A tangential incision from the mucocutaneous junction is made at the right lateral and/or left lateral site down to the subcutaneous tissue. (Fig. 86–3). Full thickness of the separated bowel is mobilized (Fig. 86–4) and sutured to the skin edges at the raised site of the incision (Fig. 86–5). This method is simple, effective, and rapid.

K. When the stoma is buried between heavy skin folds and is almost "invisible," causing much leakage around the appliance, a laparotomy is necessary. Mobilization of the bowel and relocation of the stoma is generally necessary. Retraction of the stoma is avoidable: It is important that careful attention be paid to site selection and construction. Similarly if local revision either fails or is inappropriate, a laparotomy with relocation should be offered.

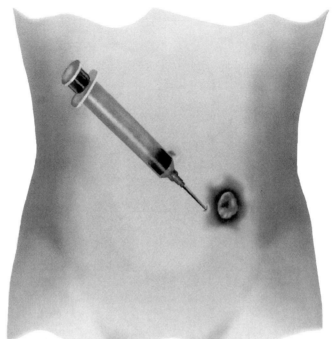

FIGURE 86–2 Infiltration of local anesthesia.

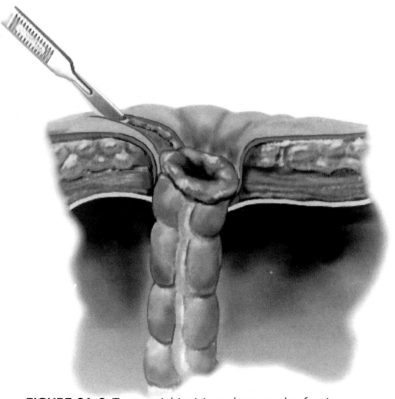

FIGURE 86–3 Tangential incision, deep to the fascia.

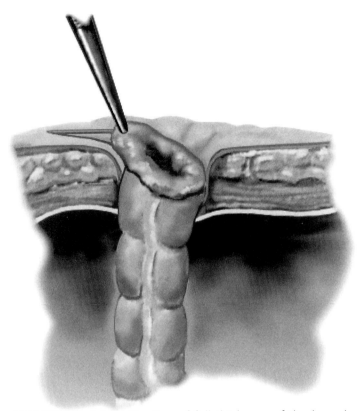

FIGURE 86–4 Mobilization of full thickness of the bowel.

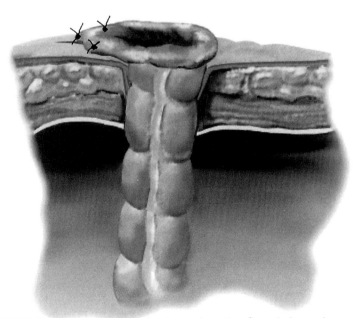

FIGURE 86–5 Suture of the bowel to the flared skin edges.

BIBLIOGRAPHY

1. Birnbaum W, Ferrier P: Complications of abdominal colostomy. *Am J Surg* 83:64–67, 1952.
2. Burns FJ: Complications of colostomy. *Dis Colon Rectum* 13:448–450, 1970.
3. MacKeigan J, Cataldo PA (eds): *Intestinal Stomas.* St. Louis: Quality Medical Publishing, 1993.
4. Mollitt DL, Malangoni MA, Balantine TVN, et al: Colostomy complications in children. *Arch Surg* 115:455–458, 1980.
5. Wexner SD, Jagelman DG. J-ileostomy and split ileostomy. In Bauer JJ, Gorfine SR, Kreel I, et al. (eds): *Colorectal Surgery Illustrated: A Focused Approach.* New York: Mosby Year Book, 1993, pp 289–294.

See also Chapters 62, 76, 86 and 87.

CHAPTER 87

Peristomal Skin Complications

Mary Lou Boyer, B.S., R.N., C.E.T.N.

Refer to Algorithm 87–1.

A. *Contact dermatitis* refers to inflammation of the skin as a result of contact with an external agent such as stool, urine, pastes, solvents, soaps or deodorants. This problem may involve a chemical irritant or an allergic reaction.

B. *Chemical irritant contact dermatitis* is the most common peristomal skin complication and is often due to poor fitting or loosening of the pouching system, which allows seepage of urine or fecal drainage onto the skin.

C. When left in contact with skin for prolonged periods of time, these agents may cause erythema, erosion, or ulcers, such contact is accompanied by itching, burning, or pain. Severe skin erosion can occur after only a few hours of contact. Once the skin is irritated, chemical products used for ostomy care, including mild soaps, may maintain or potentiate the injury.

D. Treatment for chemical irritant contact dermatitis must begin with determining the cause. One must check for peristomal fistulas and evaluate the pouching system and individual technique. Refit the patient into the proper pouching system for abdominal contour and cut to stoma shape and size. Next gently wash the skin with warm water and allow it to air-dry. Dust skin with skin barrier powder and/or skin sealant, prior to applying pouch. Even a mild skin irritation must be treated promptly to prevent serious consequences.

E. Epidermal hyperplasia, which is thickened epithelium with a grayish white warty appearance, may result from chronic prolonged contact with stool or urine.

F. This disorder is usually treated with $\frac{1}{2}$-strength vinegar or acetic acid soaks to soften the area for better faceplate application. Severe hyperplasia may require surgical debridement and possibly the use of a nonadherent pouching system until reepithelialization occurs. Relocation of the stoma may be necessary.

G. *Allergic contact dermatitis.* A person may be or become sensitive to a part of the appliance or any other product used for the care of the ostomy. Allergic

459

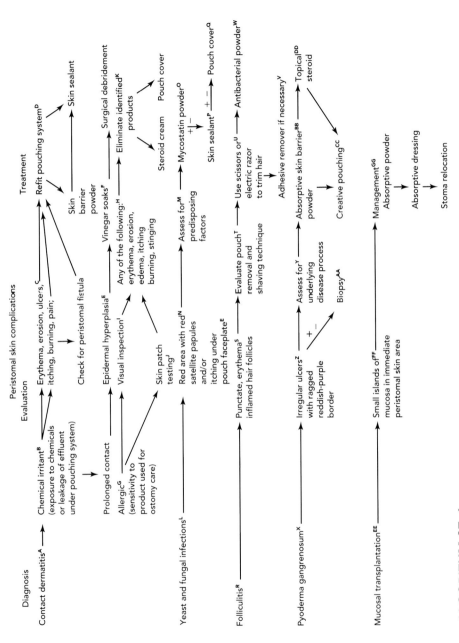

Peristomal skin complications

Diagnosis   **Evaluation**   **Treatment**

Contact dermatitis^A →

- Chemical irritant^B
  (exposure to chemicals
  or leakage of effluent
  under pouching system) → Erythema, erosion, ulcers,^C
  itching, burning, pain;

  Check for peristomal fistula → Refit pouching system^D → Skin sealant

  → Skin
  barrier
  powder

- Prolonged contact

- Allergic^G
  (sensitivity to
  product used for
  ostomy care) → Epidermal hyperplasia^E → Surgical debridement

  Visual inspection^I → Vinegar soaks^F → Eliminate identified^K
  products → Steroid cream   Pouch cover

  Skin patch
  testing^J → Any of the following:^H
  erythema, erosion,
  edema, itching
  burning, stinging

Yeast and fungal infections^L → Red area with red^N
satellite papules
and/or
itching under
pouch faceplate^E → Assess for^M
predisposing
factors → Mycostatin powder^O
+ −
→ Skin sealant^P + − → Pouch cover^Q

Folliculitis^R → Punctate, erythema^S
inflamed hair follicles → Evaluate pouch^T
removal and
shaving technique → Use scissors or^U
electric razor
to trim hair → Antibacterial powder^W

Adhesive remover if necessary^V

Pyoderma gangrenosum^X → Irregular ulcers^Z
with ragged
reddish-purple
border → Assess for^Y
underlying
disease process → Absorptive skin barrier^BB
powder → Topical^DD
steroid

+
−
Biopsy^AA → Creative pouching^CC

Mucosal transplantation^EE → Small islands of^FF
mucosa in immediate
peristomal skin area → Management^GG → Absorptive powder → Absorptive dressing → Stoma relocation

ALGORITHM 87–1

contact dermatitis may occur immediately or develop over a period of time as a delayed response.

H. The skin appears erythematous, edematous, or eroded and may be accompanied by weeping or bleeding. Allergic symptoms include itching, burning, or stinging.

I,J. Diagnosis is made by visual inspection and by skin patch tests to determine allergies. Small pieces of all possible materials are placed on the patient's abdomen opposite the stoma. Using the abdomen provides an area with the same skin thickness, skin temperature, and exposure to friction as the area where the stoma is or will be.

K. Treatment for allergic contact dermatitis includes eliminating the identified agent or at least minimizing contact between the skin and the offending agent. The inflamed area may be treated with a steroid cream. Pouch covers are helpful if the problem lies with the pouch plastic touching the skin.

L. *Yeast and fungal infections. Candida albicans* infections are a common peristomal skin complication. These organisms normally inhabit the gastrointestinal tract, but the occluded, warm, dark, moist area around the stoma provides an optimal environment for local incubation. Damaged skin is also more susceptible to Candida.

M. Systemic predisposition includes iron deficiency, diabetes, cancer, immune deficiency, myelosuppression, use of contraceptives, hypersteroidism, and use of systemic antibiotics.

N. The Candida lesion is characterized by a bright red erythematous center and a surrounding group of red satellite papules. The skin may have a whitish superficial coating and frequently will itch.

O. Local treatment consists of topical application of an antifungal powder, such as Mycostatin, with each pouch change. Excess powder must be brushed away to allow appliance to seal.

P. A skin protectant or sealant may be applied by patting or spraying over the surface of the powder and allowing it to dry prior to pouch application. The powder helps to absorb moisture and has a specific antipathogenic effect on yeast organisms. If the patient is myelosuppressed, systemic treatment may be indicated. Depending on the severity of the infection, the pouch may be left in place for 2–3 days. When the infection is severe, it should be treated daily. Treatment should be continued for several days after the area has clinically cleared; however, continued use of the antifungal agent on a prophylactic basis is not advised.

Q. If the plastic of the pouch comes in contact with the affected area, a cotton pouch cover should be used to prevent the area from becoming warm and moist.

R,S. Folliculitis is a bacterial infection characterized by punctate, erythematous, inflamed hair follicles. It is sometimes confused with a yeast infection; however, careful inspection will show that the inflammation is contained within the hair follicles. Folliculitis is caused by repeated traumatic hair removal as a result of careless pouch removal, poor shaving technique, or shaving peristomal skin too frequently. All types of trauma can cause damage to the hair follicles and the epidermis around them.

T. Thoroughly evaluate the patient's technique for pouch removal and peristomal hair removal.

U. Instruct the patient to trim peristomal hair with scissors or electric razor. Use of adhesive removers may be necessary to ease release of adhesives.

V. Adhesive removers must be thoroughly washed from skin after use.

W. In persistent cases a culture may be taken and, if necessary, an antibacterial powder prescribed.

X. *Pyoderma gangrenosum.* Pyoderma gangrenosum is believed to be a systemic skin lesion.

Y. The etiologic factors are uncertain; however, pyoderma gangrenosum may be associated with ulcerative colitis, Crohn's disease, arthritis, and malignant disorders such as myeloma and leukemia.

Z. The lesion may begin as a small pustule and progress to an irregular ulcer with a necrotic center. The base of the lesion, which is often painful, is deep red, while the ragged edges have a dusky blue to reddish-purple border. There may be single or multiple lesions that can enlarge by tunneling under the epidermis.

AA. Biopsies are usually done to exlude other skin diseases, but the appearance and clinical manifestations of the lesions are most important for diagnosis. Management of an underlying disease process generally leads to improvement of the skin lesions.

BB. Topical treatment includes keeping the area clean and using absorptive skin barrier powder.

CC. Creative pouching techniques are used to maintain pouch barrier seal.

DD. Intralesional steroid injections or topical steroid cream may aid healing.

EE. *Mucosal transplantation.* Viable intestinal mucosa may be transplanted to the abdominal skin surface when the bowel is sutured to the epidermis during stoma construction. This may cause difficulty in maintaining the pouch seal because of persistent mucous secretion.

FF. The appearance of this complication is of small islands of mucosa in the immediate peristomal skin area.

GG. Management involves use of absorptive powder or dressing to help provide a dry surface for pouch adherence. Care must be used when cleansing skin and removing pouches, as the transplanted mucosa may bleed easily when touched. Stoma relocation may be necessary in cases that are very difficult to manage.

BIBLIOGRAPHY

1. Broadwell DC, Jackson BS (eds): *Principles of Ostomy Care.* St. Louis: Mosby, 1982.

2. Hampton BG, Bryant RA (eds): *Ostomies and Continent Diversions: Nursing Management.* St. Louis: Mosby Year Book, 1992.

3. MacKeigan JM, Cataldo PA (eds): *Intestinal Stomas: Principles, Techniques, and Management.* St. Louis: Quality Medical Publishing, 1993.

4. Ng CS, Wolfsen HC, Kozarek RA, et al: Chronic parastomal ulcers: spectrum of dermatoses. *ET Nursing* 19:85–90, 1992.

5. Smith DB, Johnson DE (eds): *Ostomy Care and the Cancer Patient: Surgical and Clinical Considerations.* Orlando: Grune & Stratton, 1986.

See also Chapters 53, 85 and 86.

CHAPTER 88

Stomal Varices

Stephen M. Sentovich, M.D. and Alan G. Thorson, M.D.

Refer to Algorithm 88–1.

A. Upper or lower gastrointestinal bleeding must be differentiated from stomal bleeding that occurs either from direct mucosal trauma or trauma to variceal vessels at the mucocutaneous junction. If there is any doubt about the source of bleeding, endoscopic examination should be performed.

B. Direct pressure with or without gauze soaked in 1:100,000 epinephrine and/or suture ligation have stopped over 98% of stomal bleeds.

C. Over 50% of stoma patients with chronic ulcerative colitis and primary sclerosing cholangitis will develop stomal varices. The history may reveal other causes of portal hypertension such as alcoholic cirrhosis or metastatic liver disease. Careful physical examination of the stoma site will confirm the diagnosis by revealing visible varices or at least bluish discoloration of the peristomal skin. Laboratory evaluation should include a complete blood count, coagulation parameters, and liver function tests. A rare patient may require stomal endoscopy or a venous phase mesenteric angiogram to enable the diagnosis of stomal varices.

D. Further episodes of nonvariceal stomal bleeding can be prevented by refitting the stoma appliance to minimize local trauma.

E. After initial bleeding control with direct pressure or suture ligation, patients with stomal varices should undergo a local measure to prevent further bleeding. Particularly suited for these relatively safe procedures are patients with a short life expectancy, chronic encephalopathy, advanced cirrhosis, or metastatic liver disease. Although recurrent bleeding is common after these local therapies, life-threatening hemorrhage is rare, and these local interventions can be repeated if necessary.

F. Patients with a longer life expectancy and recurrent stomal variceal bleeding after a local procedure or patients with combined esophageal and stomal variceal bleeding should undergo either a portocaval shunt, transjugular intrahepatic portocaval shunt, or liver transplant.

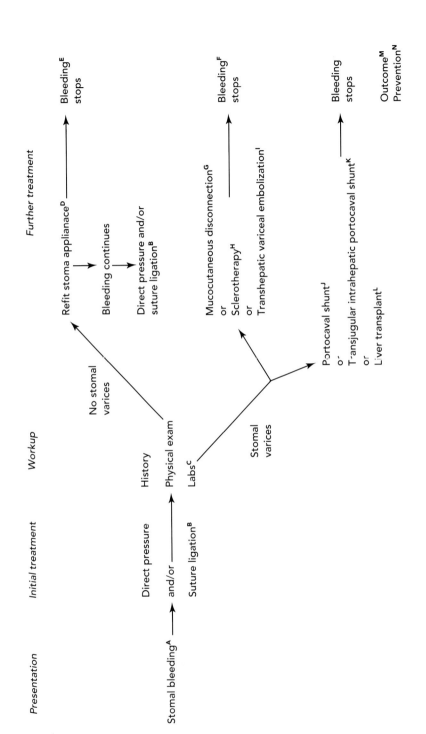

Presentation   Initial treatment   Workup   Further treatment

Stomal varices

Stomal bleeding[A] ⟶ Direct pressure
and/or ⟶ History
Suture ligation[B]

Physical exam

Labs[C]

No stomal
varices ⟶ Refit stoma applianace[D] ⟶ Bleeding[E] stops

Bleeding continues ⟶ Direct pressure and/or suture ligation[B]

Stomal
varices

Mucocutaneous disconnection[G]
or
Sclerotherapy[H]
or
Transhepatic variceal embolization[I] ⟶ Bleeding[F] stops

Portocaval shunt[J]
or
Transjugular intrahepatic portocaval shunt[K]
or
Liver transplant[L] ⟶ Bleeding stops

Outcome[M]
Prevention[N]

ALGORITHM 88–1

G. Mucocutaneous disconnection is the preferred procedure because of its low morbidity and mortality. In this procedure the stoma is disconnected from the peristomal skin and subcutaneous tissue to the fascia, thus dividing the portosystemic communications.

H. Peristomal injections of a sclerosing agent are not any more effective than is mucocutaneous disconnection and have been complicated by skin necrosis, infection, and stomal stenosis.

I. Percutaneous transhepatic variceal embolization has been occasionally performed for the control or prevention of stomal variceal bleeding. This procedure can be complicated by bleeding and may put a patient at risk for portal vein thrombosis.

J. Although no recurrent stomal bleeding has been reported after a portocaval shunt, there is no evidence that shunt surgery prolongs the survival of patients with stomal varices. Patients with stomal varices should have a nonselective portocaval shunt to decrease peristomal venous pressure since postcolectomy encephalopathy has not been reported in these patients.

K. Transjugular intrahepatic portocaval shunting has not been reported for patients with stomal varices but may be an attractive alternative in selected patients.

L. If a patient is a potential liver transplant candidate, transplantation specialty consultation is indicated prior to any biliary or portal surgery that may unnecessarily complicate future transplant surgery.

M. Adequate long-term survival data of patients with stomal varices is not available. Mean survival after the first stomal variceal bleed is about 3 years. In retrospective studies, long-term survival after shunt surgery has been better, the same, or worse than the survival of patients treated with more conservative local measures such as mucocutaneous disconnection. Thus, long-term survival is probably most dependent on the severity of the liver disease and not the number of bleeding episodes and their subsequent treatment.

N. Patients with chronic ulcerative colitis and primary sclerosing cholangitis who are to undergo colon surgery should have an ileal pouch anal or rectal anastomosis since there have been no reports of perianastomotic bleeding in these patients. In contrast, over 50% of these patients who undergo stoma surgery will develop stomal variceal bleeding.

BIBLIOGRAPHY

1. Beck DE, Fazio VW, Grundfest-Broniatowski S: Surgical management of bleeding stomal varices. *Dis Colon Rectum* 31:343–346, 1988.

2. Conte JV, Arcomano TA, Naficy MA, et al: Treatment of bleeding stomal varices: report of a case and review of the literature. *Dis Colon Rectum* 33:308–314, 1990.

3. Fucini C, Wolff BG, Dozois RR: Bleeding from peristomal varices: perspectives on prevention and treatment. *Dis Colon Rectum* 34:1073–1078, 1991.

4. Roberts PL, Martin FM, Schoetz DJ Jr, et al: Bleeding stomal varices: the role of local treatment. *Dis Colon Rectum* 33:547–549, 1990.

See also Chapter 53.

SECTION 8A

Complications
Intraoperative

CHAPTER 89

Intraoperative Ureteric Injury

Kent A. Kirby, M.D. and Charles L. Jackson, M.D.

Refer to Algorithm 89–1.

A. Iatrogenic ureteral injury can occur in open or endoscopic surgical procedures. An incidence ranging from 0.3% to 10% has been reported for colorectal surgery. The most common sites of ureteral injury include the area over the inferior mesenteric vessels, in the ovarian fossa, near the cul-de-sac where the ureter crosses the vas, near the level of the sacral promontory, at the site of the division of the lateral ligaments, and during retroperitonealization. During the latter maneuver the closure may incorporate the ureter. The surgeon should be aware of the potential for ureteric injury during surgical dissection in these areas.

B. Intraoperative recognition of ureteral injury is an important factor in patient outcome. The morbidity and mortality is significantly higher when diagnosis is delayed. Unfortunately only 25–50% of injuries are recognized at the time of surgery. The use of preoperatively placed ureteral catheters, in selected cases, although not proven to prevent injury, certainly can aid in the recognition of operative injury. In assessing intraoperative ureteral injury, the functional status of both the injured renal unit and the contralateral side must be known. This knowledge is particularly important in cases of extensive injury, where nephrectomy may be contemplated. Preoperative contrast studies including computerized tomography (CT) scan or intravenous pyelography (IVP) can assure normal renal function of the renal units. If these studies are not available an intraoperative IVP, with bolus intravenous contrast (100 cc) and subsequent abdominal flat plate film at 15 min can provide similar information. Ureteral injuries consist of either transection or ligation. If transection is suspected, administration of intravenous methylene blue or indigo carmine will confirm urinary leakage. If the diagnosis remains unclear, intraoperative IVP or even intraoperative cystoscopy and retrograde pyelography can confirm extravasation or obstruction.

C. When ureteral ligation is suspected, the entire course of the ureter in the operative field should be dissected to confirm ligation and exclude additional sites of injury. The use of cystotomy and placement of a ureteral catheter to the level of obstruction can identify the specific site of ligation.

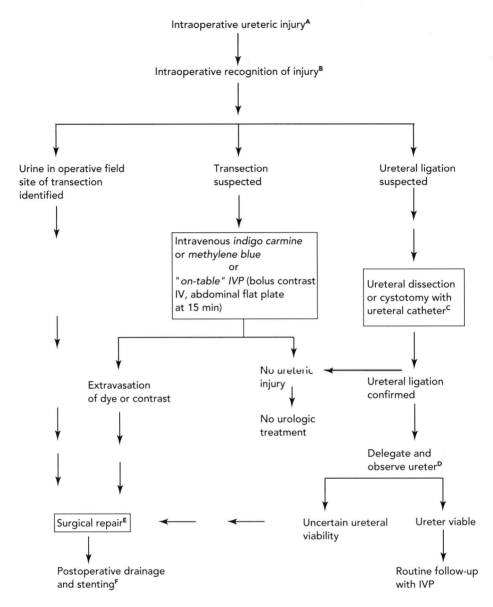

IVP = intravenous pyelography
IV = intravenous

ALGORITHM 89–1

D. Simple deligation is reasonable as a first step, particularly if a large amount of tissue is incorporated into the ligature, thus decreasing the amount of crush effect. If there are any questions regarding ureteral viability, it is advisable to proceed to surgical repair.

E. The proper surgical repair of a ureteral injury depends on the area of the ureter that has been injured and the extent of that injury. In injuries above the pelvic brim, ureteroureterostomy can be used. If necessary to reduce tension on the anastomosis, the kidney can be mobilized to gain 2–3 cm of additional length. A well-drained spatulated anastomosis with fine, absorbable, interrupted sutures should be created after initial debridement of the transected ureter. Injuries to the ureter within 5 cm of the ureterovesical junction are best managed by ureteroneocystotomy. A psoas hitch or Boari flap can be utilized if necessary to provide adequate length. Transuretero ureterostomy has been used as a method of reconstruction in cases of extensive ureteral resection in the area of the pelvic rim. The major disadvantage is the involvement of the normal contralateral ureter.

F. All repairs should be drained retroperitoneally. Ureteral stents such as the double-J stent may be inserted in all reconstructions to provide support for the anastomosis and help align the ureter while providing a conduit for urine. In difficult repairs, such as in a radiated field, the repair may be resected by supporting it with well-vascularized tissue such as an omental wrap.

BIBLIOGRAPHY

1. Lapides J, Tank ES: Urinary complications following abdominal perineal resection. *Cancer.* 28:230, 1977.
2. Fry DE, Milhalen L, Harbeecht R: Iatrogenic ureteral injury. *Arch Surg* 118:454, 1983.
3. Pearse HD, Barry JM, Fuchs EF: Intraoperative consultation for the ureter. *Urol Chin N Am* 12:923, 1985.

See also Chapters 40, 47, 56, 93 and 94.

CHAPTER 90

Splenic Injury

Mark K. Grove, M.D. and Mark E. Sesto, M.D.

Refer to Algorithm 90-1.

A. Incidental injury to the spleen occurs in 1–3% of cases in which mobilization of the splenic flexure is required. The frequency with which this complication is encountered may be increasing as abdominoperineal resection is supplanted by lower colorectal anastomoses requiring splenic mobilization. Colon resections account for one-quarter to one-half of incidental splenectomies; they are exceeded only, in some series, by gastric procedures.

B. Previous abdominal operations, neoplastic or inflammatory involvement of the spleen or its parietal attachments, and advancing age have been shown to predispose to iatrogenic splenic injury. The potential for splenic injury assumes new importance with the burgeoning use of laparoscopically assisted colonic procedures.

C. Avoiding accidental splenic injury in the conduct of colonic procedures requires adequate visualization without overzealous retraction, avoiding undue caudal traction on the splenic flexure, and early division of the splenocolic and omentosplenic peritoneal attachments prior to splenic flexure mobilization *(Figure 90–1)*.

D. The majority of intraoperative splenic injuries result from traction with avulsion of the capsule of the inferior pole (Class II injuries).

E. These injuries can frequently be managed by packing alone.

F. The application of hemostatic agents such as microcrystalline collagen and topical thrombin in minor capsular injuries has been effective in both clinical and experimental evaluations.

G. Although less frequent, bleeding from the splenic hilum (Class III) mandates full mobilization of the spleen to precisely identify the location and extent of the parenchymal injury. Attempts to control bleeding by suture ligature or electrocautery without adequate visualization should be avoided.

H. Mobilization of the spleen with a view to splenic salvage requires deliberate division of the splenophrenic, splenorenal, and splenocolic ligaments with blunt dissection of the retropancreatic plane to deliver the spleen into the operative incision. Division of the superior short gastric vessels (gastrosplenic ligament) may also be necessary.

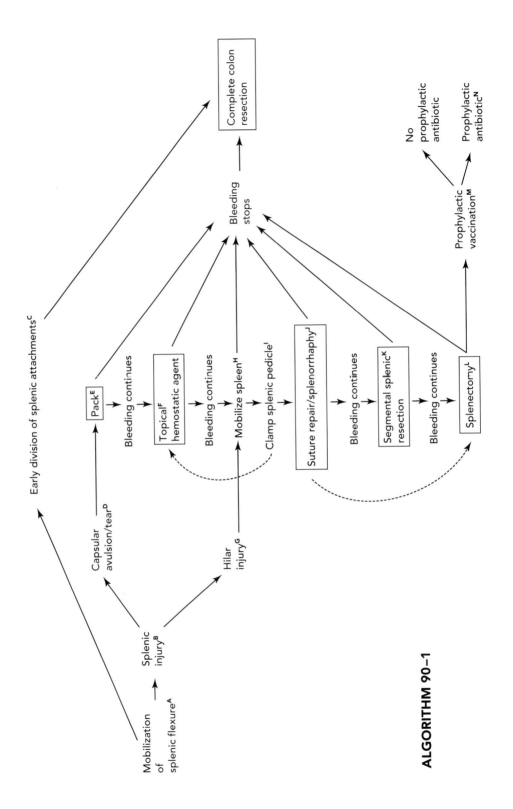

Mobilization of splenic flexure[A] → Splenic injury[B]

Splenic injury[B] → Capsular avulsion/tear[D]

Splenic injury[B] → Hilar injury[G]

Capsular avulsion/tear[D] → Early division of splenic attachments[C]

Early division of splenic attachments[C] → Complete colon resection

Capsular avulsion/tear[D] → Pack[E]

Pack[E] → Bleeding continues → Topical hemostatic agent[F]

Topical hemostatic agent[F] → Bleeding continues → Mobilize spleen[H]

Hilar injury[G] → Mobilize spleen[H]

Mobilize spleen[H] → Clamp splenic pedicle[I]

Clamp splenic pedicle[I] → Suture repair/splenorrhaphy[J]

Suture repair/splenorrhaphy[J] → Bleeding continues → Segmental splenic resection[K]

Segmental splenic resection[K] → Bleeding continues → Splenectomy[L]

Pack[E] → Bleeding stops

Topical hemostatic agent[F] → Bleeding stops

Mobilize spleen[H] → Bleeding stops

Suture repair/splenorrhaphy[J] → Bleeding stops

Segmental splenic resection[K] → Bleeding stops

Splenectomy[L] → Prophylactic vaccination[M]

Prophylactic vaccination[M] → No prophylactic antibiotic

Prophylactic vaccination[M] → Prophylactic antibiotic[N]

ALGORITHM 90–1

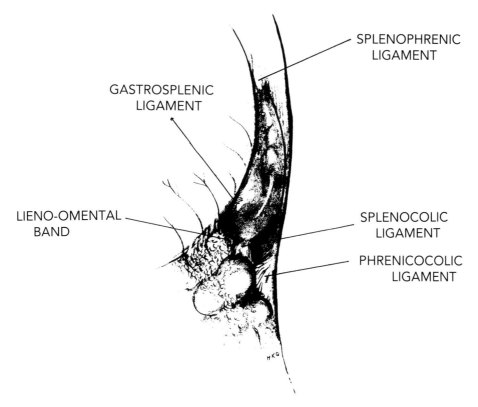

SPLENOPHRENIC
LIGAMENT

GASTROSPLENIC
LIGAMENT

LIENO-OMENTAL
BAND

SPLENOCOLIC
LIGAMENT

PHRENICOCOLIC
LIGAMENT

FIGURE 90–1 The various peritoneal, omental, and ligamentous attachments to the spleen.

I. Adequate mobilization affords the opportunity to digitally compress or clamp the hilar vessels, thereby facilitating exposure and precise control of the injury while minimizing blood loss.

J. Under controlled conditions, direct suture repair should be attempted. Fine nonabsorbable monofilament suture is preferred.

K. Inferior pole avulsions or more extensive hilar injuries may be managed by debridement or segmental splenic resection. The use of mattress sutures with or without Teflon pledgets has proved to be effective in achieving hemostasis after partial splenic resection. This maneuver is facilitated by digital splenic compression.

L. Intraoperative splenic injury has led to splenectomy in 16–40% of reported cases. Splenic salvage has been used with increasing success, however, largely as a result of improved understanding of the sequelae of splenectomy. It has been well established that colonic procedures associated with splenectomy are associated with increased morbidity (approximately 50%) and mortality (approximately 10%) compared to uncomplicated colonic resections. Similarly, the morbidity of incidental splenectomy exceeds that following splenectomy for hematologic disease or for trauma. Postoperative fever, pulmonary complications, and wound infections are particularly prevalent following incidental splenectomy. Other complications of splenectomy include pancreatic fistula, pancreatitis, thrombotic complications, and subphrenic abscess. The use of drains to prevent subphrenic collections remains controversial. Numerous factors including the condition of the patient, the elapsed and anticipated duration of the colonic procedure, the degree of blood loss, the age of the patient, and the familiarity of the operating surgeon with techniques of splenic salvage will influence the decision to proceed with expeditious splenectomy rather than to persist with attempts to control blood loss from the splenic injury. More aggressive efforts to effect splenic salvage would be appropriate in prepubertal patients. However, the risks of transfusion may negate the benefit of splenic preservation in more extensive injuries. Splenic autotransplantation has not been shown to reliably sustain splenic immune competence or to decrease the incidence of postsplenectomy infection.

M. The most compelling complication of splenectomy is the syndrome of postsplenectomy sepsis, reported to occur in 1.9–4.2% of patients after splenectomy. Children are affected roughly twice as frequently as are adults and mortality rates are higher in the pediatric age group, exceeding 50% in some reports. It is generally accepted that all patients over 2 years of age requiring splenectomy should receive prophylactic vaccination against pneumococcal infection. More recently, immunization for meningococcal and *H. influenza* vaccination has been advocated. These vaccines should ideally be administered within 72 hours of splenectomy. The response to vaccination in patients requiring systemic corticosteroids may be compromised. It seems reasonable, in such cases, to defer prophylaxis until perioperative steroid doses are minimized but prior to hospital discharge. Because of the early temporal occurrence of postsplenectomy infection, the high incidence of immunologic reaction with secondary challenges and an equivocal increase in serum immunoglobulin-G (IgG) and immunoglobulin-M (IgM) levels with reimmunization, the use of "booster" doses of polyvalent pneumococcal vaccine remains controversial.

N. Antibiotic prophylaxis (penicillin 250–500 mg/day) has been recommended for postsplenectomy patients at high risk for pneumococcal infection including those with a high likelihood of exposure, immune suppression related to chemotherapy or hematologic disease, and children under the age of 5. Therefore, it is imperative that patients after splenectomy be counseled to seek medical attention promptly at the onset of even seemingly minor febrile illnesses.

BIBLIOGRAPHY

1. Cioffiro W, Schein CJ, Gliedman ML: Splenic injury during abdominal surgery. *Arch Surg* 111:167–171, 1976.

2. Danforth DN, Thorbjarnarson B: Incidental splenectomy: a review of the literature and the New York hospital experience. *Ann Surg* 183:124–129, 1976.

3. Langevin JM, Rothenberger DA, Goldberg SM: Accidental splenic injury during surgical treatment of the colon and rectum. *Surg Gynecol Obstet* 159:139–144, 1984.

4. Schoetz DJ: Complications of surgical excision of the rectum. *Surg Clin NAM* 71:1271–1281, 1991.

5. Shaw JHF, Print CG: Postsplenectomy sepsis. *Br J Surg* 76:1074–1081, 1989.

See also Chapter 47.

CHAPTER 91

Colonoscopic Perforations

Frank Opelka, M.D.

Refer to Algorithm 91--1.

A. Major complications arise during either diagnostic or therapeutic colonoscopy causing perforation, postpolypectomy coagulation syndrome, and hemorrhage. Other complications are minor and include problems related to the mechanical bowel preparation, intravenous medications, hypoxia, and bacteremia. Perforation is the most common major complication of diagnostic colonoscopy occurring in 0.06--0.8% of diagnostic procedures.

B. The endoscopist may immediately identify the perforation during the procedure if either the peritoneal cavity or the extraluminal adipose tissue is visualized. When the perforation is not seen during the examination, the index of suspicion increases when the patient complains of abdominal pain or distension. Supine and erect abdominal roentgenograms may display the presence of air within the peritoneal cavity.

C. Delayed presentations occur with small perforations or retroperitoneal perforations. Delayed perforations create symptoms that often arise after the patient has returned home. We reported that 58% of patients (10 of 17) presented with perforations 24 hours after colonscopy. The patient may complain of a fever, persistent abdominal pain and distension, nausea, or vomiting. Retroperitoneal perforations may dissect along the root of the mesentery. The pneumoretroperitoneum extends along the aorta into the chest and cervical area, creating pneumomediastinum and cervical subcutaneous emphysema.

D. Perforations result from mechanical forces during colonoscopic insertion and from barotrauma during colonic insufflation. The mechanical forces causing perforations occur with forceful instrument insertion, endoscopic torquing with creation or withdrawal of an alpha loop, slide-by insertion technique, and insertion of a sigmoid splinting instrument. The mechanical perforations result from a direct injury at the colonoscopic tip or from colonic stretching or bowing by the endoscope at sights remote from the distal end of the scope. Most of the mechanical perforations occur in the rectosigmoid. The rectum or sigmoid are often fixed from surgical adhesions or other inflammatory conditions within the pelvis. Colon pathology that contributes to rectosigmoid fixa-

477

Colonoscopic perforations

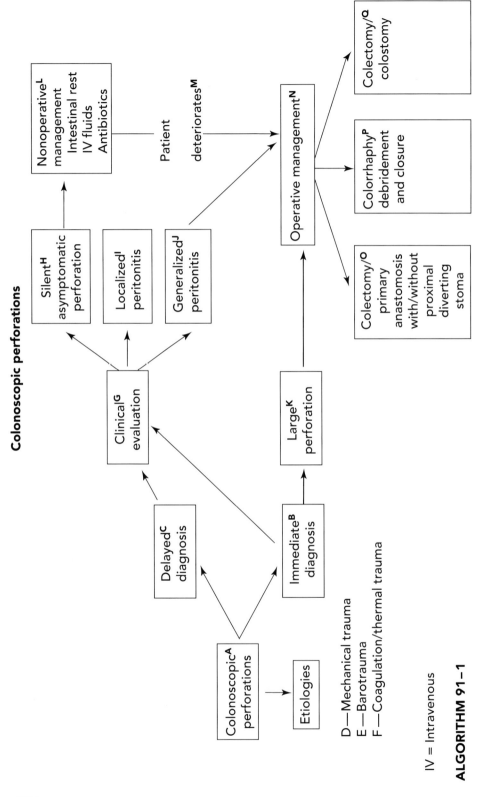

IV = Intravenous

ALGORITHM 91-1

478

tion includes ulcerated or friable tumors, stricture, inflammatory bowel disease, or diverticulitis. When anticipating excessive resistance during insertion or torquing of the scope, the endoscopist should withdraw the instrument, inspecting carefully to assure that the colon remains intact.

E. Colonic insufflation is essential during introduction of the scope and examination of the lumen of the colon. Excessive insufflation causes significant abdominal pain and discomfort and increases the difficulty of the examination. The endoscopist should limit the air insufflation to the minimum required for a safe insertion and adequate inspection of the colon. Cadaver studies reveal that the cecum is most susceptible to pneumatic perforations, followed by the transverse colon, sigmoid colon, and rectum. The injuries begin with serosal linear tears due to the luminal distension and progress to a full-thickness perforation. Clinical investigations measuring intraluminal pressures and simple diverticular rupture during colonscopy have not revealed a predisposition to pneumatic rupture. Perforation is more probably associated with endoscopy in patients with acute diverticulitis. The right colon and cecum are predisposed to barotrauma because the colonic wall is thin and the cecal diameter is large. According to Laplace's law, wall tension is directly related to the radius of a cylinder (the colon lumen). Thus, during insufflation, as the cecum distends, the wall tension of the colon increases until the serosa tears and perforations occur.

F. Perforations during therapeutic colonoscopy occur from thermal or electrical injury when using electrocautery or laser. Transmural injuries can also occur when instruments inserted through the endoscope directly perforate the bowel. The reported incidence of therapeutic perforations varies from 0.5%–3.0%. The injury can extend full thickness or remain limited to the colon wall without perforation. Several authors have diagnosed patients with colonic electrocautery injuries to have postpolypectomy coagulation syndrome. The injury is a transmural burn with serositis overlying the electrocautery site. These limited injuries cause abdominal pain and tenderness. The patients complain of a fever, nausea, and vomiting. The abdominal roentgenograms do not show any evidence of a perforation. Often, these patients are difficult to distinguish from patients with perforations. Electrocautery creates transmural injury when the current proves excessive for the coagulation technique employed. These techniques include fulguration, hot biopsy forceps, and snare excision. Wadas noted most perforations from hot biopsy forceps occurred in the right colon where the coagulation injury quickly extended through the thin colon wall. Full-thickness injuries from coagulation are related to the current density. The density is directly related to intensity and duration and diameter of the application of the electric current and inversely related to the diameter of tissue involved. Hot biopsy forceps are ideally suited to limit the diameter of application of current. The excessive duration or intensity, however, can lead to full-thickness injury. Snare electrocautery forceps are tightened during the process of tissue coagulation, thus decreasing the application diameter of current and sharply increasing the current density. This can lead to transmural coagulation and perforation.

G. Perforation is not always evident immediately after a polypectomy.

H. The patient may remain asymptomatic or slowly develop localized peritonitis over the next 4–12 hours.

I. Patients with localized peritonitis or asymptomatic perforations do not require urgent operative therapy.

J. Immediate laparotomy is indicated in patients with generalized peritonitis.

K. Perforations recognized during colonoscopy usually represent large perforations from barotrauma or mechanical injuries. These are more extensive than are electrocautery injuries and do not spontaneously seal without the risk of prolonged peritoneal soilage. Associated colon pathology contributes to the poor healing and may influence the decision to operate.

L. Nonoperative treatment with intestinal intravenous fluids, and antibiotics limit the peritonitis, allowing the perforation to seal. Several series have reported that one-third of patients presenting with perforation were successfully treated without surgery. If the colon has no underlying pathology and the mechanical bowel preparation was adequate, spontaneous healing progresses with resolution of abdominal symptoms over the next 24–48 hours.

M. If the patient deteriorates or fails to improve, operative management is indicated.

N. Large perforations identified during colonoscopy require urgent laparotomy. The surgical options include colorrhaphy, colectomy, and primary anastomosis with or without a proximal diverting stoma, and colectomy with colostomy.

O. Colorrhaphy is reserved for limited injuries not associated with any significant underlying colonic pathology. Debridement and closure of the perforation in patients with a mechanical bowel preparation limits complications associated with bowel resections.

P. Colectomy with a primary anastomosis removes perforated bowel and associated colon pathology. A proximal diverting stoma (loop ileostomy) is indicated in patients treated with resection and primary anastomosis in patients with significant peritonitis, underlying pathology, or other comorbidities. In patients with limited peritoneal soilage and exudate, a diverting proximal stoma is not necessary.

Q. Bowel resection and colostomy is used in patients with significant peritoneal soilage, operative delay, and when the underlying colonic pathology prevents a primary anastomosis.

BIBLIOGRAPHY

1. Christie JP, Marrazzo J: "Mini-perforation" of the colon—not all postpolypectomy perforations require laparotomy. *Dis Colon Rectum* 34:132–135, 1991.

2. Habr-Gama A, Waye JD: Complications and hazards of gastrointestinal endoscopy. *World J Surg* 13:193–201, 1989.

3. Kavin H, Sinicrope F, Esker AH: Management of perforation of the colon at colonscopy. *J Gastroenterol* 87:161–167, 1992.

4. Macrae FA, Tan KG, Williams CB: Towards safer colonoscopy: a report on the complications of 5000 diagnostic or therapeutic colonoscopies. *Gut* 24:376–383, 1983.

5. Wadas DD, Sanowski RA: Complications of the hot biopsy forceps technique. *Gastrointest Endosc* 33:32–37, 1987.

See also Chapters 2, 59, 66, 68, 69, 95A and 95B.

SECTION 8B

Complications
Postoperative

CHAPTER 92

Anastomotic Stricture

Mark Killingback, M.D.

Refer to Algorithm 92-1.

A. *Colon anastomoses*. Anastomotic stricture proximal to the sigmoid colon is rarely encountered except in patients with colonic Crohn's disease. A recent survey revealed that anastomotic strictures proximal to the sigmoid accounted for only 9.9% of the total reported. If present, such strictures rarely produce significant symptoms due to the more fluid consistency of the stool; therefore a narrow lumen in the colon can be tolerated. Strictures due to anastomotic fibrosis may be due to a subclinical leak or the excessive use of nonabsorbable suture material such as silk for the anastomosis. They are generally diagnosed by endoscopy or radiography.

B. Strictures due to Crohn's disease affecting the colon are seldom suitable for strictureplasty, and management is integrated with the overall aspects of the disease.

C. If treatment is indicated for symptoms, then resection of the stricture is the management of choice.

D. *Rectal anastomoses*. The American Society of Colon and Rectal Surgery survey reported that rectal anastomotic strictures occurred in 57.9% of 121 large bowel strictures. The author's experience is different as strictures have almost exclusively occurred in rectal stapled anastomoses. The most common cause of stricture has been specific to the circular staple technique. Less common is the fibrosis related to a paraanastomotic abscess associated with a major anastomotic leak that can be subclinical. Other causes are perioperative radiotherapy and local recurrence of carcinoma. There is no accepted definition of a stricture. The author defines a stricture as a lumen <17 mm (the diameter of the standard rigid sigmoidoscope and the diameter of the middle phalanx of the authors index finger). The circular staple technique has been associated with a higher anastomotic stricture incidence than any previous technique. The etiology is unproven, but imperfect mucosal healing may be an important factor. The author has conducted a prospective audit on 854 single circular

483

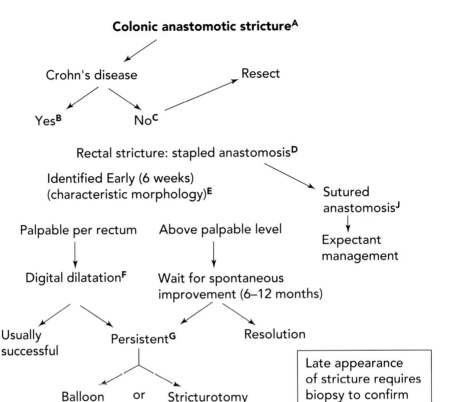

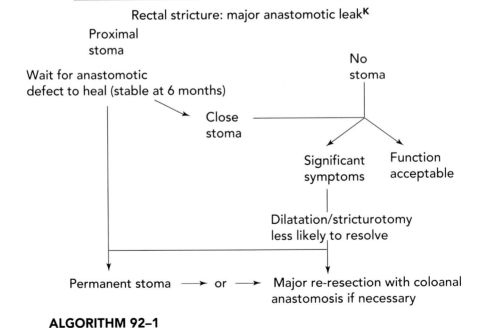

ALGORITHM 92–1

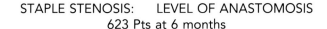

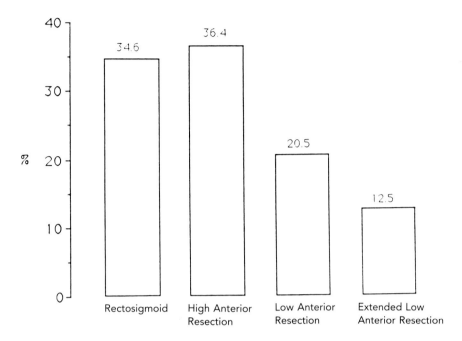

FIGURE 92-1 The incidence of stenosis at various levels.

stapled anastomoses of the rectum with almost all anastomoses tested by postoperative contrast x-ray studies.

E. Staple strictures occur early and are usually evident at the first postoperative visit (6 weeks). They do not appear subsequently if the anastomosis is satisfactory at 6 weeks. The late development of a rectal anastomotic stricture is pathognomonic of a local recurrence of carcinoma. The author's prospective study on stenosis showed a significant difference in the incidence of a stricture of intraperitoneal rectal anastomosis (35.6%) compared with extraperitoneal anastomosis (16.8%) as measured at 6 months. The incidence of stenosis at various levels is shown in Fig. 92-1. There was no relationship to adjustable closure of staples, staple diameter, proximal stoma, diverticular disease, or anastomotic leak. Obstructive symptoms related to rectal function may be present, but patients may be asymptomatic with lumen sizes of ≤ 5 mm (Fig. 92-2). Treatment of the stricture is indicated for symptoms or the inability to examine the patient with a colonoscope (13-mm diameter). In addition, a lumen <17 mm would seem to be undesirable for the patient's future evaluations.

F. Digital dilatation at the initial postoperative visit is now advocated for a stricture. This usually resolves the problem. If it does not, alternative treatments need not be applied for up to 12 months (symptoms allowing) as there is significant spontaneous resolution in 16-42% of strictures dependent on the level.

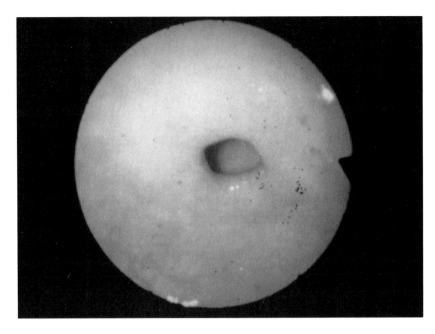

FIGURE 92–2 Stapled anastomosis <5 mm. Patient denied symptoms.

G. Endoscopic techniques are necessary for refractory strictures and those beyond the reach of the digit. Obturator dilatation with a sigmoidoscope or various metal dilators is less controlled and risks perforation and is therefore not recommended.

H. Intraluminal balloon techniques have been reported as safe and successful. The TTS (transit-time study) balloon (Microvasive®) is recommended. The technique appears to be ideal for the intraperitoneal rectal stricture.

I. Endoscopic radial incision (stricturotomy) with diathermy (Fig. 92–3) or laser using the colonoscope is an effective method, but care is needed to avoid a perforation. Resection with a urologic resectoscope can be effective, but few general or colorectal surgeons will adopt this technique. Successful resection has been reported by the use of the stapler. Major abdominal surgery to resect the stricture or permanent colostomy should not be necessary.

J. *Sutured anastomosis.* The author believes that a single layer interrupted anastomosis using absorbable suture material, for example, Vicryl, which heals primarily (as checked by early postoperative gastrograffin enema), will not stricture due to fibrosis (in the absence of radiotherapy, major colon ischemia, or recurrent disease). The inversion suture technique will result in a significant edema and reaction in the early months after operation that will always subside spontaneously and therefore should be managed conservatively.

K. *Rectal anastomotic stricture associated with a major leak.* A prolonged para-anastomotic abscess with associated fibrosis will usually produce a longer, thick, and firm stricture that is less likely to respond to intraluminal dilatation or endoscopic stricturotomy. If symptoms are significant, then abdominal re-resection is likely to be the only effective treatment. If the patient is less fit for such a technical challenge, a permanent stoma may be the appropriate option.

ENDOSCOPIC STRICTURE–OTOMY

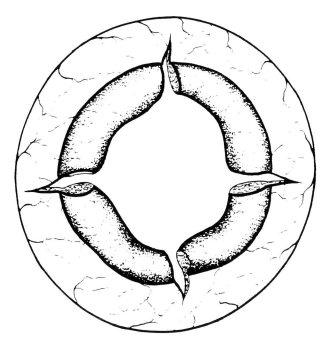

FIGURE 92–3 Endoscopic stricturotomy.

If a low anastomosis was performed initially, a coloanal anastomosis will be the only viable option to avoid a permanent stoma. In this setting, a colonic J pouch will provide superior function within the first 12–24 months after surgery.

BIBLIOGRAPHY

1. Accordi F, Sogno O, Carniato S, et al: Endoscopic treatment of stenosis following stapler anastomosis. *Dis Colon Rectum* 30:647–649, 1987.
2. Hinton G, Celestin L: A new technique for excision of recurrent anastomotic strictures of the rectum. *Ann Roy Coll Surg* 68:260–261, 1986.
3. Hunt T, Kelly M: Endoscopic transanal resection (ETAR) of colorectal strictures in stapled anastomoses. *Ann Roy Coll Surg* 76:121–122, 1994.
4. Killingback MJ: Staple stenosis. Harry E. Bacon Lectureship 1991. Annual Meeting of the American Society of Colon and Rectal Surgeons.
5. Kozarek RA: Hydrostatic balloon dilatation of gastrointestinal stenoses: a nation survey. *Gastrointest Endosc* 32:15, 1986.
6. Luchtefeld MA, Milson JW, Senagore A, et al: Colorectal anastomotic stenosis, results of a survey of the ASCRS membership. *Dis Colon Rectum* 32:733–736, 1989.

7. Polglase AL, Hughes ESR, McDermott FT, et al: A comparison of end-to-end staple and suture colorectal anastomosis in the dog. *Surg Gynecol Obstet* 152:792–796, 1981.

8. Sander R, Posl H, Spuhler A: Management of non-neoplastic stenoses of the GI tract—a further indication for Nd-YAG laser application. *Endoscopy* 16:149–151, 1984.

9. Venkatesh KS, Ramanujam PS, McGee S: Hydrostatic balloon dilatation of benign colonic anastomotic strictures. *Dis Colon Rectum* 35:789–791, 1992.

See also Chapters 47, 49, 50, 62 and 65.

CHAPTER 93

Anastomotic Leakage

E. L. Bokey, M.D. and M. J. Solomon, M.D.

Refer to Algorithm 93–1.

A. Anastomotic leakage is one of the most feared complications following bowel resection and restoration of intestinal continuity. It is usual to associate anastomatic leakage with patients who are malnourished, are immunosuppressed, or in whom local sepsis or obstruction were present at the time of surgery. However, by far the most common cause of leakage relates to surgical technique: poor blood supply, tension on the anastomosis, and inadequate or insufficient seromuscular approximation. The incidence of anastomotic leakage from intraperitoneal anastomoses is low. It is less than 1% for elective and 2% for emergency right hemicolectomy. The same statistics apply to intraperitoneal anastomoses following left-sided colectomies and high anterior resection. In contrast, anastomoses following low anterior resections (LARs) are more at risk with a reported incidence varying between 2% and 20% depending on definition of terms. The size and distance of the tumour from the dentate line influence the anastomotic leak rate; however, the stage, age, and sex of the patient do not have an adverse effect. Anastomotic leakage may be minimized by careful technique. Meticulous attention should be devoted to blood supply, anastomotic technique, and providing a tension-free anastomosis. In the case of very low anterior resection, it is advisable to mobilize the splenic flexure and further divide the inferior mesenteric vein at the inferior border of the pancreas. The use of diverting stomas proximal to a LAR is controversial. They protect against the consequences but not the occurrence of a leak. The routine use of drains has not been shown to affect the incidence of leakage, although many surgeons still use drains to drain the pelvis after a LAR.
B. In some patients the consequences of anastomotic leakage are evident with obvious clinical manifestations of generalized peritonitis.
C. After resuscitation and the administration of broad-spectrum antibiotics and the marking of all potential stoma sites, a laparotomy with peritoneal lavage is performed. If the defect is large, the proximal end of the anastomosis is

489

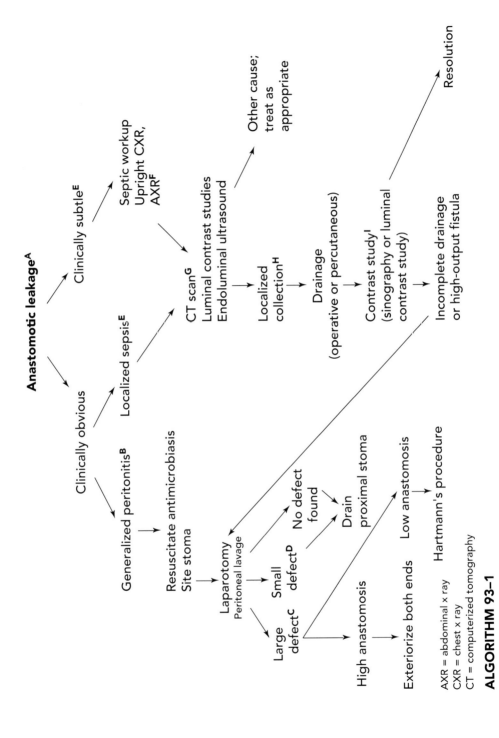

Anastomotic leakage^A

Clinically obvious

Clinically subtle^E

Generalized peritonitis^B

Localized sepsis^E

Septic workup
Upright CXR,
AXR^F

Resuscitate antimicrobiasis
Site stoma

CT scan^G
Luminal contrast studies
Endoluminal ultrasound

Other cause;
treat as
appropriate

Localized
collection^H

Laparotomy
Peritoneal lavage

Small
defect^D

No defect
found

Drain
proximal stoma

Drainage
(operative or percutaneous)

Large
defect^C

Low anastomosis

Contrast study^I
(sinography or luminal
contrast study)

High anastomosis

Hartmann's procedure

Incomplete drainage
or high-output fistula

Resolution

Exteriorize both ends

AXR = abdominal x ray
CXR = chest x ray
CT = computerized tomography

ALGORITHM 93–1

brought out as an end stoma and the distal end of the anastomosis is brought out as a mucous fistula. In the case of anterior resection the rectum can be stapled or oversewn and returned to the pelvis.

D. When the anastomotic defect is small or not obvious at operation, another therapeutic option is to establish a proximal stoma and drain the local anastomotic area.

E. Small anastomotic leaks may present as localized abscesses or peritonitis. In some patients the clinical consequences of an anastomotic leak are subtle and may manifest themselves only by nonspecific signs and symptoms.

F. A prompt evaluation for sepsis should include an upright chest x-ray (CXR) and abdominal x-ray (AXR).

G. The next studies should be luminal contrast including a water-soluble contrast agent to assess for leakage and a computerized tomography (CT) scan to assess for concurrent abdominal or pelvic abscesses.

H. Localized abscesses may spontaneously discharge or may need to be surgically or percutaneously drained under ultrasound or CT guidance. Transanal ultrasound can be helpful in the diagnosis and drainage of low pelvic anastomoses.

I. Once drainage of localized abscesses associated with anastomotic leakage has been performed, a sinogram performed at a later date will be helpful in determining the subsequent management of the fistula. Incomplete drainage of the abscess, a high-output fistula where containment of the discharge, protection of the skin and maintenance of nutrition, fluid, and electrolyte balance cannot be obtained, all require operative intervention. Stricture, obstruction, or persistent low-grade sepsis may result from untreated anastomotic leakage.

BIBLIOGRAPHY

1. Bokey EL, Chapius PH, Hughes WJ, et al: Morbidity, mortality and survival following resection for carcinoma of the rectum. *Austral NZ J Surg* 60:253–259, 1990.

2. Goligher JC, Graham NG, DeDombal FT: Anastomotic dehiscence after anterior resection of rectum and sigmoid. *Br J Surg* 57:109–118, 1970.

3. Longo WE, Milson JW, Lavery IC, et al: Pelvic abscess after colon and rectal surgery. What is optimal management? *Dis Colon Rectum* 36:936–941, 1993.

See also Chapters 41, 47, 65, 92 and 94.

CHAPTER 94

Postoperative Pelvic Abscess

Tina Ure, M.D. and Anthony M. Vernava, III, M.D.

Refer to Algorithm 94–1.

A. Postoperative pelvic abscess is a dreaded complication that may occur following any intestinal resection, but more frequently occurs after resection of the rectosigmoid for cancer, Crohn's colitis, ulcerative colitis, or diverticular disease. Regardless of etiology, the principles of treatment are adequate drainage and parenteral antibiotic therapy. The choice and timing of drainage procedure depends on the condition of the patient, the location of the abscess, and the initial response to therapy. The associated morbidity and mortality is high: 30–40% in some series. Prompt recognition and treatment are essential for successful outcome.

B. Pelvic abscess usually results from either an anastomotic dehiscence, contamination during surgery, or inadequate hemostasis; often the cause is never found. Patients with coexisting medical illnesses such as insulin-dependent diabetes, chronic renal failure, cirrhosis, chronic obstructive pulmonary disease, previous radiation, or immunosuppression (such as in patients taking steroids for inflammatory bowel disease) are subject to development of septic complications. While anastomotic leak is frequently the cause, a pelvic abscess can also occur after proctectomy without restoration of intestinal continuity.

C. A pelvic abscess may occur in the postoperative period several days to weeks following operation. Early symptoms include fever, pain, persistent or recurrent ileus, abdominal distention, intestinal obstruction, intractable diarrhea, generalized listlessness, or manifest lethargy. Leukocytosis is the most common laboratory finding, although it may not manifest if the patient is taking high-dose exogenous steroids; metabolic acidosis may be identified in some cases. A less common presentation is that of shock or renal, pulmonary, or hepatic failure.

D. Early diagnosis is aided by a high index of suspicion and investigation of subtle symptoms, or recognition that the patient is failing to progress in the usual time course for recuperation. Careful physical examination of the abdomen or

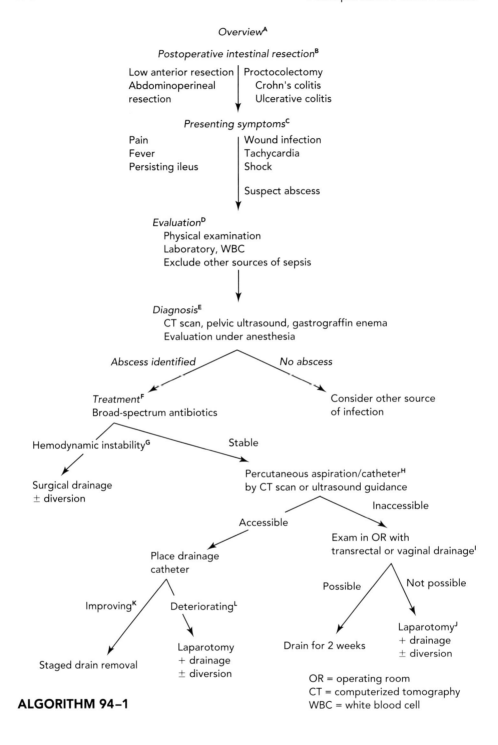

Overview[A]

Postoperative intestinal resection[B]

Low anterior resection | Proctocolectomy
Abdominoperineal | Crohn's colitis
resection | Ulcerative colitis

Presenting symptoms[C]

Pain | Wound infection
Fever | Tachycardia
Persisting ileus | Shock

Suspect abscess

Evaluation[D]
Physical examination
Laboratory, WBC
Exclude other sources of sepsis

Diagnosis[E]
CT scan, pelvic ultrasound, gastrograffin enema
Evaluation under anesthesia

Abscess identified   No abscess

Treatment[F]   Consider other source
Broad-spectrum antibiotics   of infection

Hemodynamic instability[G]   Stable

Surgical drainage
± diversion   Percutaneous aspiration/catheter[H]
                                   by CT scan or ultrasound guidance

                                                          Inaccessible

                              Accessible
                                                    Exam in OR with
                                                    transrectal or vaginal drainage[I]

                    Place drainage
                    catheter
                                        Possible   Not possible

Improving[K]   Deteriorating[L]

                                                              Laparotomy[J]
                                                              + drainage
                    Laparotomy   Drain for 2 weeks   ± diversion
                    + drainage
Staged drain removal + diversion

ALGORITHM 94–1   OR = operating room
                                       CT = computerized tomography
                                       WBC = white blood cell

perineum may reveal new or increased tenderness fullness to palpation, or drainage from a wound. In the absence of physical findings, other causes for symptoms should be evaluated by chest roentgenograms, urine analysis, sputum samples, and routine fever evaluation.

E. Computerized tomography (CT) scan, pelvic ultrasound, or gastrograffin enema most often demonstrates the suspected pelvic abscess. CT correctly diagnosed an abscess in 78 of 79 patients (98% sensitivity) and correctly excluded abscesses in 31 of 32 patients (specificity 97%). When identified, an abscess appears as a circumscribed area of uniform low CT attenuation or as an extraluminal fluid collection. Oral contrast should be given whenever possible so that the bowel containing the contrast is more easily distinguished from the abscess cavity. Ultrasound has nearly as high sensitivity and specificity rates (93.3% and 98.6%, respectively); additionally ultrasound has the advantage of being relatively inexpensive, portable, and noninvasive. CT- or ultrasound-guided aspiration of the pelvic fluid should be performed to confirm the presence of pus, identify organisms, and test for antibiotic susceptibility. Contrast enema studies may demonstrate extravasation of dye or displacement of bowel by a mass effect; while not widely used, a diagnostic accuracy of 88% is reported. If imaging techniques fail to identify any suspicious fluid collections, a search for other causes for the patient's illness or failure to progress should be undertaken. Finally, examination under anesthesia may be required to establish a diagnosis if imaging techniques are equivocal.

F. Broad-spectrum antibiotic therapy should be instituted as soon as the diagnosis of pelvic abscess is made. Coverage should be directed toward enteric flora including *Escherichia coli, Bacteroides fragilis, Enterococcus species,* which are the organisms most commonly found in intraabdominal abscesses. Of paramount importance in conjunction with antimicrobial treatment is the basic principle of adequate drainage. Methods of drainage include formal laparotomy, transperineal (per rectum or vagina) drainage, or CT-guided percutaneous catheter drainage.

G. Expeditious operative drainage is indicated in patients who are unstable. The decision to perform fecal diversion is based on the presence of septicemia, gross peritonitis, or enterocutaneous fistula.

H. CT- or ultrasound-guided percutaneous drainage should be the initial therapeutic maneuver in hemodynamically stable patients without evidence of generalized peritonitis. Percutaneous drainage in these patients appears as efficacious as open drainage.

I. Patients with accessible fluid collections may be candidates for transrectal or transvaginal drainage. In appropriate patients this method of drainage may be preferable to either percutaneous or open methods.

J. Abscesses in a location not amenable to percutaneous or transrectal or transvaginal drainage are best treated by open surgical drainage.

K. Following percutaneous catheter placement, the patient is continued on appropriate antibiotics, and evaluated frequently for response to therapy. Reimaging with CT scan should be done at intervals of 5–7 days to check the position of the catheter to maintain optimal location. This protocol also allows for evaluation of the adequacy of fluid drainage, as well as the interval development of new abscesses.

L. If at any time the patient's condition deteriorates, or fails to improve after an appropriate period of time, then one should suspect inadequate drainage with a persistent abscess and pelvic sepsis. Additional drainage performed via laparotomy may be required, and fecal diversion should be reconsidered.

BIBLIOGRAPHY

1. Bohnen JMA, Mustard RA, Oxholm SE, et al: APACHE II score and abdominal sepsis. *Arch Surg* 123:225–229, 1988.
2. Glass CA, Cohn I: Drainage of intra-abdominal abscess: a comparison of surgical and computerized tomography guided catheter drainage. *Am J Surg* 147:315–317, 1984.
3. Hemming A, Davis NL, Robins RD: Surgical versus percutaneous drainage of intra-abdominal abscesses. *Am J Surg* 161:593–595, 1991.
4. Johnson WB, Gerzof SG, Robbins AH, et al: Treatment of abdominal abscesses: comparative evaluation of operation drainage versus percutaneous catheter drainage guided by computed tomography or ultrasound. *Ann Surg* 194:510–520, 1981.
5. Koehler PR, Moss AA: Diagnosis of intra-abdominal and pelvic abscesses by computerized tomography. *JAMA* 244:4952, 1980.
6. Levison MA, Zeigler D: Correlation of APACHE II score, drainage technique, and outcome in postoperative intra-abdominal abscess. *Surg Gynecol Obstet* 172:89–94, 1991.
7. Longo WE, Milsom JW, Lavery IC, et al: Pelvic abscess after colon and rectal surgery — what is optimal management? *Dis Colon Rectum* 36:936–941, 1993.
8. Lurie K, Plazk L, Deveney CW: Intra-abdominal abscess in the 1980's. *Surg Clin N Am* 67:621–632, 1987.
9. Taylor KJW, Sullivan DC, Wassan JF, et al: Ultrasound and gallium for the diagnosis of abdominal and pelvic abscesses. *Gastrointest Radiol* 3:294–296, 1978.

See also Chapters 47 and 93.

CHAPTER 95A

Postpolypectomy Hemorrhage

Frank G. Opelka, M.D. and David H. Gibbs, M.D.

Refer to Algorithm 95A-1.

A. Colonoscopy is the most accurate diagnostic modality available for the evaluation of the colon. Postpolypectomy hemorrhage is the most common major complication, with an incidence of 0.20–1.0%. However, the majority of hemorrhagic complications are minor, occur at the time of polypectomy, and can be colonoscopically controlled. We define "major hemorrhage" as postpolypectomy bleeding requiring admission to the hospital and diagnostic intervention.

B. Major postpolypectomy hemorrhage is either immediate and identified in the endoscopy suite; or delayed, with the patient presenting within 2–15 days of a colonoscopy. Initial evaluation includes ascertaining vital signs and establishing the hemodynamic stability of the patient. All patients require intravenous fluid support, placement of a Foley catheter, and a laboratory profile for hemoglobin, platelet count, and a coagulation profile. A nasogastric intubation and aspiration excludes massive upper gastrointestinal bleeding prior to further investigations of the lower gastrointestinal tract. Ongoing volume resuscitation depends on the patient's general condition and response to the resuscitation efforts.

C. After stabilization, the anus, rectum, and distal colon are examined to exclude a distal site of bleeding such as hemorrhoids, fissures, or fistulas. Complete anoscopy and proctoscopy allow for adequate evacuation of all clots and blood to assess the anus and rectum for hemorrhage. If the distal exam is normal, colonoscopy may reveal a proximal source.

D. Colonoscopy has limited use in assessment of a lower gastrointestinal (GI) bleed. Often, the blood obscures endoscopic visualization and increases the risk of insertion injury, rendering colonoscopy suboptimal for the treatment of postpolypectomy hemorrhage. However, in certain instances, repeat colon-

497

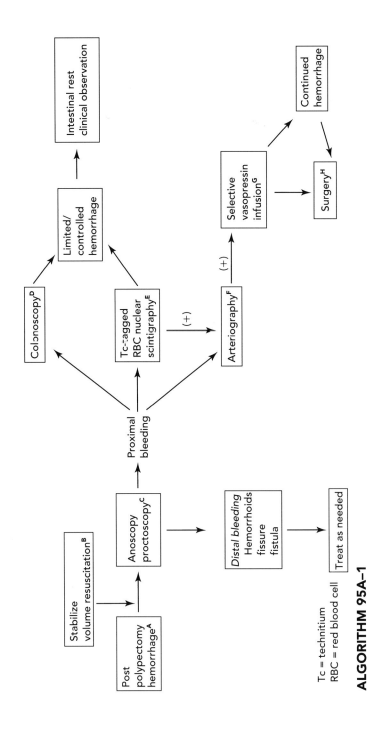

ALGORITHM 95A–1

Tc = technitium
RBC = red blood cell

oscopy for minimal bleeding or to resnare a pedunculated polyp stalk may prove more cost-effective than extensive diagnostic evaluations, especially since the location of the bleeding may be known in advance.

E. Scintigraphy with technetium-labeled red blood cells (Tc^{99}-tagged red blood cell scan) detects massive hemorrhage or mild to moderate hemorrhage (bleeding rates = 0.1–0.5 cc/min) and can localize the site of bleeding. If the scintigram demonstrates extravasation in the early images, arteriography is indicated. Negative scans or delayed extravasation depict minimal bleeding that will resolve with supportive volume replacement and intestinal rest.

F. Arteriography is indicated in any patient with hemodynamic instability who does not respond to the initial resuscitation or in patients with early positive scintigrams. Extravasation during arteriography represents significant hemorrhage, >1.0 cc/min. If the scintigram is positive and the arteriogram is negative, the patient requires 24-hour intensive care observation. The vascular access sheath should remain in place during this period to allow for urgent access to repeat arteriography if the patient demonstrates recurrent or episodic hemorrhage.

G. Selective vasopressin infusion (0.1–0.4 units/min) is the mainstay of arteriographic control of lower GI hemorrhage. It is a useful therapy in postpolypectomy hemorrhage that is demonstrated during arteriography. Vasopressin requires continuous intensive care monitoring for hypertension, angina, cardiac arrhythmias, or abdominal pain. Once the hemorrhage is controlled, the therapy is weaned over 8–12 hours. Repeat arteriography is indicated only if the question of persistent hemorrhage arises because of continued hematochezia or melena.

H. Although surgery is rarely indicated for control of postpolypectomy hemorrhage, there are instances in which it may become necessary. The usual circumstance is failure of all other measures to control hemorrhage. Infrequently, hemorrhage occurs in patients in whom surgery is necessary to treat the primary colonic condition. In this instance, surgery may supersede the previously mentioned therapeutic interventions.

BIBLIOGRAPHY

1. Dent TL: Evaluation of the bleeding patient. *Surg Gynecol Obstet* 151:817, 1980.

2. Gibbs DH, Opelka FG, Beck DE, et al: Post polypectomy lower gastrointestinal hemorrhage. *Dis Colon Rectum* (in press).

3. Jensen DM, Machicado GA: Diagnosis and treatment of severe hematochezia. The role of urgent colonoscopy after purge. *Gastroenterology* 95:1569–1574, 1988.

4. Nivatvongs S: Complications in colonoscopic polypectomy. An experience with 1555 polypectomies. *Dis Colon rectum* 29:825–830, 1986.

5. Opelka FG, Timmcke AE: Management of bleeding diverticulosis. *Seminars Colon Rectal Surg* 1:109–115, 1990.

6. Rosen L, Bub DS, Reed JF III, et al: Hemorrhage following colonoscopic polypectomy. *Dis Colon Rectum* 36:1126–1131, 1993.

See also Chapters 2, 10, 66, 69, 91 and 95B.

CHAPTER 95B

Postpolypectomy Hemorrhage

Thomas B. Blake, III, M.D. and Paul R. Williamson, M.D.

Refer to Algorithm 95B-1.

A. The reported incidence ranges from 0.3% to 6.1%
B. "Immediate bleeding" is defined as bleeding visualized immediately after the polypectomy. It is usually the result of inadequate coagulation of the pedicle or improper snare technique.
C. "Delayed bleeding" is defined as bleeding that occurs any time after polypectomy from 20 min to several weeks. It is usually secondary to detachment of the eschar coagulum.
D. Local measures are performed to control visible bleeding.
E. Resnare stalk if adequate stalk is present and strangulate it for 20 mins. This maneuver may be repeated if bleeding reoccurs.
F. Coagulation is performed after the stalk resnared if bleeding persists: It is performed using short-burst coagulation current without cutting through the stalk. Small stalks may be grasped with insulated biopsy forceps and coagulated. Complication of full-thickness burn can occur.
G. A sclerotherapy needle is used to inject epinephrine in 1:10,000 concentration around the bleeding site followed by irrigation with cold water and/or application of a heater probe or coagulation using graspers or snares.
H. The heater probe is applied in various pulses of 15 J using a 2.4-mm heater probe to the edge and the base of bleeding site. As cautery, it may cause a full-thickness burn.
I. Sucralfate has been used for "oozing" after polypectomy. One gram of sucralfate (Marion Merrell Dow, Inc.) is dissolved in 30 cc of water and sucralfate suspension is irrigated over the bleeding site. The proposed mechanism of action is that the negatively charged polyanions of sucralfate bind to the positively charged proteins in the damaged mucosa, forming polyvalent bridges.

501

Postpolypectomy hemorrhage

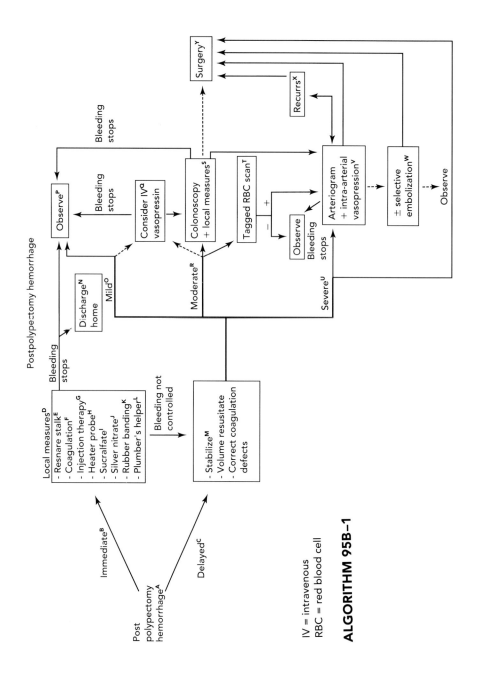

IV = intravenous
RBC = red blood cell

ALGORITHM 95B–1

J. Scrapings from silver nitrate applicator sticks (Foster Medical Corporation) are loaded in biopsy forceps and the bleeding site is grasped depositing the silver nitrate. This measure may be repeated until control is obtained. Silver nitrate acts as a chemical cautery by precipitating tissue proteins and is not absorbed. It may be useful in the thin walled cecum.

K. Rubber-band application is useful for bleeding sites within reach of the hemorrhoid bander. The bleeding site is grasped and rubber bands are applied over the site. Endoscopic appliers are available, although published experience with this modality is minimal.

L. "Plumber's Helper" or Frankeldt polypectomy grasping forceps by *V. Mueller,* are used to grasp the bleeding site via a rigid sigmoidoscopy and twisted. The instrument is taped in place and the scope is removed over the grasper. After 19–20 hours, the site is reinspected by sliding the scope over the grasper. If bleeding has subsided, it is untwisted and slowly removed.

M. Bleeding not controlled by local measures dictates admission to the hospital with close observation and stabilization by fluid resuscitation and transfusion as needed with correction of coagulation abnormalities. Serial hemoglobin and hematocrits are followed (see paragraph P).

N. The patient may be discharged home depending on clinical assessment, ease of control of bleeding, and stability during the procedure. The patient is instructed to seek medical attention if signs or symptoms of bleeding develop.

O. The majority of bleeding stops with conservative treatment and bowel rest.

P. Observation includes nothing per mouth, intravenous (IV) hydration, and serial drawing of hemoglobins and hematocrits. If vital signs remain stable without clinical bleeding with hemoglobin and hematocrits stabilized, diet is resumed. The patient may still be observed in hospital for 24–48 hours after resumption of diet.

Q. Vasopressin used intravenously as an initial rate of 0.2 units/min with cessation of bleeding has been reported. It is used the same way as in upper gastrointestinal (GI) bleeding with the dose tapered over 24 hours.

R. Moderate bleeding is continued despite stabilization and resuscitation.

S. Colonoscopy is performed in unprepped bowel or after rapid prep with enemas or gastric lavage with polyethyleneglycol. Once a bleeding site is visualized, local measures are tried.

T. Tagged red blood cell (RBC) scan may be used to demonstrate the source of bleeding. The difficulty is in demonstrating an exact site of bleeding; colonoscopy may be more helpful.

U. Severe bleeding that is life-threatening or unresponsive to supportive measures or attempts at colonoscopic hemostasis require >4–6 unit transfusion over 24–36 hours.

V. Intraarterial vasopressin is an alternative to emergency colon resection in high-risk surgical patients. The bleeding site is usually localized at the time of colonoscopy, decreasing the time required for diagnostic arteriography. Transcatheter infusion of vasopressin is started at 0.2–0.4 units/min with repeat angiography within 20–30 minutes. The dosage may be increased as long as physical findings of ischemia and side effects are not present. If bleeding has stopped, the dose is tapered over 24 hours. The patient requires monitoring for hypertension, electrolyte imbalance, fluid retention, and transient cardiac arrhythmias.

W. Superselective embolization may be attempted but has potential for bowel infarction with a requirement for more extensive bowel resection. It may play a role in preoperative control of life-threatening hemorrhage.

X. "Recurrent bleeding" is that in which the patient is clinically stable but begins to rebleed after tapering of intraarterial vasopressin. Consider restarting vasopressin for additional 24 hours or proceed to surgery.

Y. Surgery may be required if all other measures are not successful and the patient has required a 4-6 unit transfusion, and is not a candidate for vasopressin therapy. The aim is to control bleeding by either oversewing the bleeding site or by resection. The type of surgical intervention should be dictated by the pathology and the bleeding site.

BIBLIOGRAPHY

1. Alberti-Flor JJ, Hernandez ME, Ferrer JP: Combined injection and thermal therapy in the management of early post-polypectomy bleeding. *Am J Gastroenterol* 87:1681-1682, 1992.

2. Anseline PF, Fazio VW: Management of massive postpolypectomy hemorrhage: report of a technique. *Dis Colon Rectum* 25:251-253, 1982.

3. Bronner MH, Yantis PL: Intracolonic sucralfate suspension for postpolypectomy hemorrhage. *Gastrointest Endosc* 32:362-363, 1986.

4. Carlyle DR, Goldstein HM: Angiographic management of bleeding following transcolonoscopic polypectomy. *Am J Digestive Dis* 20:1196-1201, 1975.

5. Dill JE: Vasopressin in post polypectomy bleeding (letter). *Gastrointest Endosc* 33:399, 1987.

6. Ghazi A, Grossman M: Complications of colonoscopy and polypectomy. *Surg Clin N Am* 62:889-896, 1982.

7. Nitvatvongs S: Complications in colonoscopic polypectomy. An experience with 1,555 polypectomies. *Dis Colon Rectum* 29:825-830, 1986.

8. Opelka F: Colonoscopic complications. 1994 core subjects. The American Society of Colon & Rectal Surgeons 93rd annual meeting. Orlando, May 237, 1994.

9. Petroski D: Postpolypectomy hemorrhage managed by chemical cautery. *Gastrointest Endosc* 28:94-95, 1982.

10. Rex DK, Lewis BS, Wayne JD: Colonoscopy and endoscopic therapy for delayed postpolypectomy hemorrhage. *Gastrointest Endosc* 38:127-129, 1992.

11. Robinson DL, Spokas FJ, Smith DC: Banding technique for hemostasis of postpolypectomy bleeding. *Iowa Med* 77:117-118, 1987.

12. Rosen L, Bub DS, Reed JF 3rd, et al: Hemorrhage following colonoscopic polypectomy. *Dis Colon Rectum* 36:1126-1131, 1993.

13. Sanchez FW, Rogers JM, Vujic I, et al: Transcatheter control of postpolypectomy hemorrhage. *Gastrointest Radiol* 11:254-256, 1986.

See also Chapters 2, 10, 66, 69, 91 and 95A.

INDEX